Emerging Comorbidities in Heart Failure

Editors

ANTONIO CITTADINI
HECTOR O. VENTURA

CARDIOLOGY CLINICS

www.cardiology.theclinics.com

May 2022 • Volume 40 • Number 2

ELSEVIER

1600 John F. Kennedy Boulevard • Suite 1800 • Philadelphia, Pennsylvania, 19103-2899

http://www.theclinics.com

CARDIOLOGY CLINICS Volume 40, Number 2
May 2022 ISSN 0733-8651, ISBN-13: 978-0-323-96161-5

Editor: Joanna Collett
Developmental Editor: Karen Justine Solomon

Cardiology Clinics (ISSN 0733-8651) is published quarterly by Elsevier Inc., 360 Park Avenue South, New York, NY 10010-1710. Months of issue are February, May, August, and November. Business and Editorial Offices: 1600 John F. Kennedy Blvd., Ste. 1800, Philadelphia, PA 19103-2899. Customer Service Office: 3251 Riverport Lane, Maryland Heights, MO 63043. Periodicals postage paid at New York, NY and additional mailing offices. Subscription prices are $370.00 per year for US individuals, $948.00 per year for US institutions, $100.00 per year for US students and residents, $458.00 per year for Canadian individuals, $967.00 per year for Canadian institutions, $480.00 per year for international individuals, $967.00 per year for international institutions, $100.00 per year for Canadian students/residents and $220.00 per year for international students/residents. To receive student/resident rate, orders must be accompanied by name of affiliated institution, data of term, and the *signature* of program/residency coordinator on institution letterhead. Orders will be billed at individual rate until proof of status is received. Foreign air speed delivery is included in all *Clinics* subscription prices. All prices are subject to change without notice. **POSTMASTER:** Send address changes to *Cardiology Clinics*, Elsevier Health Sciences Division, Subscription Customer Service, 3251 Riverport Lane, Maryland Heights, MO 63043. **Customer Service: 1-800-654-2452 (U.S. and Canada); 314-447-8871 (outside U.S. and Canada). Fax: 314-447-8029. E-mail: journalscustomerservice-usa@elsevier.com (for print support); journalsonlinesupport-usa@elsevier.com (for online support).**

Reprints. For copies of 100 or more, of articles in this publication, please contact the Commercial Reprints Department, Elsevier Inc., 360 Park Avenue South, New York, NY 10010-1710. Tel.: 212-633-3874; Fax: 212-633-3820; E-mail: reprints@elsevier.com.

Cardiology Clinics is also published in Spanish by McGraw-Hill Interamericana Editores S. A., P.O. Box 5-237, 06500, Mexico D. F., Mexico; in Portuguese by Reichmann and Alfonso Editores Rio de Janeiro, Brazil; and in Greek by Dimitrios P. Lagos, 8 Pondon Street, GR115-28 Ilissia, Greece.

Cardiology Clinics is covered in *MEDLINE/PubMed (Index Medicus), Excerpta Medica, The Cumulative Index to Nursing and Allied Health Literature* (CINAHL).

Contributors

EDITORIAL BOARD

JAMIL A. ABOULHOSN, MD, FACC, FSCAI
Director, Ahmanson/UCLA Adult Congenital Heart Center, Streisand/American Heart Association Endowed Chair, Divisions of Cardiology and Pediatric Cardiology, David Geffen School of Medicine at UCLA, Los Angeles, California, USA

DAVID M. SHAVELLE, MD, FACC, FSCAI
Associate Professor, Keck School of Medicine of USC, Director, General Cardiovascular Fellowship Program, Director, Cardiac Catheterization Laboratory, LAC + USC Medical Center, Division of Cardiovascular Medicine, University of Southern California, Los Angeles, California, USA

TERRENCE D. WELCH, MD, FACC
Associate Professor of Medicine and Medical Education, Director, Cardiovascular Fellowship Program, Section of Cardiovascular Medicine, Dartmouth-Hitchcock Heart and Vascular Center, Lebanon, New Hampshire, USA; Geisel School of Medicine at Dartmouth, Hanover, New Hampshire, USA

AUDREY H. WU, MD, MPH
Associate Professor, Advanced Heart Failure and Transplant Program, Division of Cardiovascular Medicine, Department of Medicine, University of Michigan, Ann Arbor, Michigan, USA

EDITORS

ANTONIO CITTADINI, MD
Professor of General Internal Medicine, Department of Translational Medical Sciences, Federico II University, Naples, Italy

HECTOR O. VENTURA, MD
Section Head, Cardiomyopathy and Heart Transplantation, Professor, Department of Cardiovascular Diseases, John Ochsner Heart and Vascular Institute, Ochsner Clinic Foundation, The University of Queensland Ochsner Clinical School, Faculty of Medicine, The University of Queensland, New Orleans, Louisiana, USA

AUTHORS

STEFAN D. ANKER, MD, PhD
Division of Cardiology and Metabolism, Department of Cardiology (CVK), Berlin-Brandenburg Center for Regenerative Therapies (BCRT), German Centre for Cardiovascular Research (DZHK) Partner Site Berlin, Charité Universitätsmedizin Berlin, Berlin, Germany

ROSS ARENA, PhD
Professor, Department of Physical Therapy, College of Applied Health Sciences, University of Illinois at Chicago, Chicago, Illinois, USA;

TotalCardiology Research Network, Calgary, Alberta, Canada

NICHOLAS J. BARONE, BS
Office of the Medical Director, Montefiore Medical Center, Bronx, New York, USA

STEFANIA BASILI, MD
Department of Translational and Precision Medicine, Sapienza University of Rome, Policlinico Umberto I, Rome, Italy

NICOLA BENJAMIN, MSc
Centre for Pulmonary Hypertension, Thoraxklinik at Heidelberg University Hospital, Translational Lung Research Center Heidelberg (TLRC), Member of the German Center for Lung Research (DZL), Heidelberg, Germany

DENNIS BERNIEH, PhD
Department of Cardiovascular Sciences, NIHR Leicester Cardiovascular Biomedical Research Centre, University of Leicester, Glenfield Hospital, Leicester, United Kingdom

EDUARDO BOSSONE, MD, PhD, FCCP, FESC, FACC
Division of Cardiology, AORN A Cardarelli Hospital, Naples, Italy

MALCOLM BURGESS, MD
Department of Cardiology, Aintree Hospital, Liverpool, United Kingdom

SALVATORE CARBONE, PhD
Assistant Professor, Department of Kinesiology & Health Sciences, College of Humanities & Sciences, Department of Internal Medicine, Division of Cardiology, VCU Pauley Heart Center, Virginia Commonwealth University, Richmond, Virginia, USA

SHABANA CASSAMBAI, PhD
Department of Cardiovascular Sciences, NIHR Leicester Cardiovascular Biomedical Research Centre, University of Leicester, Glenfield Hospital, Leicester, United Kingdom

ANTONIO CITTADINI, MD
Professor of General Internal Medicine, Department of Translational Medical Sciences, Federico II University, Naples, Italy

ANDREW L. CLARK, MA, MD, FRCP
Department of Cardiology, Castle Hill Hospital, Hull York Medical School, University of Hull, Kingston upon Hull, United Kingdom

JOHN G.F. CLELAND, MD, FRCP, FESC, FACC
Robertson Institute of Biostatistics and Clinical Trials Unit, University of Glasgow, Glasgow, United Kingdom

AMANDA C. CONIGLIO, MD
Department of Medicine, Duke University School of Medicine, Durham, North Carolina, USA

MARIA ROSA COSTANZO, MD, FACC, FAHA, FESC
Medical Director, Heart Failure Research, Advocate Heart Institute, Medical Director, Edward Hospital Center for Advanced Heart Failure, Naperville, Illinois, USA

ROBERTA D'ASSANTE, PhD
Research Fellow, Department of Translational Medical Sciences, Federico II University, Naples, Italy

SARA DANZI, PhD
Associate Professor, Department of Biological Sciences and Geology, Queensborough Community College, City University of New York, Bayside, New York, USA

KATHERINE E. DI PALO, PharmD, FAHA
Office of the Medical Director, Montefiore Medical Center, Bronx, New York, USA

ANDREW ELAGIZI, MD
Cardiovascular Fellow, John Ochsner Heart and Vascular Institute, Ochsner Clinical School, The University of Queensland School of Medicine, New Orleans, Louisiana, USA

EKKEHARD GRÜNIG, MD, PhD
Centre for Pulmonary Hypertension, Head of Pulmonary Hypertension Unit, Thoraxklinik at Heidelberg University Hospital, Translational Lung Research Center Heidelberg (TLRC), Member of the German Center for Lung Research (DZL), Heidelberg, Germany

MUHAMMAD ZUBAIR ISRAR, PhD
Department of Cardiovascular Sciences, NIHR Leicester Cardiovascular Biomedical Research Centre, University of Leicester, Glenfield Hospital, Leicester, United Kingdom

IRWIN KLEIN, MD
Professor of Medicine, NYU School of Medicine, Melville, New York, USA

CARL J. LAVIE, MD
Professor, John Ochsner Heart and Vascular Institute, Ochsner Clinical School-The University of Queensland School of Medicine, New Orleans, Louisiana, USA

GREGORY Y.H. LIP, MD
Liverpool Centre for Cardiovascular Science, University of Liverpool and Liverpool Heart and Chest Hospital, Liverpool, United Kingdom; Aalborg Thrombosis Research Unit, Department of Clinical Medicine, Aalborg University, Aalborg, Denmark

ALBERTO-MARIA MARRA, MD
IRCSS SDN, Naples, Italy

ROBERT J. MENTZ, MD
Department of Medicine, Duke University School of Medicine, Duke Clinical Research Institute, Durham, North Carolina, USA

MARTINA MINIERO, MD
Specialist Trainee, Department of Translational Medical Sciences, Federico II University, Naples, Italy

RAFFAELE NAPOLI, MD
Associate Professor of General Internal Medicine, Department of Translational Medical Sciences, Federico II University, Naples, Italy

MOHAMMED OBEIDAT, BMBS, BSc (Hons), MRCP (UK)
Department of Cardiology, Aintree Hospital, Liverpool, United Kingdom

PIERPAOLO PELLICORI, MD, FESC
Robertson Institute of Biostatistics and Clinical Trials Unit, University of Glasgow, Glasgow, United Kingdom

VALERIA RAPARELLI, MD, PhD
Department of Experimental Medicine, Sapienza University of Rome, Policlinico Umberto I, Rome, Italy; McGill University Health Centre Research Institute, Centre for Outcomes Research and Evaluation, Montreal, Quebec, Canada

FABRIZIO RECCHIA, MD
Department of Translational and Precision Medicine, Sapienza University of Rome, Policlinico Umberto I, Rome, Italy

GIULIO FRANCESCO ROMITI, MD
Department of Translational and Precision Medicine, Sapienza University of Rome, Policlinico Umberto I, Rome, Italy

ANDREA SALZANO, MD, MRCP
Department of Cardiovascular Sciences, NIHR Leicester Cardiovascular Biomedical Research Centre, University of Leicester, Glenfield Hospital, Leicester, United Kingdom

TORU SUZUKI, MD, PhD, FRCP
Department of Cardiovascular Sciences, NIHR Leicester Cardiovascular Biomedical Research Centre, University of Leicester, Glenfield Hospital, Leicester, United Kingdom

MIROSLAVA VALENTOVA, MD, PhD
Department of Cardiology and Pneumology, University Medical Center Göttingen, Göttingen, Germany; DZHK (German Centre for Cardiovascular Research), Partner Site Göttingen, Germany

HECTOR O. VENTURA, MD
Section Head, Cardiomyopathy and Heart Transplantation, Professor, Department of Cardiovascular Diseases, John Ochsner Heart and Vascular Institute, Ochsner Clinic Foundation, The University of Queensland Ochsner Clinical School, Faculty of Medicine, The University of Queensland, New Orleans, Louisiana, USA

GIACOMO VISIOLI, MD
Department of Sense Organs, Sapienza University of Rome, Policlinico Umberto I, Rome, Italy

STEPHAN VON HAEHLING, MD, PhD
Department of Cardiology and Pneumology, University Medical Center Göttingen, Göttingen, Germany; DZHK (German Centre for Cardiovascular Research), Partner Site Göttingen, Germany

MAX WONG, PhD
Department of Cardiovascular Sciences, NIHR Leicester Cardiovascular Biomedical Research Centre, University of Leicester, Glenfield Hospital, Leicester, United Kingdom

YOSHIYUKI YAZAKI, MD
Department of Cardiovascular Sciences, NIHR
Leicester Cardiovascular Biomedical Research
Centre, University of Leicester, Glenfield
Hospital, Leicester, United Kingdom

ANDREA ZITO, MS
Department of Translational and Precision
Medicine, Sapienza University of Rome,
Policlinico Umberto I, Rome, Italy

Contents

The effects of hyperthyroidism and hypothyroidism on the heart and cardiovascular system are well documented. It has also been shown that various forms of heart disease including but not limited to congenital, hypertensive, ischemic, cardiac surgery, and heart transplantation cause an alteration in thyroid function tests including a decrease in serum liothyronine (T_3). This article discusses the basic science and clinical data that support the hypothesis that these changes pose pathophysiologic and potential novel therapeutic challenges.

Chronic heart failure (CHF) is a complex syndrome characterized by symptoms and signs supported by different forms of cardiac impairment. The link between multiple hormonal and metabolic derangements and the development of CHF and the beneficial effects seen with hormonal replacement therapy suggest that a reduction of anabolic pathways might contribute to the onset of CHF. Therefore, an imbalance between anabolic and catabolic forces could be responsible for the development of CHF. There are sufficient evidence to support the screening in patients with CHF of hormonal deficiencies and their correction with replacement therapy.

A novel pathophysiological model of interest is the association between heart failure (HF) and the gastrointestinal system, the 'gut hypothesis'. The choline and carnitine metabolic by-product, Trimethylamine N-oxide (TMAO) is one of the more prominent molecules associated with the link between HF and the gut. Indeed, TMAO levels are increased in HF populations and higher TMAO levels are associated with poor prognosis, whereas low TMAO levels either at baseline/follow up confer better prognosis. Considering that TMAO levels seem not to be affected by guideline-HF treatment, this model could represent a novel and independent therapeutic target for HF.

Heart failure (HF) and chronic obstructive pulmonary disease (COPD) are both common causes of breathlessness and often conspire to confound accurate diagnosis and optimal therapy. Risk factors (such as aging, smoking, and obesity) and clinical presentation (eg, cough and breathlessness on exertion) can be very similar, but the treatment and prognostic implications are very different. This review discusses the diagnostic challenges in individuals with exertional dyspnea. We also highlight the prevalence, clinical relevance and therapeutic implications of a concurrent diagnosis of COPD and HF.

Sleep-disordered breathing (SDB), including obstructive sleep apnea, central sleep apnea (CSA), and Cheyne-Stokes respiration, is common in patients with heart failure (HF) and associated with lower left ventricular ejection fraction (EF), increased arrhythmia burden, and increased mortality. Continuous positive airway pressure therapy improves short-term and long-term outcomes in HF patients. Adaptive servoventilation (ASV) therapy in patients with low-EF HF with predominant CSA is not recommended. Ongoing trials are evaluating whether ASV will have a role in SDB treatment. Phrenic nerve stimulation is an emerging treatment option that has shown promising outcomes. All HF patients should be screened for SDB.

Pulmonary hypertension (PH) often complicates chronic left-sided heart failure, with a remarkable impact on quality of life, exercise capacity, and survival. PH in chronic left-sided heart failure (PH-LHD) is not only caused by backward transmission of pressures but also involves impairment of atrial function, inflammation, and vasoconstriction. Once the left atrium loses its reservoir capacity, usually pulmonary vascular resistances increase. Right atrial dilation commonly represents the first sign of PH-LHD, before right ventricle dilatation and systolic dysfunction develop, leading to right heart insufficiency, and ultimately, right heart failure.

Cardiac cachexia is a co-morbidity of heart failure (HF) defined by a non-edematous weight loss of $\geq$6% within the previous 6–12 months. Cachexia affects about 10–39% patients with HF and occurs typically in advanced stages of HF, especially in the presence of congestive right ventricular dysfunction. This review elucidates the approaches and pitfalls in the diagnosis of cachexia. It summarizes the prevalence and impact of cardiac cachexia. It also discusses changes in body composition over the course of HF and provides an overview of the mechanisms involved in wasting in HF.

Overweight and obesity adversely impact cardiac structure and function, affecting systolic and diastolic ventricular function. Epidemiologic studies have documented an obesity paradox in large heart failure cohorts, where overweight and obese individuals with established heart failure have a better short- and medium-term prognosis compared with leaner patients; this relationship is strongly impacted by level of cardiorespiratory fitness. There are implications for therapies aimed at increasing lean mass as well as weight loss and improvements in quality of diet for the prevention and treatment of heart failure and concomitant obesity to improve cardiorespiratory fitness.

Abnormal fluid handling leads to physiologic abnormalities in multiple organ systems. Deranged hemodynamics, neurohormonal activation, excessive tubular sodium reabsorption, inflammation, oxidative stress, and nephrotoxic medications are important drivers of harmful cardiorenal interactions in patients with heart failure. Accurate quantitative measurement of fluid volume is vital to individualizing therapy for such patients. Blood volume analysis and pulmonary artery pressure monitoring seem the most reliable methods for assessing fluid volume and guiding decongestive therapies. Still the cornerstone of decongestive therapy, diuretics' effectiveness decreases with progression of heart failure. Extracorporeal ultrafiltration, an alternative to diuretics, has been shown to reduce heart-failure events.

Hypertension is possibly the most powerful, modifiable risk factor for the development of heart failure. Chronic hypertension drives cardiac remodeling within the left ventricle resulting in hypertensive heart disease, which ultimately manifests as heart failure. Early detection and appropriate management are necessary to prevent heart failure as well as other cardiovascular diseases. Achieving blood pressure goals in conjunction with using evidence-based treatments can improve clinical outcomes for patients with comorbid hypertension and heart failure.

Heart failure (HF) and atrial fibrillation (AF), increasingly common in the aging population, are closely related and commonly found together. This article explores the relationship between AF and HF and the thromboembolic effect of these diseases. Morbidity and mortality are increased when the 2 conditions are seen together. Stroke risks are significant with AF and all subtypes of HF. This article suggests that all patients with AF and HF should be considered for anticoagulation. Current evidence suggests that non–vitamin K antagonist oral anticoagulants are effective and safe in AF and HF in comparison with warfarin.

Understanding the role of sex- and gender-related factors, when dealing with a global growing epidemic such as heart failure, is a much needed and unmet goal for health care providers and scientists in order to design targeted strategies, aimed at improving both clinical and patient reported outcomes measures in women and men with heart failure. The present review provides an overview of the current available evidence on sex- and gender-related differences in heart failure.

The occurrence of depression, anxiety, and insomnia is strikingly high in patients with heart failure and is linked to increased morbidity and mortality. However, symptoms are frequently unrecognized and the integration of mental health into cardiology care plans is not routine. This article describes the prevalence, identification, and treatment of common comorbid psychological disorders.

CARDIOLOGY CLINICS

SERIES OF RELATED INTEREST

Cardiac Electrophysiology Clinics
Available at: https://www.cardiacep.theclinics.com/
Clinics in Chest Medicine
Available at: https://www.chestmed.theclinics.com/
Heart Failure Clinics
Available at: https://www.heartfailure.theclinics.com/
Interventional Cardiology Clinics
Available at: https://www.interventional.theclinics.com/

THE CLINICS ARE AVAILABLE ONLINE!
Access your subscription at:
www.theclinics.com

Preface
Emerging Comorbidities in Heart Failure

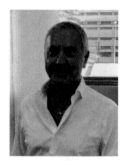

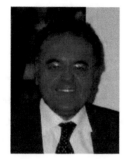

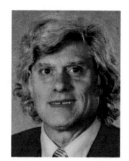

Antonio Cittadini, MD   Eduardo Bossone, MD, PhD   Hector O. Ventura, MD

Editors

Heart failure (HF), a complex clinical syndrome characterized by cardinal symptoms and signs, represents an intriguing clinical challenge for cardiologists and physicians, considering its increase in prevalence, incidence, hospitalizations, and death[1]; furthermore, the recent COVID-19 outbreak created novel needs in the everyday clinical practice, with the necessity of ideate new strategies of management.[2] In this context, HF patients display several chronic coexisting diseases,[3] strongly impacting on morbidity, mortality, and health-related quality of life.[4,5] In addition, the presence of comorbidities determines a more complex clinical management leading to increasing health care costs (**Fig. 1**).[6]

The purpose of the present issue of *Cardiology Clinics* is to review several comorbidities (ie, noncardiac and cardiac), with the aim of helping clinicians in the everyday management of HF patients.

NONCARDIAC COMORBIDITIES

Growing evidence suggests that HF patients displaying a hormone disarrangement are characterized by impaired cardiovascular performance and poor prognosis.[7–10] Recently, this hypothesis has been confirmed by data from the T.O.S.CA. registry,[11,12] with patients affected by multiple hormone and metabolic deficiency syndrome (defined as 2 or more hormone deficiencies) experienced the worst outcome. In this regard, Danzi and colleagues and Napoli and colleagues reviewed in the present issue the role of thyroid hormones, growth hormone, testosterone, and insulin in HF, also in consideration of their potential therapeutic role.[13–16] A novel HF pathophysiologic model, the so-called gut hypothesis (ie, the interplay between HF and the gastrointestinal system), has been reviewed by Salzano and colleagues; specifically, the choline/carnitine derived metabolite trimethylamine *N*-oxide, strictly linked to the Western diet,[17,18] appears to be a novel risk predictor as well as a promising therapeutic target in HF.[19–21] A recently emerged paradigm shift in HF pathophysiology is the interaction between right HF and pulmonary circulation.[22,23] Indeed, disorders such as chronic obstructive pulmonary disease, sleep breathing disorders, and pulmonary hypertension (ie, when right heart-

Cardiol Clin 40 (2022) xi–xiv
https://doi.org/10.1016/j.ccl.2022.02.001
0733-8651/22/© 2022 Published by Elsevier Inc.

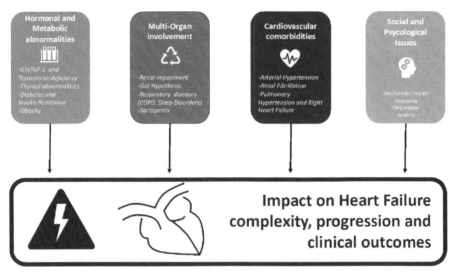

Fig. 1. Impact of emerging comorbidities on HF. (*Modified from* Cittadini A, Bossone E, Ventura HO. Emerging comorbidities in heart failure. Heart Fail Clin 2020;16(1):xiii-xv.)

pulmonary circulation unit is impaired) play a central role in HF progression,[3,6,24] as reviewed by Pellicori and colleagues, Coniglio and colleagues, and Marra and colleagues. Intriguingly, right ventricular dysfunction is also linked to cardiac cachexia and sarcopenia, critical turning points in the context of HF, as Valentova and colleagues exposed in their review. In addition, the role of the "obesity paradox" in chronic heart failure has been reviewed by Carbone and colleagues. Specifically, a paradoxical decrease in mortality in those with higher body mass index has been observed in HF patients, in the context of the so-called reverse epidemiology.[25] Finally, the amount of renal impairment is a keystone in clinical decision making in HF patients.[26,27] In this regard, Costanzo described the cardiorenal syndrome, focusing on the importance of accurate quantitative measurement of fluid volume in patients with HF.

CARDIOVASCULAR COMORBIDITIES

In the present issue, Di Palo and colleagues discuss arterial hypertension (ie, "blood pressure paradox"). Indeed, whereas in most of cardiovascular disease high blood pressure has an adverse prognostic role[28,29]; in HF, the optimal target of blood pressure remains a matter of debate. Furthermore, clinicians are challenged by the management of antithrombotic treatment in patients with coexisting HF and atrial fibrillation[30]; Obeidat and colleagues, reviewing the role of direct oral anticoagulant, highlight their safety and effectiveness also in HF.

Sex and gender integration still remains an unmet need in research and clinic,[31–33] and HF is no exception, as Romiti and colleagues describe in this issue.

Finally, as highlighted by Di Paolo and colleagues, clinicians should take care also of psychological comorbidities of HF, including depression, anxiety, and insomnia, considering their important burden on patients' quality of life.

In conclusion, we are confident that the perspectives reported in this issue of *Cardiology Clinics* will help clinicians and physician to best understand and manage these comorbidities in HF patients.

Antonio Cittadini, MD
Department of Translational Medical Sciences,
Federico II University
Via S Pansini 5, Naples 80131, Italy

Eduardo Bossone, MD, PhD
Division of Cardiology
AORN A Cardarelli Hospital
Via A Cardarelli 9, Naples 80131, Italy

Hector O. Ventura, MD
John Ochsner Heart and Vascular Institute
Ochsner Clinical Foundation
1514 Jefferson Highway
New Orleans, LA 70121, USA

The University of Queensland Ochsner Clinical
School
The University of Queensland
New Orleans, LA, USA

E-mail addresses:
antonio.cittadini@unina.it (A. Cittadini)
ebossone@hotmail.com (E. Bossone)
hventura@ochsner.org (H.O. Ventura)

REFERENCES

1. Tsao CW, Aday AW, Almarzooq ZI, et al. Heart disease and stroke statistics–2022 update: a report from the American Heart Association. Circulation 2022;145(8):e153–639. https://doi.org/10.1161/CIR.0000000000001052 CIR0000000000001052.

2. Salzano A, D'Assante R, Stagnaro FM, et al. Heart failure management during COVID-19 outbreak in Italy. Telemedicine experience from a heart failure university tertiary referral centre. Eur J Heart Fail 2020;22(6):1048–50. https://doi.org/10.1002/ejhf.1911.

3. Streng KW, Nauta JF, Hillege HL, et al. Non-cardiac comorbidities in heart failure with reduced, mid-range and preserved ejection fraction. Int J Cardiol 2018;271:132–9.

4. Wolsk E, Claggett B, Køber L, et al. Contribution of cardiac and extra-cardiac disease burden to risk of cardiovascular outcomes varies by ejection fraction in heart failure. Eur J Heart Fail 2018;20:504–10.

5. Radhoe SP, Veenis JF, Linssen GCM, et al. Diabetes and treatment of chronic heart failure in a large real-world heart failure population. ESC Heart Fail 2022;9:353–62.

6. Iorio A, Senni M, Barbati G, et al. Prevalence and prognostic impact of non-cardiac co-morbidities in heart failure outpatients with preserved and reduced ejection fraction: a community-based study. Eur J Heart Fail 2018;20:1257–66.

7. Arcopinto M, Salzano A, Giallauria F, et al. Growth hormone deficiency is associated with worse cardiac function, physical performance, and outcome in chronic heart failure: insights from the T.O.S.CA. GHD Study. PLoS One 2017;12:e0170058.

8. Arcopinto M, Salzano A, Bossone E, et al. Multiple hormone deficiencies in chronic heart failure. Int J Cardiol 2015;184:421–3.

9. Salzano A, Marra AM, Ferrara F, et al. Multiple hormone deficiency syndrome in heart failure with preserved ejection fraction. Int J Cardiol 2016;225:1–3.

10. Marra AM, Arcopinto M, Bobbio E, et al. An unusual case of dilated cardiomyopathy associated with partial hypopituitarism. Intern Emerg Med 2012;7(suppl 2):S85–7.

11. Cittadini A, Salzano A, Iacoviello M, et al. Multiple hormonal and metabolic deficiency syndrome predicts outcome in heart failure: the T.O.S.CA. Registry. Eur J Prev Cardiol 2021;28:1691–700.

12. Bossone E, Arcopinto M, Iacoviello M, et al. Multiple hormonal and metabolic deficiency syndrome in chronic heart failure: rationale, design, and demographic characteristics of the T.O.S.CA. Registry. Intern Emerg Med 2018;13:661–71.

13. Salzano A, Marra AM, Arcopinto M, et al. Combined effects of growth hormone and testosterone replacement treatment in heart failure. ESC Heart Fail 2019;6(6):1216–21. https://doi.org/10.1002/ehf2.12520.

14. Salzano A, D'Assante R, Lander M, et al. Hormonal replacement therapy in heart failure: focus on growth hormone and testosterone. Heart Fail Clin 2019;15:377–91.

15. Salzano A, Marra AM, D'Assante R, et al. Growth hormone therapy in heart failure. Heart Fail Clin 2018;14:501–15.

16. Arcopinto M, Salzano A, Isgaard J, et al. Hormone replacement therapy in heart failure. Curr Opin Cardiol 2015;30:277–84.

17. Cassambai S, Salzano A, Yazaki Y, et al. Impact of acute choline loading on circulating trimethylamine N-oxide levels. Eur J Prev Cardiol 2019;26(17):1899–902. https://doi.org/10.1177/2047487319831372, 2047487319831372.

18. Yazaki Y, Aizawa K, Israr MZ, et al. Ethnic differences in association of outcomes with trimethylamine N-oxide in acute heart failure patients. ESC Heart Fail 2020;7(5):2373–8. https://doi.org/10.1002/ehf2.12777.

19. Salzano A, Israr MZ, Yazaki Y, et al. Combined use of trimethylamine N-oxide with BNP for risk stratification in heart failure with preserved ejection fraction: findings from the DIAMONDHFpEF study. Eur J Prev Cardiol 2020;27(19):2159–62. https://doi.org/10.1177/2047487319870355, 2047487319870355.

20. Yazaki Y, Salzano A, Nelson CP, et al. Geographical location affects the levels and association of trimethylamine N-oxide with heart failure mortality in BIOSTAT-CHF: a post-hoc analysis. Eur J Heart Fail 2019;21(10):1291–4. https://doi.org/10.1002/ejhf.1550.

21. Israr MZ, Bernieh D, Salzano A, et al. Association of gut-related metabolites with outcome in acute heart failure. Am Heart J 2021;234:71–80.

22. Marra AM, Sherman AE, Salzano A, et al. Right side of the heart pulmonary circulation unit involvement in left-sided heart failure: diagnostic, prognostic, and therapeutic implications. Chest 2022;161(2):535–51. https://doi.org/10.1016/j.chest.2021.09.023.

23. D'Alto M, Marra AM, Severino S, et al. Right ventricular-arterial uncoupling independently predicts survival in COVID-19 ARDS. Crit Care 2020;24:670.

24. Marra AM, Egenlauf B, Ehlken N, et al. Change of right heart size and function by long-term therapy with riociguat in patients with pulmonary arterial hypertension and chronic thromboembolic pulmonary hypertension. Int J Cardiol 2015;195:19–26.

25. Aimo A, Januzzi JL, Vergaro G, et al. Revisiting the obesity paradox in heart failure: per cent body fat as predictor of biomarkers and outcome. Eur J Prev Cardiol 2019;26(16):1751–9. https://doi.org/10.1177/2047487319852809, 2047487319852809.

26. Melgaard L, Overvad TF, Skjøth F, et al. Risk of stroke and bleeding in patients with heart failure and chronic kidney disease: a nationwide cohort study. ESC Heart Fail 2018;5:319–26.

27. Mullens W, Damman K, Harjola VP, et al. The use of diuretics in heart failure with congestion—a position statement from the Heart Failure Association of the European Society of Cardiology. Eur J Heart Fail 2019;21:137–55.

28. Ventura HO, Lavie CJ. Hypertension: management and measurements. Curr Opin Cardiol 2018;33: 375–6.

29. Stewart MH, Lavie CJ, Ventura HO. Future pharmacological therapy in hypertension. Curr Opin Cardiol 2018;33:408–15.

30. Carlisle MA, Fudim M, DeVore AD, et al. Heart failure and atrial fibrillation, like fire and fury. JACC Heart Fail 2019;7:447–56.

31. Marra AM, Benjamin N, Eichstaedt C, et al. Gender-related differences in pulmonary arterial hypertension targeted drugs administration. Pharmacol Res 2016;114:103–9.

32. Salzano A, Demelo-Rodriguez P, Marra AM, et al. A focused review of gender differences in antithrombotic therapy. Curr Med Chem 2017;24:2576–88.

33. Giannoulis MG, Boroujerdi MA, Powrie J, et al. Gender differences in growth hormone response to exercise before and after rhGH administration and the effect of rhGH on the hormone profile of fit normal adults. Clin Endocrinol (Oxf) 2005;62:315–22.

Thyroid Abnormalities in Heart Failure

Sara Danzi, PhD[a], Irwin Klein, MD[b],*

KEYWORDS

- Triiodothyronine • T_3 • Nonthyroidal illness • Cardiac • Thyroid hormone • Low T_3 syndrome
- Cardiovascular

KEY POINTS

- Thyroid hormone metabolism is altered in chronic heart failure, after myocardial infarction, after cardiac surgery, and in acute and chronic illness.
- A variety of clinical and physiologic factors suggest that the low levels of T_3 that result from altered thyroid hormone metabolism have adverse consequences similar to that of classical hypothyroidism suggesting a low T_3 syndrome, or nonthyroidal Illness. This low T_3 syndrome is a strong prognostic, independent predictor of death in patients with acute and chronic heart disease.
- T_3 regulates many important genes in the cardiac myocyte. Low T_3 states that accompany cardiac disease states alter gene expression similar to that seen in hypothyroidism.
- In patients with heart failure, the decrease in serum T_3 concentration is proportional to the severity of the heart disease as assessed by the New York Heart Association (NYHA) functional classification.
- When serum T_3 levels are low, total and low-density lipoprotein (LDL) cholesterol and apolipoprotein B levels rise. The increase is proportional to the increase in serum TSH.

INTRODUCTION

More than 200 years ago Caleb Hillier Parry, an English physician, described a woman with goiter and palpitations whose "each systole shook the whole thorax." He was the first to suggest the notion that there was a connection between diseases of the heart and enlargement of the thyroid gland.[1] Thyroid dysfunction including hyperthyroidism and hypothyroidism is common and may affect 15% of women and a smaller percentage of men. As such it would be anticipated that many patients seen in the practice of cardiology would be affected by thyroid disease, either diagnosed or not. Often, however, this association is not considered in the evaluation and management of patients with hypercholesterolemia, hypertension, heart failure, and arrhythmias. The challenge to the cardiologist therefore is (1) to recognize the cardiovascular signs and symptoms of hyperthyroidism and hypothyroidism even in their most subtle presentations, (2) to be familiar with appropriate testing to confirm the clinical suspicion, and (3) to initiate therapy either alone or when appropriate in conjunction with an endocrinologist.[2]

The clinical manifestations of thyroid dysfunction include significant effects on the heart and cardiovascular system. In fact, the cardiovascular abnormalities are some of the most characteristic clinical signs and symptoms of hyperthyroidism including, but not limited to, tachycardia, atrial fibrillation, systolic hypertension, and

This article originally appeared in *Heart Failure Clinics*, Volume 16, Issue 1, January 2020.
Disclosure Statement: I. Klein is an advisor to LioTriDevelopment Corp. S. Danzi has nothing to disclose.
[a] Department of Biological Sciences and Geology, Queensborough Community College, City University of New York, 222-05 56th Avenue, Bayside, NY 11364, USA; [b] NYU School of Medicine, 555 Broadhollow Road, Suite 229, Melville, NY 11747, USA
* Corresponding author.
E-mail address: iklein@northwell.edu

hyperdynamic precordium.[2,3] Hypothyroidism has the opposite effects. Hypothyroidism contributes to, or may cause de novo, many of the conditions seen in cardiology practice including hypercholesterolemia, diastolic hypertension, statin myopathy, and left ventricular diastolic dysfunction leading to heart failure with preserved ejection fraction (**Table 1**). The recognition of the role of thyroid disease in these patients is especially important because in almost every case, restoration of a euthyroid state with thyroid hormone replacement results in improvement or normalization of the cardiovascular abnormality. Heart failure itself can result in reduced serum levels of active thyroid hormone (low T_3 syndrome),[4] and similar to that seen in hypothyroidism, can further impair cardiac function. We discuss the role of changes in thyroid hormone metabolism that may arise in patients with no prior history of primary thyroidal illness but as a result of cardiovascular disease.

THYROID DISEASE

Thyroid disease states, often arise as a result of a genetic predisposition to the autoimmune diathesis giving rise to either Graves or Hashimoto disease. Hypothyroidism is the most common form of thyroid dysfunction and this prevalence increases with advancing age. In contrast hyperthyroidism is significantly less common with the onset characteristically (but not exclusively) occurring in women around the childbearing years. The prevalence of thyroid dysfunction is five to seven times more common in women than men; not surprising given the autoimmune cause of both conditions. There are a sufficient number of sensitive and specific thyroid function tests to establish a diagnosis of either hyperthyroidism (overt or subclinical) or hypothyroidism (overt or subclinical) with a high degree of precision. As such most Societies recommend that physicians use routine laboratory testing (thyroid-stimulating hormone [TSH]) to conform with aggressive case finding.[5] This is especially relevant to the practice of cardiology and many commonly used International Classification of Diseases-10 codes support thyroid function testing.[1–3]

THYROID HORMONE METABOLISM
Thyroid Hormone Regulation

Thyroid hormones produced by the thyroid gland include tetraiodothyronine (T_4) and triiodothyronine (T_3). The gland produces primarily T_4 ($\sim 85\%$) and significantly less T_3 ($\sim 15\%$), although T_3 is the active form of the hormone. The conversion of T_4, a prohormone, to T_3 takes place in the tissues of specific organs and most of the available serum T_3 is provided by enzymatic deiodination of T_4 in the liver and kidney. The enzyme, 5'-monodeiodinase, removes one iodine atom from T_4 to produce T_3. Factors that impair the activity of this enzyme lead to decreased levels of T_3 in the serum and therefore, in dependent tissues.

Thyroid hormone production is regulated by a negative feedback loop. The hypothalamus produces thyrotropin-releasing hormone, which stimulates the anterior pituitary to produce thyrotropin, or TSH. TSH acts on the thyroid gland to release thyroid hormones, T_4 and T_3. It is primarily T_4 that feeds back to the pituitary to decrease production of TSH. Insufficient deiodination of T_4 to T_3 can cause levels of T_3 to be low, when TSH and T_4 are within the normal range (discussed later).

Thyroid Function Testing

There are highly sensitive and specific tests for hyperthyroidism and hypothyroidism. Commonly used tests include serum measures of thyrotropin (TSH), T_4 (total and free), and T_3. A single TSH test

Table 1
Changes in cardiovascular function associated with thyroid disease

	Normal	Hyperthyroid	Hypothyroid
SVR (dyne s cm^{-5})	1500–1700	700–1200	2100–2700
Heart rate (bpm)	72–84	88–130	60–80
% EF	60	>60	<60
IVRT (ms)	60–80	25–40	>80
Cardiac output (L/min)	5.8	>7.0	<4.5
Blood volume (% normal)	100	105.5	84.5

Abbreviation: EF, ejection fraction; IVRT, isovolumic relaxation time; SVR, systemic vascular resistance.

Adapted from Klein I, Ojamaa K. Thyroid hormone and the cardiovascular system. N Engl J Med. 2001;344:502; with permission.

in a nonhospitalized patient is sufficient to establish a diagnosis with low levels of TSH (<0.01 UIU/L) showing pituitary suppression, indicating hyperthyroidism and elevated levels greater than 10 UIU/L indicating primary thyroidal failure. Confirmatory measures of T_4 and T_3 solidify the diagnosis. However, in milder (subclinical) disease states the levels of T_4 may be normal.

The clinical importance of this testing is not only to provide laboratory data to validate a suspected diagnosis but perhaps more importantly safe, effective and inexpensive treatments are available for both conditions.[1–4] Thus the young woman with palpitations, the middle-aged man with the acute onset of atrial fibrillation, or the elderly man with new-onset hypercholesterolemia and myopathy are equally likely to benefit from TSH testing.[2]

EFFECT OF T_3 ON THE CARDIAC MYOCYTE
Cellular Action of T_3

The heart is sensitive to changes in serum T_3. This has been demonstrated by rapid changes in T_3-mediated cardiac gene expression as serum T_3 levels decline in an animal model (**Fig. 1**).[6] Cardiac tissue does not appreciably convert T_4 to T_3; therefore, the heart is dependent on available serum T_3. The monocarboxylate transporters MCT8 and MCT10 are highly specific for thyroid hormones and are the primary thyroid hormone transporters for cardiac myocytes. Although MCT8 and MCT10 facilitate uptake and efflux of

T_4 and T_3 in experimental cell systems, our data suggest that T_4 is not transported into the heart.[7] MCT10 has greater affinity for T_3 than T_4 and has a greater capacity to transport T_3 than MCT8.[8]

The transcriptional actions of T_3 are mediated by nuclear receptor proteins (TRs) that bind to specific thyroid hormone response elements in the upstream region of T_3-responsive genes.[9] These nuclear receptors, which include isoforms of TR-α and TR-β, activate expression of positively regulated genes in the presence of T_3 and in the absence of T_3, repress transcription.

Thyroid hormone also has extranuclear nongenomic effects on the cardiac myocyte and on the systemic vasculature. These T_3-mediated effects include changes in various membrane ion channels for sodium, potassium, and calcium; effects on adenine nucleotide translocator-1 in the mitochondrial membrane; and a variety of intracellular signaling pathways in the heart and vascular smooth muscle cells.[10] Together, the nongenomic and genomic effects of T_3 act to regulate cardiac function and cardiovascular hemodynamics.

T_3-Regulated Cardiac Genes

T_3 is an important regulator of cardiac gene expression and the list of T_3-mediated genes that are altered in heart failure is almost identical to the changes in gene expression in overt hypothyroidism.[11] These include the genes that encode the contractile proteins, α-myosin heavy chain (MHC) and β-MHC, the sodium calcium exchanger (NCX1), the sarcoplasmic reticulum calcium ATPase (SERCA2), phospholamban, and the β-adrenergic receptor. The net effect of these alterations in gene expression is to alter cardiac contractility, calcium cycling, and diastolic relaxation of the myocardium. α-MHC, the fast myosin, is positively regulated by thyroid hormone, whereas the slow myosin ATPase, β-MHC, is negatively regulated. The SERCA2 pump functions to sequester calcium in the sarcoplasmic reticulum during the relaxation phase of myocyte contraction, because calcium is required for the contraction phase. Phospholamban is a membrane protein that negatively regulates SERCA2 function. SERCA2 is positively regulated by thyroid hormone and phospholamban is negatively regulated. These two proteins play a critical role in diastolic function. Changes in the relative amounts of these proteins and the state of phosphorylation of phospholamban may account for altered diastolic function in heart failure and thyroid disease (**Fig. 2**).[12]

Both MCT8 and MCT10, the iodothyronine specific transporters, are also negatively regulated by thyroid hormone (**Table 2**).[7]

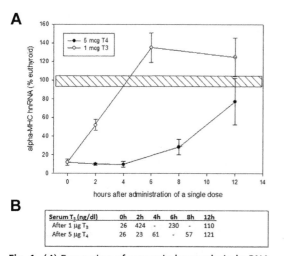

Fig. 1. (A) Expression of α-myosin heavy chain hnRNA levels (as % euthyroid) in hypothyroid rats after administration of a single dose of T_3 (1 μg) or T_4 (5 μg). (B) Corresponding serum T_3 levels (ng/dL) for same experiment described in A. hnRNA, heterogeneous nuclear RNA, the first product of transcription, or prespliced primary transcript; MHC, myosin heavy chain.

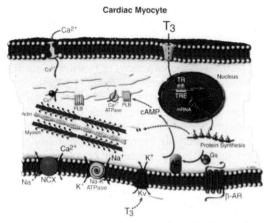

Cardiac Myocyte

Fig. 2. The cellular pathways and mechanisms of action of thyroid hormone (T_3) on the cardiac myocyte. T_3 has genomic and nongenomic effects on the cardiac myocyte. Genomic mechanisms involve T_3 binding to TRs, which regulate transcription of specific cardiac genes. Nongenomic mechanisms include direct modulation of membrane ion channels (*dashed arrows*). AC, adenylyl cyclase; b-AR, b-adrenergic receptor; Gs, guanine nucleotide binding protein; Kv, voltage-gated potassium channels; NCX, sodium calcium exchanger; PLB, phospholamban; TRE, thyroid hormone response element. (*From* Klein I, Danzi S. Thyroid disease and the heart. Circulation. 2007;116(15):1726; with permission.)

T_3 EFFECTS ON CARDIOVASCULAR HEMODYNAMICS

Thyroid hormone acts directly on the heart and vasculature and indirectly to influence cardiovascular hemodynamics. The net result is that contractility is enhanced and vascular resistance is decreased in response to thyroid hormone action, whereas in the absence of sufficient thyroid hormone, contractility is decreased and resistance is increased. This is caused by direct effects of T_3 on tissue thermogenesis, system vascular resistance, and cardiac chronotropy and inotropy, resulting in changes in blood volume and cardiac output (**Fig. 3**).[2]

In hyperthyroidism, cardiac contractility is enhanced and cardiac output and resting heart rate are increased. Systolic and diastolic functions are enhanced and the decrease in system vascular resistance decreases afterload. The enhanced cardiovascular hemodynamics leads to increased blood flow and tissue perfusion. The clinical manifestations of hyperthyroidism include atrial arrhythmias in older patients along with tachycardia, widened pulse pressure, and dyspnea on exertion.[13]

In hypothyroidism, signs are opposite to those of hyperthyroidism and are more subtle, but may include bradycardia, diastolic hypertension, and a narrowed pulse pressure. Cardiac contractility is decreased and systemic vascular resistance is increased. As in the clinically hypothyroid patient, the characteristic hemodynamic profile of heart failure includes a low cardiac output caused by impaired cardiac contractility, and an elevated systemic vascular resistance.[4]

T_3 seems to reduce systemic vascular resistance by direct effects on vascular smooth muscle cells and through changes in the vascular endothelium. Nongenomic actions target membrane ion channels and endothelial nitric oxide synthase. Increased endothelial nitric oxide production may result, in part, from the T_3-mediated effects on the protein kinase akt pathway either via nongenomic or genomic mechanisms. Nitric oxide synthesized in endothelial cells then acts in a paracrine manner on adjacent vascular smooth muscle cells to facilitate vascular relaxation. Relaxation of vascular smooth muscle leads to decreased arterial resistance and pressure, which thereby increases cardiac output.[14–16]

Nonthyroidal Disease

In contrast to primary thyroid disease, over the last three decades there has been the recognition that there are a variety of nonthyroidal disease states that can alter measures of thyroid function. Because these were first characterized by normal levels of TSH (the prime measure of thyroid hormone metabolism) in the face of low levels of liothyronine (T_3) these were referred to as euthyroid

Table 2 Effect of T_3 on cardiac-specific genes	
Positively Regulated	**Negatively Regulated**
α-Myosin heavy chain	β-Myosin heavy chain
Sarcoplasmic reticulum Ca^{2+}-ATPase	Phospholamban
Na^+/K^+ ATPase	Adenylyl cyclase catalytic subunits
$β_1$-Adrenergic receptor	Thyroid hormone receptor alpha-1
Atrial natriuretic hormone	Na^+/Ca^{2+} exchanger
Voltage-gated potassium channels	Thyroid hormone transporters (MCT8, MCT10)
	Adenine nucleotide translocase-1 (ANT1)

From Danzi S, Klein I. Thyroid disease and the cardiovascular system. Endocrinol Metab Clin North Am. 2014;43:518; with permission.

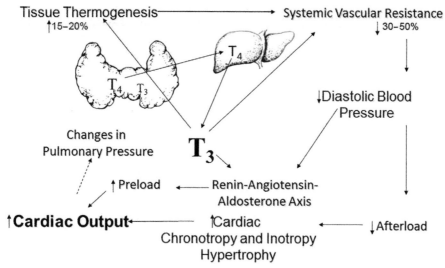

Fig. 3. Effects of thyroid hormone on cardiovascular hemodynamics. The individual changes for hyperthyroidism are noted for each parameter. The effects of hypothyroidism are diametrically opposite. (*Adapted from* Klein I, Danzi S. Thyroid disease and the heart. Circulation. 2007;116(15):1727; with permission.)

sick states. However, a variety of clinical and physiologic factors suggested that the low levels of T_3 had adverse consequences similar to that of classical hypothyroidism, leading to an alternative designation of "nonthyroidal illnesses" (NTI).

To investigate this at the preclinical level our laboratory adopted the energy-restricted rodent model to simulate the low T_3 level in otherwise euthyroid animals. Various physiologic and biochemical measures of thyroid and cardiovascular functional activity were compared with animals rendered classically hypothyroid by thyroidectomy. Both groups of animals were treated with replacement doses of T_4 or T_3 and at sacrifice, thyroid function tests were measured and left ventricular contractility was assessed in the Langendorf isolated perfused heart model (**Fig. 4**).[17] The NTI animals displayed impaired inotropic and lusitropic changes identical to the hypothyroid hearts. In vivo treatment with replacement doses of T_3 but not T_4 treatment restored the NTI animals to control euthyroid functional levels. Based on analysis of gene expression from the myocytes of these five groups of animals it was shown that these changes arose at the classical nuclear transcriptional level well known as the site of action for T_3.[18]

Cardiovascular Diseases as Causes of Nonthyroidal Illness

Thyroid hormone metabolism, specifically the deiodination of T_4, is decreased in chronic heart failure, after myocardial infarction, after cardiac surgery, and in acute and chronic illness. Recent studies have characterized the changes in thyroid

hormone metabolism that accompany a variety of cardiovascular disease states.[2,19,20] In patients with heart failure, the decrease in serum T_3 concentration is proportional to the severity of the heart disease as assessed by the New York Heart Association functional classification.[4,19,21,22] This seems to result from a cytokine-mediated inhibition in the normal hepatic conversion of T_4 to the active T_3 and is well characterized as part of the spectrum of NTI or the low T_3 syndrome.[23,24] Interleukin-6 and tumor necrosis factor-α levels are increased in the low T_3 syndrome.[25] The effect on serum T_3 seems to result from a cytokine-induced blockade of 5-monodeiodinase synthesis and activity.[26] There is ample evidence that multiple mechanisms contribute to the low T_3 syndrome. In more severe cases, serum T_4 may also be decreased and the term NTI may be used to

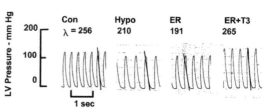

Fig. 4. Effect of the low T_3 syndrome on cardiac contractile function. Con, control; ER + T3, energy restricted with T3 treatment; ER, energy restricted; Hypo, hypothyroid; LV, left ventricular. (*From* Katzeff HL, Powell SR, Ojamaa K. Alterations in cardiac contractility and gene expression during low-T3 syndrome: prevention with T3. Am J Physiol. 1997;273:E951–E953; with permission.)

describe the same syndrome.[27] This low T_3 syndrome is a strong prognostic, independent predictor of death in patients with acute and chronic heart disease.[19,20,28] In human and animal studies, T_3 replacement in heart failure improved left ventricular function and restored myocyte gene expression to euthyroid levels, similar to that seen in the treatment of hypothyroidism. These low T_3 levels may contribute further to impaired diastolic function in patients with preserved and reduced ejection fraction.[29–33]

Although TSH levels may remain normal, serum levels of total T_3 fall in proportion to the severity of heart failure and also serve as a predictor of poor outcome. Similarly, low T_3 levels, despite normal TSH, are associated with worse outcomes after cardiac surgery.[33] It is interesting to speculate that these low levels of T_3 may contribute further to impaired diastolic function in patients with preserved and reduced ejection fraction.[4,11,29] Whether thyroid hormone–based therapies, including T_3 or novel thyroid hormone analogues, prove useful, especially in patients with heart failure with preserved ejection fraction, remains to be established (**Fig. 5**).

B-type natriuretic peptide (BNP) is a hormone produced by the heart and released in response to changes in pressure inside the heart, which can be related to heart failure and other cardiac problems. In a recent, large study of patients in a primary care setting, BNP was found to be a predictor of all-cause mortality.[34] The N-terminal pro-BNP (NT-proBNP) levels are easily measured, objective markers of cardiac function and are used to diagnose heart failure, including diastolic dysfunction. Selvaraj and colleagues[29] demonstrated an association of serum T_3 with BNP and severe left ventricular diastolic dysfunction in heart failure with preserved ejection fraction. As T_3 levels decrease, NT-proBNP levels increase. There is an inverse correlation between BNP levels and heart failure. Levels goes up when heart failure develops or gets worse, and levels goes down when heart failure is stable. Although low T_3 levels have been shown to be independent predictors of all-cause and cardiac mortalities among critically ill patients with heart failure, the combination of high NT-proBNP with low T_3 levels predict a worse long-term outcome.[35]

THYROID HORMONE EFFECTS ON LIPID METABOLISM

Thyroid hormone alters the lipid profile, specifically to decrease serum cholesterol levels. Therefore, in hypothyroidism, similar to heart failure, total and low density lipoprotein (LDL) cholesterol and apolipoprotein B levels rise. The increase is proportional to the increase in serum TSH.[36] A recent study demonstrated that after thyroidectomy for thyroid cancer, treatment of hypothyroid patients with levothyroxine resulted in a reduction of cardiac lipid content and improved cardiac index.[37]

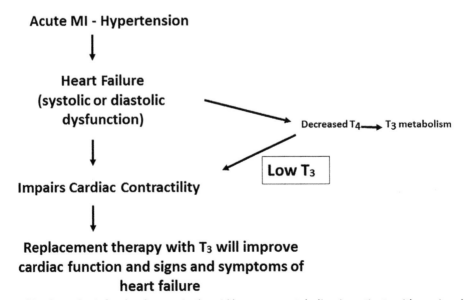

Acute MI - Hypertension

↓

Heart Failure (systolic or diastolic dysfunction)

Decreased T_4 → T_3 metabolism

Low T_3

↓

Impairs Cardiac Contractility

↓

Replacement therapy with T_3 will improve cardiac function and signs and symptoms of heart failure

Fig. 5. A working hypothesis for the changes in thyroid hormone metabolism in patients with varying degrees of heart failure that can contribute to progression of impaired cardiac contractility. MI, myocardial infarction. (*Adapted from* Klein I, Danzi S. Thyroid hormone treatment to mend a broken heart. J Clin Endocrinol Metab. 2008;93:1173; with permission.)

Cholesterol Metabolism

Increased LDL cholesterol occurs in the setting of hypothyroidism and in proportion to the rise in serum TSH levels.[36,37] Thyroid hormone alters cholesterol metabolism through a variety of mechanisms, including a decrease in LDL receptor expression but perhaps more importantly a decrease in biliary excretion. The cholesterol-lowering effect of thyroid hormone in patients with hypothyroidism was originally described in 1930. LDL is the principal lipoprotein that is reduced; the reduction is induced by increased hepatic clearance caused by increased expression of the hepatic LDL-receptor gene. In rodents, thyromimetic compounds also accelerate clearance of cholesterol by the liver by increasing the high-density lipoprotein receptor called scavenger receptor B1 (SR-B1), increasing the activity of cholesterol 7α-hydroxylase and increasing fecal excretion of cholesterol and bile acids. Previous attempts to mimic these actions with thyroid hormone metabolites and analogues have confirmed their cholesterol-lowering properties. Further support for the role of thyroid hormone in the regulation of cholesterol metabolism comes from a recent study that describes a liver-selective thyroid hormone agonist, eprotirome, that can synergistically lower cholesterol levels in statin-treated patients.[38] Not only was LDL significantly decreased, but a rather unique ability to lower Lp(a), an especially atherogenic lipid particle, was seen.

Statin-Induced Myopathy

Hypothyroidism is well known to produce a skeletal muscle myopathy associated with cramps; stiffness; decreased muscle endurance; and in severe cases, pseudohypertrophy and pseudomyotonia. The deep tendon reflexes are delayed and serum creatine kinase (CK) levels can be markedly increased to 20 times normal with a predominately MM isoform pattern. All abnormalities resolve with thyroid hormone replacement.[39] HMG-CoA reductase inhibitors (statins) can also produce a myopathic syndrome as many as 10% of patients with a clinical spectrum extending from mild cramping to full blown rhabdomyolysis. The overlap between hypothyroid myopathy and statin-induced myopathy is characterized in **Table 3**. It has been the experience of our group and others that patients with hypothyroidism are at increased risk of developing a statin-induced myopathy.[40] This point is especially clinically relevant because patients with hypothyroidism are likely to have some degree of endogenous hypercholesterolemia and be candidates for lipid-lowering therapy. It may be that T_4 treatment alone can accomplish the desired effect.[40]

Thyroid Hormone–Based Treatment of Heart Failure

Current treatment of heart failure requires multiple medications including β-adrenergic blocking drugs, angiotensin-converting enzyme inhibitors, aldosterone antagonists, digitalis, and diuretics. Within the last 2 years two new Food and Drug Administration–approved medications have entered the market. Angiotensin receptor-neprilysin inhibitor (Entresto), a combination of sacubitril and valsartan, and a novel channel inhibitor of the sinoatrial node (Corlanor) are now available for treatment of patients with symptomatic heart failure. Despite maximum medical therapy, mortality remains high and novel treatment strategies are actively sought. One field of investigation is that of gene therapy in which a variety of viral vectors encoding specific cardiac regulatory and structural proteins are directed to the impaired myocyte. Because calcium uptake and release by the sarcoplasmic reticulum is frequently impaired in heart failure, the ability to increase

Table 3 Muscle disease syndromes	
Statin-Induced	**Hypothyroid-Related**
Myopathy: any associated disease Myalgia: muscle aches/weakness without CK elevation Myositis: symptoms plus elevated CK Rhabdomyolysis: symptoms plus markedly elevated CK levels	Myalgia: nonspecific muscle symptoms, cramping, especially nocturnal, variable CK level Myopathy: impaired endurance usually with CK elevation; pseudomyotonia Hoffmann syndrome: impaired function; pseudohypertrophy, often marked CK elevations

CK, creatine kinase.
From Rush J, Danzi S, Klein I. Role of thyroid disease in the development of statin-induced myopathy. The Endocrinologist. 2006;16(5):279–85; with permission.

SERCA or to lower its inhibitory regulator phospholamban are attractive targets for genetic manipulation. Studies of the cellular mechanisms of thyroid hormone action described previously on the cardiac myocyte have demonstrated that similar to the hypothyroid myocardium, treatment of the failing heart with T_3 produces a similar and desirable change in the cardiac phenotype. Other thyroid hormone responsive genes, which may play a role in the improved cardiac contractile function, include β_1-adrenergic receptor, stimulatory guanine nucleotide binding proteins (G_s), α-MHC, sodium-calcium exchanger, and perhaps the voltage-gated potassium channels (K_v). Because most patients who die of heart failure do so as the result of a ventricular arrhythmia, a positive effect on K_v expression leading to a shortening of the QT interval on the electrocardiogram is therapeutically desirable.

Perhaps most importantly is the observation from many studies, that T_3 treatment does not produce untoward effects when administered in either physiologic or short-term pharmacologic doses to patients with concomitant cardiac disease.[41] There have been no reported episodes of supraventricular arrhythmias, increases in heart rate, or worsening of cardiac ischemia in any of the reported series to date. To restore serum T_3 levels to normal, investigations have used short-term intravenous administration of drug. Although potentially useful in acute studies, this does not address the more relevant question of long-term therapy. Thus, any long-term studies undertaken to establish safety and efficacy of T_3 treatment of heart failure need to use a formulation of T_3 not currently available. The clinical reality that such patients will already be treated with β-adrenergic blockade provides a combination of treatments with therapeutic synergy.

REFERENCES

1. Klein I, Danzi S. Thyroid disease and the heart. Curr Probl Cardiol 2016;41:65–92.
2. Klein I. Endocrine disorders and cardiovascular disease. In: Bonow RO, Mann DL, Zipes DP, et al, editors. Braunwald's heart disease. 10th edition. St. Louis, MO: WB Saunders and Company; 2014. p. 1793–808 [Chapter 81].
3. Klein I, Danzi S. Thyroid disease and the heart. Circulation 2007;116(15):1725–35.
4. Ascheim DD, Hryniewicz K. Thyroid hormone metabolism in patients with congestive heart failure: the low triiodothyronine state. Thyroid 2002;12(6):511–5.
5. Hennessey JV, Klein I, Woeber K, et al. Aggressive case finding: a clinical strategy for the documentation of thyroid dysfunction. Ann Intern Med 2015;163(4):311–2.
6. Danzi S, Ojamaa K, Klein I. Triiodothyronine-mediated myosin heavy chain gene transcription in the heart. Am J Physiol Heart Circ Physiol 2003;284:H2255–62.
7. Danzi S, Klein I. Thyroid hormone and the cardiovascular system. Med Clin North Am 2012;96:257–68.
8. Dumitrescu AM, Liao XH, Weiss RE, et al. Tissue-specific thyroid hormone deprivation and excess in monocarboxylate transporter (Mct) 8-deficient mice. Endocrinology 2009;150:4450–8.
9. Dillmann WH. Cellular action of thyroid hormone on the heart. Thyroid 2002;12:447–52.
10. Davis PJ, Davis FB. Nongenomic actions of thyroid hormone on the heart. Thyroid 2002;12:459–66.
11. Danzi S, Klein I. Changes in thyroid hormone metabolism and gene expression in the failing heart: therapeutic implications. In: Iervasi G, Pingitore A, editors. Thyroid and heart failure, from pathophysiology to clinics. Milan, Italy: Springer-Verlag; 2009. p. 97–107 [Chapter 10].
12. Kiss E, Jakab G, Kranias EG, et al. Thyroid-hormone-induced alterations in phospholamban protein expression: regulatory effects on sarcoplasmic reticulum Ca2+ transport and myocardial relaxation. Circ Res 1994;75:245–51.
13. Shimizu T, Koide S, Noh JY, et al. Hyperthyroidism and the management of atrial fibrillation. Thyroid 2002;12:489–93.
14. Park K, Dai H, Ojamaa K, et al. Direct vasomotor effect of thyroid hormones on rat skeletal muscle resistance arteries. Anesth Analg 1997;85:734–8.
15. Taddei S, Caraccio N, Virdis A, et al. Impaired endothelium-dependent vasodilatation in subclinical hypothyroidism: beneficial effect of levothyroxine therapy. J Clin Endocrinol Metab 2003;88:3731–7.
16. Kuzman JA, Gerdes AM, Kobayashi S, et al. Thyroid hormone activates Akt and prevents serum starvation-induced cell death in neonatal rat cardiomyocytes. J Mol Cell Cardiol 2005;39:841–4.
17. Katzeff HL, Powell SR, Ojamaa K. Alterations in cardiac contractility and gene expression during low-T3 syndrome: prevention with T3. Am J Physiol 1997; 273:E951–6.
18. Klein I, Ojamaa K. Thyroid hormone and the cardiovascular system. N Engl J Med 2001;344:501–9.
19. Iervasi G, Pingitore A, Landi P, et al. Low-T3 syndrome: a strong prognostic predictor of death in patients with heart disease. Circulation 2003;107:708–13.
20. Cerillo AG, Storti S, Kallushi E, et al. The low triiodothyronine syndrome: a strong predictor of low cardiac output and death in patients undergoing coronary artery bypass grafting. Ann Thorac Surg 2014;97(6):2089–95.
21. Hamilton AM. Prevalence and clinical implications of abnormal thyroid hormone metabolism in advanced heart failure. Ann Thorac Surg 1993;56:S48–53.

22. Hamilton MA, Stevenson LW, Luu M, et al. Altered hormone metabolism in advanced heart failure. J Am Coll Cardiol 1990;16:91–5.

23. Boelen A, Maas MA, Lowik CW, et al. Induced illness in interleukin-6 (IL-6) knock-out mice: causal role of IL-6 in the development of the low 3,5,3'-triiodothyronine syndrome. Endocrinology 1996;137:5250–4.

24. Danzi S, Klein I. Thyroid disease and the cardiovascular system. Endocrinol Metab Clin North Am 2014; 43:517–28.

25. Yu J, Koenig RJ. Induction of type 1 iodothyronine deiodinase to prevent the nonthyroidal illness syndrome in mice. Endocrinology 2006;147:3580–5.

26. Lubrano V, Pingitore A, Carpi A, et al. Relationship between triiodothyronine and proinflammatory cytokines in chronic heart failure. Biomed Pharmacother 2010;64:165–9.

27. De Vries EM, Fliers E, Boelen A. The molecular basis of the non-thyroidal illness syndrome. J Endocrinol 2015;225:R67–81.

28. Zhang B, Peng W, Wang C, et al. A low fT3 level as a prognostic marker in patients with acute myocardial infarctions. Intern Med 2012;51:3009–15.

29. Selvaraj S, Klein I, Danzi S, et al. Association of serum triiodothyronine with B-type natriuretic peptide and severe left ventricular diastolic dysfunction in heart failure with preserved ejection fraction. Am J Cardiol 2012;110(2):234–9.

30. Klein I, Danzi S. Thyroid hormone treatment to mend a broken heart. J Clin Endocrinol Metab 2008;93: 1172–4.

31. Pingitore A, Galli E, Barison A, et al. Acute effects of triiodothyronine (T3) replacement therapy in patients with chronic heart failure and low-T3 syndrome: a randomized, placebo-controlled study. J Clin Endocrinol Metab 2008;93:1351–8.

32. Henderson K, Danzi S, Paul JT, et al. Physiological replacement of T_3 improves left ventricular function in an animal model of myocardial infarction-induced congestive heart failure. Circ Heart Fail 2009;2:243–52.

33. Iervasi G, Molinaro S, Landi P, et al. Association between increased mortality and mild thyroid dysfunction in cardiac patients. Arch Intern Med 2007;167: 1526–32.

34. Hejl JL, Grand MK, Siersma V, et al. Brain natriuretic peptide in plasma as predictor of all-cause mortality in a large Danish primary health care population suspected of heart failure. Clin Chem 2018;64(12): 1723–31.

35. Chuang C-P, Jong Y-S, Wu C-Y, et al. Impact of triiodothyronine and N-terminal pro-B-type natriuretic peptide on the long-term survival of critically ill patients with acute heart failure. Am J Cardiol 2014; 113:845–50.

36. Cappola AR, Ladenson PW. Hypothyroidism and atherosclerosis. J Clin Endocrinol Metab 2003;88: 2438–44.

37. Scherer T, Wolf P, Winhofer Y, et al. Levothyroxine replacement in hypothyroid humans reduces myocardial lipid load and improves cardiac function. J Clin Endocrinol Metab 2014;99:E2341–6.

38. Ladenson PW, Kristensen JD, Ridgway EC, et al. Use of the thyroid hormone analogue eprotirome in statin-treated dyslipidemia. N Engl J Med 2010; 362(10):906–16.

39. Lando HM, Burman KD. Two cases of statin-induced myopathy caused by induced hypothyroidism. Endocr Pract 2008;14:726–31.

40. Rush J, Danzi S, Klein I. Role of thyroid disease in the development of statin-induced myopathy. Endocrinologist 2006;16(5):279–85.

41. Danzi S, Klein I. Alterations in thyroid hormones which accompany cardiovascular disease. Clin Thyroidol 2009;21:3–5.

Anabolic Deficiencies in Heart Failure
Ready for Prime Time?

Raffaele Napoli, MD[a], Roberta D'Assante, PhD[a], Martina Miniero, MD[a],
Andrea Salzano, MD, MRCP (London)[b], Antonio Cittadini, MD[a],*

KEYWORDS

- Chronic heart failure • HFrEF • HFpEF • Multiple hormonal deficiency • Insulin resistance
- Testosterone • GH/IGF 1 axis • Thyroid hormone

KEY POINTS

- Many patients with chronic heart failure show some hormonal deficiency that might worsen morbidity and mortality.
- Chronic heart failure development might be explained by the imbalance between catabolic and anabolic pathways present in the disease.
- Multiple hormonal deficiency is associated with a relevant worsening of prognosis in patients with chronic heart failure and patients should be screened for it.
- Replacement hormonal therapy in patients with chronic heart failure has shown promising beneficial results.

INTRODUCTION

Heart failure (HF) is a syndrome defined based on clinical symptoms and signs due to cardiac abnormalities, either structural and/or functional.[1] Until a few years ago, an impairment of systolic function, that is, reduction of ejection fraction (EF), was considered essential in the definition of the disease. Nowadays, an emerging importance is attributed to HF with normal or only slightly reduced EF, but abnormal ventricle relaxation. Such a condition, defined HF with preserved EF (HFpEF), has modified and seriously complicated the interpretation of the mechanisms behind the onset of chronic HF (CHF). The 2 conditions ultimately may overlap in individual patients and are almost invariably present in the advanced stage of CHF. The mechanisms behind the development of CHF with reduced EF (HFrEF) and HFpEF can be different.[2] From the epidemiologic point of view and compared with HFrEF, the HFpEF is more rapidly increasing its occurrence and is more frequently associated with chronic metabolic abnormalities of patients.[2,3] Drawing an exact line rigidly separating the 2 forms of HF is difficult. However, experimental data suggest that whereas HFrEF is initially characterized by the necrosis of cardiomyocytes and the subsequent collagen deposition occurs mainly to fulfill the void due to the cell death, in HFpEF the pathologic insult appears to involve primarily the endothelial cells and collagen deposition is located in the spaces

This article originally appeared in *Heart Failure Clinics*, Volume 16, Issue 1, January 2020.

Disclosure Statement: Dr A. Salzano receives research grant support from CardioPath, Department of Advanced Biomedical Sciences, Federico II University, Naples, Italy, UniNa and Compagnia di San Paolo in the frame of the STAR program.

[a] Department of Translational Medical Sciences, Federico II University, Via S Pansini 5, 80131 Naples, Italy;
[b] Diagnostic and Nuclear Research Institute, IRCCS SDN, Via E Gianturco 113, 80142 Naples, Italy
* Corresponding author.
E-mail address: cittadin@unina.it
twitter: @RaffaeleGNapoli (R.N.)

between the cardiomyocytes.[2] In advanced HF, with the evolution of the disease, the combination of cardiomyocyte necrosis, endothelial dysfunction, and diffuse collagen deposition coexist in the same heart. The mechanisms ultimately leading to the development of HF start many years before the clinical syndrome appears and the diagnosis can be made. Therefore, of great interest would be to identify and clarify the mechanisms behind the 2 clinical forms of the disease to counteract precociously and efficaciously the onset of the disease.

Based mainly on the data deriving from the study of HFrEF, a model for the development of HF was designed. According to this model, following myocardial injury, heart function is impaired and fails to fulfill the hemodynamic needs. An adaptive response, aimed to sustain cardiac performance, mainly systolic function, is triggered. Such response is characterized by activation of the sympathetic nervous system (SNS), renin-angiotensin-aldosterone system (RAAS), endothelin, inflammatory cytokine, and so on. Whereas in the short-term this response can be useful to improve heart performance, in the long-term becomes maladaptive, leading to the worsening of heart function.[4] This interpretation of the sequence of events leading finally to overt HF has supported a model of treatment based on the contrast to the activation of these maladaptive pathways. Accordingly, treatment with, for example, beta-blockers, angiotensin-converting enzyme inhibitors, angiotensin receptor blockers, and aldosterone receptor blockers, has proved their efficacy in patients with CHF either in terms of morbidity or mortality.[4,5] However, 2 main considerations suggest that the neurohormonal activation model does not completely fulfill the needs for the treatment of HF. First, although in recent years therapy led to an improved prognosis of patients with HF, the progression of the disease still represents a heavy unbearable burden of the treatment. The data available show that the survival of patients with HF is still low and mortality is higher than many types of cancer.[5] In addition, the number of patients discharged from hospitals with the diagnosis of HF has steadily increased in the past 2 decades, suggesting that the actual therapy, although effective, cannot satisfy all the needs of the treatment of CHF.[6] A second important point should be considered. Whereas the therapy based on the neurohormonal model has proved its efficacy in patients with HFrEF, no positive results in terms of survival are available with regard to the treatment of HFpEF. Therefore, additional mechanisms must be considered with regard to

the development of CHF, particularly HFpEF. Furthermore, HFpEF is rapidly increasing in terms of incidence and prevalence and is going to become the leading form of HF, driven likely by the wide diffusion of chronic metabolic abnormalities, like obesity, that are linked to the disease.[1,2,4–6] Therefore, a novel conceptual framework is necessary to guide a new therapeutic approach.

In several conditions of hormonal abnormalities, we can observe an increased risk of CHF, suggesting that the hormonal milieu might play a role in the maintenance of a healthy heart. It has been demonstrated for many hormones that the impairment of hormonal action may induce functional disturbances of the heart and lead to worse survival.[7–13] In addition, the frequent association between chronic metabolic diseases, such as diabetes or obesity, and CHF, particularly HFpEF, suggests that multiple hormonal and metabolic derangements can be involved in the development of CHF. Consistently, in patients with CHF, many hormonal deficiencies have been demonstrated to be present at high frequency, often coexisting in the same patient. When the reduction of the levels of multiple hormones occurs in the same individual, the prognosis of CHF becomes much worse.[14] However, not only should we consider the deficiency of hormonal stimulation when the levels of circulating hormones are reduced, but also when, in presence of normal, or even increased levels of them, the hormonal activity is compromised. Insulin resistance (IR) is a classic example of this condition. Circulating levels of insulin can be higher than normal, but its tissue activity reduced, resulting in a sort of hormonal deficiency for the target cells. When the possibility of multiple hormonal deficiency has been considered and its impact evaluated, situations of hormonal resistance have been ignored.[14] Therefore, the data available show only the least impact of multiple hormonal deficiencies in CHF.

Therefore, the possibility arises that, together with the activation of catecholamines, endothelin, RAAS system, and so forth, characterized by the stimulation of catabolic pathways, the reduction of anabolic stimuli sustained by hormones may contribute to the onset and development of CHF. In addition, as previously discussed, chronic metabolic diseases are associated with the development of CHF, particularly HFpEF. Such a picture has led to the definition of a hormonal-metabolic model that considers CHF as a multiple hormonal deficiency syndrome.[15–17] Multiple mechanisms might be present behind the multifaceted CHF syndrome. Rather than the isolated activation of a series of hormones and cytokines with catabolic activity, the imbalance between catabolic and anabolic stimulation might represent a model for a complex and serious syndrome like CHF and provide support to new therapeutic approaches.

In the current work, we discuss the role played by the perturbation of hormonal activity in the context of CHF risk and the data available regarding hormonal treatment in patients with CHF.

INSULIN RESISTANCE AND CHRONIC HEART FAILURE

The risks of diabetes and CHF are strictly linked. Compared with control populations, diabetic patients, both type 1 and type 2, have an increased risk of developing CHF and patients with CHF show a higher prevalence of diabetes.[18,19] Diabetic cardiomyopathy has been identified to indicate a condition of metabolic, functional, and structural abnormalities present in diabetic patients independent from coronary heart disease and hypertension. In the past few years, IR, a condition critically present in diabetic patients, but not exclusive to them, has been considered a mechanism possibly responsible for the development of CHF.[20] IR is widely diffuse in the population, particularly in obese and hypertensive patients, but can be present also in apparently healthy subjects. Sedentary life style, incorrect eating, and drugs can promote IR. Interestingly, more than 30% of patients with CHF are insulin resistant and more than 50% have diabetes or IR.[19] IR can predict the development of CHF, as demonstrated by a study in healthy elder patients who showed a higher risk of CHF when IR was present,[21] and correlates with the severity of CHF.[19,22] In addition, in patients with CHF, the presence of IR is associated with poor survival.[9] On the other hand, the link between IR and CHF can be bidirectional: not only can the presence of IR increase the risk of CHF, but also the presence of CHF can aggravate IR, as suggested by data in animals.[23] Endothelial dysfunction, skeletal muscle loss, and physical inactivity, cytokine increase, SNS overactivity, and circulating free fatty acid elevation, are all factors potentially responsible for the worsening of IR in patients with CHF. IR might affect cardiac function through different mechanisms. When IR is present in patients with CHF, heart metabolism becomes inflexible and the capability of using glucose by the cardiomyocyte, which represents a compensatory metabolic adaptation to unfavorable conditions, is severely impaired.[24]

In the whole population, IR can be managed by lifestyle interventions. The life style interventions potentially useful are weight control and physical activity. In patients with CHF, weight control or reduction must be handled carefully for the incumbent risk of cachexia, a frequent and serious complication of CHF. Unfortunately, the only trial in CHF looking at the effect of physical activity on mortality, the HF ACTION trial, has demonstrated no beneficial effect of exercise training on survival.[25] Many drugs used for the treatment of diabetes can improve IR. However, the insulin sensitizers thiazolidinediones, that directly contrast IR, have shown to increase the risk of developing CHF, even in the absence of diabetes.[26] Metformin in an animal model of CHF, improves cardiac function and performance very powerfully.[27] A recent careful review of the available data demonstrated that the risk of lactic acidosis with the use of metformin in patients with CHF is not substantiated by the data and that the drug can represent the drug of choice in patients with diabetes and CHF, at least for those with HFrEF.[28,29] Other drugs used for the treatment of diabetes may directly or indirectly affect IR. Particularly promising for their potential use in patients with CHF were those acting on the levels of the hormone glucagonlike peptide-1 (GLP-1), either through an inhibition of the enzyme degrading the native hormone, the dipeptidyl peptidase IV (DPP-IV) inhibitors, or the GLP-1 receptor agonists, analogues of the native hormone. The hopes of positive action on CHF were based on a few preliminary data showing that both in experimental animal models of CHF[23] or in patients with severe CHF,[30] GLP-1 administration improved left ventricular function. Unfortunately, either approaches used in the treatment of diabetes to increase circulating GLP-1 or its analogues have shown some pitfalls or did not confirm the hopes. During the trials with DPP-IV inhibitors, saxagliptin demonstrated an alarming increase in the risk of hospitalization for HF,[31] whereas alogliptin showed a 19%, not significant, increase in the same risk.[32] The trials with GLP-1 receptor agonists have all shown absence of any effect on HF hospitalization, reassuring that their use is safe with regard the risk of CHF. Furthermore, when liraglutide or albiglutide were specifically tested to evaluate their effects on HF hospitalization, survival, or changes in EF, the results were discouraging.[33,34] Great hopes for the treatment of CHF derive from the trials in diabetic patients using SGLT2 inhibitors, the gliflozines.[35–38] All of them, invariably, demonstrated a strong reduction of hospitalization for HF, even in patients who, at baseline, did not have CHF. It is well known that these drugs can act on IR and skeletal muscle glucose transport likely through the reduction of blood glucose concentration.[39,40] However, the mechanisms behind the surprising effects of these drugs on the cardiac function seems to be independent from their ability to control blood glucose concentration. The mechanism of blood glucose reduction of these drugs relies on their inhibition of glucose reabsorption by the kidney. This action is strictly dependent on the filtration rate: when estimated glomerular filtration rate (eGFR) is lower than 45 mL/1.8 m^2 per minute, the blood glucose control is virtually absent. In the CREDENCE trial, which recruited even patients with very low eGFR, canagliflozin was still able to show its effects on renal and cardiac protection,[38] indicating that mechanisms other than glucose control are responsible for the relevant effects of these drugs. Several mechanisms have been proposed to explain the beneficial action of these drugs on HF hospitalization: improvement in ventricular loading conditions through a reduction in preload (secondary to natriuresis, osmotic diuresis) and afterload (reduction in blood pressure and improvement in vascular function), improvement in cardiac metabolism and bioenergetics, myocardial Na+/H+ exchange inhibition, reduction of necrosis and cardiac fibrosis, alteration in adipokines, cytokine production, and epicardial adipose tissue mass.[41] The fact that the mechanisms of action of these drugs on many organs appear to be independent from glucose control has provided support to the hypothesis that they may act also in patients without diabetes. Many trials have started looking at the effect of SGLT2 inhibitors in patients with CHF, with or without diabetes and will be completed in the next few months. Very interestingly, almost all the trials focus on both HFrEF and HFpEF, trying to investigate whether different response to gliflozins can be seen in the 2 conditions.

GROWTH HORMONE/INSULINLIKE GROWTH FACTOR-1 DEFICIENCY IN CHRONIC HEART FAILURE

The growth hormone (GH) and insulinlike growth factor 1 (IGF-1) axis plays a relevant role in preserving the functions of the heart.[42,43] Its activity sustains myocardial architecture and preserves capillary density, calcium regulatory proteins and inhibits fibrosis, protecting against ischemia-reperfusion and mechanical stretching.[44–46] GH and IGF-1 inhibit apoptosis and favor the production of nitric oxide from the endothelial cells, favoring vasodilation and preserving from

atherosclerosis.[47–52] IGF-1 improves myocardial contractility,[53] whereas GH increases skeletal muscle protein content,[54] the latter potentially involved in contrast to skeletal muscle cachexia associated with CHF.

Very interestingly, 30% of patients with CHF present with GH deficiency (GHD).[55,56] Either reduced release or peripheral GH resistance, somatostatin overactivity, drug interference, impoverished nutritional status, or cytokine increase might potentially explain GH deficiency.[56–60] Normal GH activity appears to be relevant for good health, as GHD induces an increase in cardiovascular mortality.[61] From the clinical point of view, patients with GHD show increased vascular resistance, reduced exercise capacity, and abnormal cardiac function.[62,63] Among patients with CHF, GHD is associated with worse clinical status and increased all-cause mortality, presence of left ventricular (LV) remodeling, lower physical performance, and increased N-terminal pro b-type natriuretic peptide levels.[13] In addition, the patients show higher depression scores and impaired quality of life.[13] The presence of GH deficiency in these patients is associated with many structural and functional cardiac abnormalities, such as larger LV volumes with elevated wall stress, higher filling pressures, impairment of right ventricle function, worse cardiopulmonary performance, and reduced ventilatory efficiency.

With regard to the effect of changes in circulating IGF-1 plasma levels on heart function and structure, the data show some inconsistency. Reduced plasma levels of IGF-1 are associated with an increased risk of developing CHF and can predict cardiovascular mortality and ischemic heart disease.[64–66] Compared with healthy controls, circulating IGF-1 plasma levels can be unchanged, lower, or even higher in patients with CHF.[67–70] However, in this population, low levels of IGF-1 have been linked to worse survival, greater neurohormonal and cytokine activation, reduced skeletal muscle performance, and endothelial dysfunction.[7,13,17,51,71]

Many studies in animal models have focused on the effects of treatments with GH, IGF-1, or GH releasing peptide on cardiac function, peripheral vascular resistance, and survival, and have shown positive effects.[55,72–74] The effect of GH treatment in patients with CHF has been the purpose of several studies in the past 2 decades. Unfortunately, the results have been inconsistent.[51,75–86] Overall, when all the data are analyzed together, GH treatment appears to improve cardiac function in patients with CHF.[87] In particular, LVEF improves and systemic vascular resistance is reduced together with beneficial reduction of LV diastolic diameter and increase in LV wall thickness. GH treatment resulted also in improved exercise duration, peak oxygen uptake, LVEF, cardiac output, systemic vascular resistance, and New York Heart Association class level.[88]

The different results obtained in different trials on GH treatment of patients with CHF might be due to differences in therapy applied. On the other hand, the GH/IGF-1 patient profile might be important for the response to the treatment with GH, suggesting that patient selection can be relevant to obtain the beneficial results. Recently we evaluated the role played by the presence of GHD on the effects of GH *replacement* therapy in patients with CHF. Six months of GH replacement therapy improved LVEF, peak oxygen uptake, exercise duration, flow-mediated vasodilation, and the quality of life score, whereas decreased circulating N-terminal pro-brain natriuretic peptide levels.[55] When we reevaluated the patients during a 4-year follow-up study, we observed that treatment with GH in patients with CHF induced the reduction of both LV end-diastolic and end-systolic volume indexes, circumferential wall stress, and the increase in LVEF, suggesting the activation of the reverse remodeling of the LV. Although this was not a prespecified endpoint, the combined outcome of death from any cause or hospitalization due to CHF worsening was also sensibly reduced.[89] Therefore, GHD seems to be a condition necessary to obtain a consistent beneficial response in patients with CHF.

CHRONIC HEART FAILURE AND ABNORMAL TESTOSTERONE ACTIVITY

Data are available connecting circulating testosterone plasma levels and cardiovascular diseases.[90] On one hand, male gender, characterized by higher levels of testosterone, is associated with an increased risk of CVD.[91] Consistently, clinical and experimental data associate androgens and a pro-atherogenic cluster of cardiovascular risk factors.[92–96] On the other hand, many studies have rather associated *low* levels of androgens and incipient atherosclerosis[97] or cardiovascular diseases and worse survival.[98–100]

Dehydroepiandrosterone sulfate (DHEA-S), a relevant androgen in humans, exerts a direct action on the cardiovascular system.[101,102] Interacting with its receptors, located on the cardiomyocyte, testosterone may induce protein synthesis and cell hypertrophy[103] and regulate myocardial contractility, by the way of different mechanisms, that is, acting on L-type Ca^{+2} channel, Na^{+2}/Ca^{+2} exchanger, b1-adrenoceptors, or

myosin heavy chain subunits.[104,105] These receptors regulate intracellular Ca^{+2} flux in endothelial and vascular smooth muscle cells.[106] Moreover, through the inhibition of the production of nicotinamide adenine dinucleotide phosphate oxidase, testosterone protects against angiotensin II-induced vascular remodeling and controls superoxide production.[107] With aging, circulating testosterone and DHEA-S levels decline.[108,109] The natural progressive reduction of androgen levels contributes to sarcopenia, visceral adiposity, and osteopenia. Although a universally accepted definition of testosterone deficiency is lacking, several studies have shown that testosterone deficiency, or reduction of serum testosterone, in elderly individuals is associated with poor survival.[98,99] With regard to CHF, 25% of patients have low plasma levels of testosterone.[67,110–112] It is plausible that such reduction might contribute to the impairment of skeletal muscle function and exercise tolerance[113] and to the poor survival.[114–116]

When testosterone is administered in animal models, physiologic cardiac growth without increase in collagen deposition could be observed,[117] whereas in a model of ischemia-reperfusion injury, testosterone preserved cardiomyocytes by activating ATP-sensitive K channels and upregulating cardiac alpha(1)-adrenoceptors.[118] In a preliminary study, in a group of male patients with CHF, testosterone given orally as a single dose of 60 mg decreased peripheral vascular resistance and afterload, improving cardiac output.[119] In another study in 20 male patients with CHF, compared with placebo, intramuscular testosterone therapy (100 mg every 2 weeks for 12 weeks) improved the 6-minute walking distance and the Minnesota Living with Heart Failure Questionnaire.[114] A more robust randomized controlled trial (RCT) in 76 men with CHF treated with testosterone (5 mg/d administered by an adhesive skin patch) or placebo for 12 months failed to show structural or functional changes of the heart.[120] However, a significant increase in walking distance was observed, together with the shift of at least one New York Heart Association class for more of a quarter of the patients treated with testosterone compared with placebo.

The fact that the effect of testosterone on skeletal muscle structure and strength might play a relevant role in the treatment of CHF receives support from several clinical studies. Intramuscular testosterone treatment of 70 elderly patients with CHF for 12 weeks induced a significant increase of peak Vo_2 and ventilatory efficiency. Of great interest in this RCT is the observation that testosterone improved skeletal muscle strength, by slowing down its deterioration, and insulin sensitivity. This finding was confirmed by another recent study.[121] The improvement of muscle deterioration might limit exercise fatigue.[122] In addition, testosterone improved peak oxygen consumption, leg strength, and response to quality of life questionnaire in male patients with CHF and low testosterone status.[123] The positive effects of testosterone (transdermal, 300-mg patch, applied twice/week for 6 months) on exercise performance, measured as 6-minute walking distance and peak oxygen consumption, and on insulin sensitivity seen in men have been confirmed also in 36 women with CHF involved in a placebo-controlled RCT.[124] The absence of structural and functional changes of the heart in patients with CHF treated with testosterone, but the presence of functional and clinical improvements suggest that the hormone potentially acts through mechanisms independent from a direct action on the heart. In theory, testosterone action on skeletal muscle might justify the improvement in patient performance and health. In conclusion, testosterone administration did not induce heart structure modifications, but improved cardiovascular and skeletal muscle performance, suggesting that the action of testosterone in patients with CHF could be due to peripheral mechanisms.

ROLE OF THYROID HORMONES IN CHRONIC HEART FAILURE

The capability of thyroid hormones (TH) to regulate cardiovascular function is well known. In hypothyroidism or hyperthyroidism, cardiovascular functions are profoundly affected, both heart rhythm and function, by changes in TH serum concentration. TH can affect heart activity through different mechanisms, acting directly on the heart structure or by its action on the circulatory system.[125–127] TH can control the contractile response of the heart by regulating the expression of proteins involved.[8] Thyroid disease is associated with changes in cardiac output and contractility and peripheral vascular resistance. Even in the presence of severe abnormalities of hemodynamics, rapid treatment of hypothyroidism or hyperthyroidism is followed by the return to normal cardiovascular functions.[126,128] The cardiovascular apparatus appears to be very sensitive to even small changes in the concentration of TH, as suggested by the effect of subclinical derangements of TH on survival.[129,130] Studies in patients with CHF have shown that oral TH given at low dose (0.1 mg/d of T4) increases LVEF and improves exercise tolerance.[131] Consistently, T3 administration induces an increase in cardiac output in a few hours,[132,133] whereas potently and rapidly improves endothelial function in healthy humans following intra-arterial administration.[125] The effects of TH on peripheral circulation has important implications for patients with CHF, as an improved peripheral perfusion may potentially improve exercise tolerance.

SUMMARY

CHF is a complex syndrome characterized by symptoms and signs supported by different forms of cardiac impairment, that is, HFrEF or HFpEF. The current treatment approach of CHF is founded on the neurohormonal activation model. This model is based on the concept that a maladaptive catabolic response to myocardial injury is responsible for the development of the disease and that the purpose of the therapy is to counteract such response. Although this approach has proved its efficacy by reducing morbidity and mortality in patients with HFrEF, there is no demonstration that HFpEF is equally responsive. In addition, mortality and morbidity in CHF remain high. Therefore, alternative approaches might be needed. The link between hormonal and metabolic derangements and the development of CHF and the beneficial effects seen with hormonal replacement therapy has suggested that a reduction of anabolic pathways might contribute to the onset of CHF.[134–136] From this point of view, rather than the exclusive abnormality of the catabolic pathway supposed with the neurohormonal activation model, an imbalance between anabolic and catabolic forces could be responsible of the development of CHF. New trials should actively explore the relevance of this approach. However, there are sufficient data to support the screening in patients with CHF of hormonal deficiencies and their correction with replacement therapy. In this context, the results of the T.O.SC.A. Registry, a prospective multicenter observational study designed to investigate the prognostic impact of Multiple Hormonal Deficiencies in CHF[137] will shed light on the real prevalence and clinical impact of hormone deficiency in HF.

REFERENCES

1. Ponikowski P, Voors AA, Anker SD, et al. 2016 ESC Guidelines for the diagnosis and treatment of acute and chronic heart failure. Eur Heart J 2016;37: 2129–200.

2. Paulus WJ, Tschöpe C. A novel paradigm for heart failure with preserved ejection fraction. J Am Coll Cardiol 2013;62:263–71.

3. Steinberg BA, Zhao X, Heidenreich PA, et al. Trends in patients hospitalized with heart failure and preserved left ventricular ejection fraction: prevalence, therapies, and outcomes. Circulation 2012;126:65–75.

4. Braunwald E. Heart failure. JACC Heart Fail 2013; 1:1–20.

5. Roger VL, Weston SA, Redfield MM, et al. Trends in heart failure incidence and survival in a community-based population. JAMA 2004;292:344–50.

6. Benjamin EJ, Muntner P, Alonso A, et al. Heart disease and stroke statistics—2019 update: a report from the American Heart Association. Circulation 2019;139:e56–528.

7. Niebauer J, Pflaum CD, Clark AL, et al. Deficient insulin-like growth factor I in chronic heart failure predicts altered body composition, anabolic deficiency, cytokine and neurohormonal activation. J Am Coll Cardiol 1998;32:393–7.

8. Iervasi G, Pingitore A, Landi P, et al. Low-T3 syndrome: a strong prognostic predictor of death in patients with heart disease. Circulation 2003;107: 708–13.

9. Doehner W, Rauchhaus M, Ponikowski P, et al. Impaired insulin sensitivity as an independent risk factor for mortality in patients with stable chronic heart failure. J Am Coll Cardiol 2005;46:1019–26.

10. Marra AM, Arcopinto M, Bobbio E, et al. An unusual case of dilated cardiomyopathy associated with partial hypopituitarism. Intern Emerg Med 2012; 7(Suppl 2):S85–7.

11. Arcopinto M, Salzano A, Bossone E, et al. Multiple hormone deficiencies in chronic heart failure. Int J Cardiol 2015;184:421–3.

12. Marra AM, Arcopinto M, Salzano A, et al. Detectable interleukin-9 plasma levels are associated with impaired cardiopulmonary functional capacity and all-cause mortality in patients with chronic heart failure. Int J Cardiol 2016;209:114–7.

13. Arcopinto M, Salzano A, Giallauria F, et al. Growth hormone deficiency is associated with worse cardiac function, physical performance, and outcome in chronic heart failure: insights from the T.O.S.CA. GHD Study. PLoS One 2017;12(1):e0170058.

14. Jankowska EA, Biel B, Majda J, et al. Anabolic deficiency in men with chronic heart failure: prevalence and detrimental impact on survival. Circulation 2006;114:1829–37.

15. Saccà L. Heart failure as a multiple hormonal deficiency syndrome. Circ Heart Fail 2009;2:151–6.

16. Salzano A, Marra AM, Ferrara F, et al. Multiple hormone deficiency syndrome in heart failure with preserved ejection fraction. Int J Cardiol 2016;225: 1–3.

17. Arcopinto M, Salzano A, Isgaard J, et al. Hormone replacement therapy in heart failure. Curr Opin Cardiol 2015;30:277–84.

18. McAllister DA, Read SH, Kerssens J, et al. Incidence of hospitalization for heart failure and case-fatality among 3.25 million people with and without diabetes mellitus. Circulation 2018;138: 2774–86.

19. Suskin N, McKelvie RS, Burns RJ, et al. Glucose and insulin abnormalities relate to functional capacity in patients with congestive heart failure. Eur Heart J 2000;21:1368–75.

20. Saccà L, Napoli R. Insulin resistance in chronic heart failure: a difficult bull to take by the horns. Nutr Metab Cardiovasc Dis 2009;19(5):303–5.

21. Ingelsson E, Sundstrom J, Arnlov J, et al. Insulin resistance and risk of congestive heart failure. JAMA 2005;294:334–41.

22. Swan JW, Anker SD, Walton C, et al. Insulin resistance in chronic heart failure: relation to severity and etiology of heart failure. J Am Coll Cardiol 1997;30:527–32.

23. Nikolaidis LA, Elahi D, Hentosz T, et al. Recombinant glucagon-like peptide-1 increases myocardial glucose uptake and improves left ventricular performance in conscious dogs with pacing-induced dilated cardiomyopathy. Circulation 2004;110: 955–61.

24. Witteless RM, Fowler MN. Insulin-resistant cardiomyopathy clinical evidence, mechanisms, and treatment options. J Am Coll Cardiol 2008;51: 93–102.

25. O'Connor CM1, Whellan DJ, Lee KL, et al. Efficacy and safety of exercise training in patients with chronic heart failure: HF-ACTION randomized controlled trial. JAMA 2009;301:1439–50.

26. Gerstein HC, Yusuf S, Bosch J, et al. Effect of rosiglitazone on the frequency of diabetes in patients with impaired glucose tolerance or impaired fasting glucose: a randomised controlled trial. Lancet 2006;368:1096–105.

27. Cittadini A, Napoli R, Monti MG, et al. Metformin prevents the development of chronic heart failure in the SHHF rat model. Diabetes 2012;201: 944–53.

28. Masoudi FA, Inzucchi SE, Wang Y, et al. Thiazolidinediones, metformin, and outcomes in older patients with diabetes and heart failure: an observational study. Circulation 2005;111:583–90.

29. Ponikowski P, Voors AA, Anker SD, et al. ESC Guidelines for the diagnosis and treatment of acute and chronic heart failure: the task force for the diagnosis and treatment of acute and chronic heart failure of the European Society of Cardiology (ESC). Developed with the special contribution of the Heart Failure Association (CHFA) of the ESC. Eur J Heart Fail 2016;18:891–975.

30. Sokos GG, Nikolaidis LA, Mankad S, et al. Glucagon-like peptide-1 infusion improves left ventricular ejection fraction and functional status in

patients with chronic heart failure. J Card Fail 2006; 12:694–9.

31. Scirica BM, Bhatt DL, Braunwald E, et al. Saxagliptin and cardiovascular outcomes in patients with type 2 diabetes mellitus. N Engl J Med 2013;369: 1317–26.

32. White WB, Cannon CP, Heller SR, et al. Alogliptin after acute coronary syndrome in patients with type 2 diabetes. N Engl J Med 2013;369:1326–35.

33. Jorsal A, Kistorp C, Holmager P, et al. Effect of liraglutide, a glucagon-like peptide-1 analogue, on left ventricular function in stable chronic heart failure patients with and without diabetes (LIVE)-a multicentre, double-blind, randomised, placebo-controlled trial. Eur J Heart Fail 2017;19:69–77.

34. Lepore JJ, Olson E, Demopoulos L, et al. Effects of the novel long-acting GLP-1 agonist, albiglutide, on cardiac function, cardiac metabolism, and exercise capacity in patients with chronic heart failure and reduced ejection fraction. JACC Heart Fail 2016; 4:559–66.

35. Zinman B, Wanner C, Lachin JM, et al. Empagliflozin, cardiovascular outcomes, and mortality in type 2 diabetes. N Engl J Med 2015;373:2117–8.

36. Neal B, Perkovic V, Mahaffey KW, et al. Canagliflozin and cardiovascular and renal events in type 2 diabetes. N Engl J Med 2017;376:644–57.

37. Wiviott SD, Raz I, Bonaca MP, et al. Dapagliflozin and cardiovascular outcomes in type 2 diabetes. N Engl J Med 2018. https://doi.org/10.1056/ NEJMoa1812389.

38. Perkovic V, Jardine MJ, Neal B, et al. Canagliflozin and renal outcomes in Type 2 diabetes and nephropathy. N Engl J Med 2019. https://doi.org/10. 1056/NEJMoa1811744.

39. Rossetti L, Smith D, Shulman GI, et al. Correction of hyperglycemia with phlorizin normalizes tissue sensitivity to insulin in diabetic rats. J Clin Invest 1987;79:1510–5.

40. Napoli R, Hirshman MF, Horton ES. Mechanisms and time course of impaired skeletal muscle glucose uptake in streptozocin diabetic rats. J Clin Invest 1995;95:427–37.

41. Verma S, McMurray JJV. SGLT2 inhibitors and mechanisms of cardiovascular benefit: a state-of-the-art review. Diabetologia 2018;61:2108–17.

42. Sacca' L, Fazio S. Cardiac performance: growth hormone enters the race. Nat Med 1996;2:29–31.

43. Saccà L. Growth hormone therapy for heart failure: swimming against the stream. J Card Fail 1999;5: 269–75.

44. Cittadini A, Stromer H, Katz SE, et al. Differential cardiac effects of growth hormone and insulin-like growth factor-1 in the rat. A combined in vivo and in vitro evaluation. Circulation 1996;93:800.

45. Stromer H, Palmieri EA, De Groot MC, et al. Growth hormone- and pressure overload-induced cardiac

hypertrophy evoke different responses to ischemia-reperfusion and mechanical stretch. Growth Horm IGF Res 2006;16:29–40.

46. Bruel A, Oxlund H. The effect of growth hormone on rat myocardial collagen. Growth Horm IGF Res 1999;9:123–30.

47. Cittadini A, Grossman JD, Napoli R, et al. Growth hormone attenuates early left ventricular remodeling and improves cardiac function in rats with large myocardial infarction. J Am Coll Cardiol 1997;29: 1109–16.

48. D'Assante R, Napoli R, Salzano A, et al. Human heart shifts from IGF-1 production to utilization with chronic heart failure. Endocrine 2019. https:// doi.org/10.1007/s12020-019-01993-y.

49. Boger RH. Role of nitric oxide in the haemodynamic effects of growth hormone. Growth Horm IGF Res 1998;8:163–5.

50. Merola B, Longobardi S, Sofia M, et al. Lung volumes and respiratory muscle strength in adult patients with childhood- or adult-onset growth hormone deficiency: effect of 12 months' growth hormone replacement therapy. Eur J Endocrinol 1996;135:553–8.

51. Napoli R, Guardasole V, Matarazzo M, et al. Growth hormone corrects vascular dysfunction in patients with chronic heart failure. J Am Coll Cardiol 2002; 39:90–9.

52. Napoli R, Guardasole V, Angelini V, et al. Acute effects of growth hormone on vascular function in human subjects. J Clin Endocrinol Metab 2003;88: 2817–20.

53. Cittadini A, Ishiguro Y, Stromer H, et al. Insulin-like growth factor-1 but not growth hormone augments mammalian myocardial contractility by sensitizing the myofilament to Ca2þ through a wortmannin-sensitive pathway: studies in rat and ferret isolated muscles. Circ Res 1998;83: 50–9.

54. Napoli R, Cittadini A, Chow JC, et al. Chronic growth hormone treatment in normal rats reduces post-prandial skeletal muscle plasma membrane GLUT1 content, but not glucose transport or GLUT4 expression and localization. Biochem J 1996;315:959–63.

55. Cittadini A, Saldamarco M, Marra AM, et al. Growth hormone in patients with chronic heart failure and beneficial effects of its correction. J Clin Endocrinol Metab 2009;94:3329–36.

56. Broglio F, Benso A, Gottero C, et al. Patients with dilated cardiomyopathy show reduction of the somatotroph responsiveness to GHRH both alone and combined with arginine. Eur J Endocrinol 2000;142:157–63.

57. Broglio F, Fubini A, Morello M, et al. Activity of GH/ IGF-I axis in patients with dilated cardiomyopathy. Clin Endocrinol (Oxf) 1999;50:417–30.

58. Saccà L, Napoli R, Cittadini A. Growth hormone, acromegaly, and heart failure: an intricate triangulation. Clin Endocrinol (Oxf) 2003;59:660–71.

59. Mann DL, Bristow MR. Mechanisms and models in heart failure. The biomechanical model and beyond. Circulation 2005;111:2837–49.

60. Colao A. The GH-IGF-I axis and the cardiovascular system: clinical implications. Clin Endocrinol (Oxf) 2008;69:347–58.

61. Rosen T, Bengtsson BA. Premature mortality due to cardiovascular disease in hypopituitarism. Lancet 1990;336:285–8.

62. Saccà L. Growth hormone: a newcomer in cardiovascular medicine. Cardiovasc Res 1997;36:3–9.

63. Colao A, Di Somma C, Cuocolo A, et al. The severity of growth hormone deficiency correlates with the severity of cardiac impairment in 100 adult patients with hypopituitarism: an observational, case-control study. J Clin Endocrinol Metab 2004; 89:5998–6004.

64. Juul A, Scheike T, Davidsen M, et al. Low serum insulin-like growth factor 1 is associated with increased risk of ischemic heart disease: a population-based case-control study. Circulation 2002;106:939–44.

65. Vasan RS, Sullivan LM, D'Agostino RB, et al. Serum insulin-like growth factor I and risk for heart failure in elderly individuals without a previous myocardial infarction: the Framingham Heart Study. Ann Intern Med 2003;139:642–8.

66. Laughlin GA, Barrett-Connor E, Criqui MH, et al. The prospective association of serum insulin-like growth factor I (IGF-I) and IGF-binding protein-1 levels with all cause and cardiovascular disease mortality in older adults: the Rancho Bernardo Study. J Clin Endocrinol Metab 2004; 89:114–20.

67. Anker SD, Chua TP, Ponikowski P, et al. Hormonal changes and catabolic/anabolic imbalance in chronic heart failure: the importance for cardiac cachexia. Circulation 1997;96:526–34.

68. Al-Obaidi MK, Hon JFK, Stubbs PJ, et al. Plasma insulin-like growth factor-1 elevated in mild-to-moderate but not severe heart failure. Am Heart J 2001;142:e10.

69. Anwar A, Gaspoz JM, Pampallona S, et al. Effect of congestive heart failure on the insulin-like growth factor-1 system. Am J Cardiol 2002;90: 1402–5.

70. Andreassen M, Caroline Kistorp C, Raymond I, et al. Plasma insulin-like growth factor I as predictor of progression and all cause mortality in chronic heart failure. Growth Horm IGF Res 2009;19: 486–90.

71. Petretta M, Colao A, Sardu C, et al. NT-proBNP, IGF-I and survival in patients with chronic heart failure. Growth Horm IGF Res 2007;17:288–96.

72. Yang R, Bunting S, Gillett N, et al. Growth hormone improves cardiac performance in experimental heart failure. Circulation 1995;92:262–7.

73. Duerr RL, McKirnan MD, Gim RD, et al. Cardiovascular effects of insulin-like growth factor-1 and growth hormone in chronic left ventricular failure in the rat. Circulation 1996;93:2188–96.

74. Ryoke T, Gu Y, Mao L, et al. Progressive cardiac dysfunction and fibrosis in the cardiomyopathic hamster and effects of growth hormone and angiotensin-converting enzyme inhibition. Circulation 1999;100:1734–40.

75. Fazio S, Sabatini D, Capaldo B, et al. A preliminary study of growth hormone in the treatment of dilated cardiomyopathy. N Engl J Med 1996;334:809–14.

76. Frustaci A, Gentiloni N, Russo MA. Growth hormone in the treatment of dilated cardiomyopathy. N Engl J Med 1996;335:672–3.

77. Genth-Zotz S, Zotz R, Geil S, et al. Recombinant growth hormone therapy in patients with ischemic cardiomyopathy: effects on hemodynamics, left ventricular function, and cardiopulmonary exercise capacity. Circulation 1999;99:18–21.

78. Isgaard J, Bergh CH, Caidahl K, et al. A placebo-controlled study of growth hormone in patients with congestive heart failure. Eur Heart J 1998;19: 1704–11.

79. Osterziel KJ, Strohm O, Schuler J, et al. Randomised, double-blind, placebo-controlled trial of human recombinant growth hormone in patients with chronic heart failure due to dilated cardiomyopathy. Lancet 1998;351:1233–7.

80. Jose VJ, Zechariah TU, George P, et al. Growth hormone therapy in patients with dilated cardiomyopathy: preliminary observations of a pilot study. Indian Heart J 1999;51:183–5.

81. Smit JW, Janssen YJ, Lamb HJ, et al. Six months of recombinant human GH therapy in patients with ischemic cardiac failure does not influence left ventricular function and mass. J Clin Endocrinol Metab 2001;86:4638–43.

82. Spallarossa P, Rossettin P, Minuto F, et al. Evaluation of growth hormone administration in patients with chronic heart failure secondary to coronary artery disease. Am J Cardiol 1999;84:430–3.

83. Perrot A, Ranke MB, Dietz R, et al. Growth hormone treatment in dilated cardiomyopathy. J Card Surg 2001;16:127–31.

84. Acevedo M, Corbalan R, Chamorro G, et al. Administration of growth hormone to patients with advanced cardiac heart failure: effects upon left ventricular function, exercise capacity, and neurohormonal status. Int J Cardiol 2003;87:185–91.

85. Adamopoulos S, Parissis JT, Paraskevaidis I, et al. Effects of growth hormone on circulating cytokine network, and left ventricular contractile performance and geometry in patients with idiopathic

dilated cardiomyopathy. Eur Heart J 2003;24: 2186–96.

86. Cittadini A, Ines Comi L, Longobardi S, et al. A preliminary randomized study of growth hormone administration in Becker and Duchenne muscular dystrophies. Eur Heart J 2003;24:664–72.

87. Le Corvoisier P, Hittinger L, Chanson P, et al. Cardiac effects of growth hormone treatment in chronic heart failure: a metanalysis. J Clin Endocrinol Metab 2007;92:180–5.

88. Tritos NA, Danias PG. Growth hormone therapy in congestive heart failure due to left ventricular systolic dysfunction: a meta-analysis. Endocr Pract 2008;14:40–9.

89. Cittadini A, Marra A, Arcopinto M, et al. Growth hormone replacement delays the progression of chronic heart failure combined with growth hormone deficiency. JACC Heart Fail 2013;1: 325–30.

90. Khaw KT, Dowsett M, Folkerd E, et al. Endogenous testosterone and mortality due to all causes, cardiovascular disease, and cancer in men: European prospective investigation into cancer in Norfolk (EPIC-Norfolk) Prospective Population Study. Circulation 2007;116:2694–701.

91. Criqui MH. Epidemiology of atherosclerosis: an updated overview. Am J Cardiol 1986;57:18C–23C.

92. Dubey RK, Oparil S, Imthurn B, et al. Sex hormones and hypertension. Cardiovasc Res 2002; 53:688–708.

93. Ng MK, Quinn CM, McCrohon JA, et al. Androgens up-regulate atherosclerosis- related genes in macrophages from males but not females: molecular insights into gender differences in atherosclerosis. J Am Coll Cardiol 2003;42:1306–13.

94. McCrohon JA, Jessup W, Handelsman DJ, et al. Androgen exposure increases human monocyte adhesion to vascular endothelium and endothelial cell expression of vascular cell adhesion molecule-1. Circulation 1999;99:2317–22.

95. Muller M, van der Schouw YT, Thijssen JH, et al. Endogenous sex hormones and cardiovascular disease in men. J Clin Endocrinol Metab 2003;88: 5076–86.

96. Adams MR, Williams JK, Kaplan JR. Effects of androgens on coronary artery atherosclerosis and atherosclerosis-related impairment of vascular responsiveness. Arterioscler Thromb Vasc Biol 1995;15:562–70.

97. Mäkinen J, Järvisalo MJ, Pöllänen P, et al. Increased carotid atherosclerosis in andropausal middle-aged men. J Am Coll Cardiol 2005;45: 1603–8.

98. Haring R, Völzke H, Steveling A, et al. Low serum testosterone levels are associated with increased risk of mortality in a population-based cohort of men aged 20-79. Eur Heart J 2010;31:1494–501.

99. Laughlin GA, Barrett-Connor E, Bergstrom J. Low serum testosterone and mortality in older men. J Clin Endocrinol Metab 2008;93:68–75.

100. Malkin CJ, Pugh PJ, Morris PD, et al. Low serum testosterone and increased mortality in men with coronary heart disease. Heart 2010;96:1821–5.

101. Komesaroff PA. Unravelling the enigma of dehydroepiandrosterone: moving forward step by step. Endocrinology 2008;149:886–8.

102. Tivesten A, Vandenput L, Carlzon D, et al. Dehydroepiandrosterone and its sulfate predict the 5-year risk of coronary heart disease events in elderly men. J Am Coll Cardiol 2014;64:1801–10.

103. Marsh JD, Lehmann MH, Ritchie RH, et al. Androgen receptors mediate hypertrophy in cardiac myocytes. Circulation 1998;98:256–61.

104. Golden KL, Marsh JD, Jiang Y, et al. Gonadectomy of adult male rats reduces contractility of isolated cardiac myocytes. Am J Physiol Endocrinol Metab 2003;285:E449–53.

105. Golden KL, Marsh JD, Jiang Y, et al. Gonadectomy alters myosin heavy chain composition in isolated cardiac myocytes. Endocrine 2004;24:137–40.

106. Liu PY, Death AK, Handelsman DJ. Androgens and cardiovascular disease. Endocr Rev 2003;24: 313–40.

107. Ikeda Y, Aihara K, Yoshida S, et al. Androgen-androgen receptor system protects against angiotensin II-induced vascular remodeling. Endocrinology 2009;150:2857–64.

108. Lapauw B, Goemaere S, Zmierczak H, et al. The decline of serum testosterone levels in community-dwelling men over 70 years of age: descriptive data and predictors of longitudinal changes. Eur J Endocrinol 2008;159:459–68.

109. Kaufman JM, Vermeulen A. The decline of androgen levels in elderly men and its clinical and therapeutic implications. Endocr Rev 2005; 26:833–76.

110. Moriyama Y, Yasue H, Yoshimura M, et al. The plasma levels of dehydroepiandrosterone sulfate are decreased in patients with chronic heart failure in proportion to the severity. J Clin Endocrinol Metab 2000;85:1834–40.

111. Kontoleon PE, Anastasiou-Nana MI, Papapetrou PD, et al. Hormonal profile in patients with congestive heart failure. Int J Cardiol 2003;87:179–83.

112. Malkin CJ, Jones TH, Channer KS. Testosterone in chronic heart failure. Front Horm Res 2009;37: 183–96.

113. Iellamo F, Rosano G, Volterrani M. Testosterone deficiency and exercise intolerance in heart failure: treatment implications. Curr Heart Fail Rep 2010;7: 59–65.

114. Pugh PJ, Jones RD, West JN, et al. Testosterone treatment for men with chronic heart failure. Heart 2004;90:446–7.

115. Malkin CJ, Channer KS, Jones TH. Testosterone and heart failure. Curr Opin Endocrinol Diabetes Obes 2010;17:262–8.
116. Volterrani M, Rosano G, Iellamo F. Testosterone and heart failure. Endocrine 2012;42:272–7.
117. Nahrendorf M, Frantz S, Hu K, et al. Effect of testosterone on post-myocardial infarction remodeling and function. Cardiovasc Res 2003;57:370–8.
118. Tsang S, Wu S, Liu J, et al. Testosterone protects rat hearts against ischaemic insults by enhancing the effects of alpha(1)-adrenoceptor stimulation. Br J Pharmacol 2008;153:693–709.
119. Pugh PJ, Jones TH, Channer KS. Acute haemodynamic effects of testosterone administration in men with heart failure. Eur Heart J 2002;23:28.
120. Malkin CJ, Pugh PJ, West JN, et al. Testosterone therapy in men with moderate severity heart failure: a double-blind randomized placebo controlled trial. Eur Heart J 2006;27:57–64.
121. Mirdamadi A, Garakyaraghi M, Pourmoghaddas A, et al. Beneficial effects of testosterone therapy on functional capacity, cardiovascular parameters, and quality of life in patients with congestive heart failure. Biomed Res Int 2014;39:24–32.
122. Caminiti G, Volterrani M, Iellamo F, et al. Effect of long-acting testosterone treatment on functional exercise capacity, skeletal muscle performance, insulin resistance, and baroreflex sensitivity in elderly patients with chronic heart failure a double-blind, placebo-controlled, randomized study. J Am Coll Cardiol 2009;54:919–27.
123. Stout M, Tew GA, Doll H, et al. Testosterone therapy during exercise rehabilitation in male patients with chronic heart failure who have low testosterone status: a double-blind randomized controlled feasibility study. Am Heart J 2012;164:893–901.
124. Iellamo F, Volterrani M, Caminiti G, et al. Testosterone therapy in women with chronic heart failure: a pilot double-blind, randomized, placebo-controlled study. J Am Coll Cardiol 2010;56:1310–6.
125. Napoli R, Guardasole V, Angelini V, et al. Acute effects of triiodothyronine on endothelial function in human subjects. J Clin Endocrinol Metab 2007;92:250–4.
126. Napoli R, Guardasole V, Zarra E, et al. Impaired endothelial- and nonendothelial-mediated vasodilation in patients with acute or chronic hypothyroidism. Clin Endocrinol (Oxf) 2010;72:107–11.
127. Napoli R, Biondi B, Guardasole V, et al. Impact of hyperthyroidism and its correction on vascular reactivity in humans. Circulation 2001;104:3076–80.
128. Klein I, Danzi S. Thyroid disease and the heart. Circulation 2007;116:1725–35.
129. Biondi B, Fazio S, Palmieri EA, et al. Left ventricular diastolic dysfunction in patients with subclinical hypothyroidism. J Clin Endocrinol Metab 1999;84:2064–7.
130. Iervasi G, Molinaro S, Landi P, et al. Association between increased mortality and mild thyroid dysfunction in cardiac patients. Arch Intern Med 2007;167:1526–32.
131. Moruzzi P, Doria E, Agostoni PG. Medium-term effectiveness of L-thyroxine treatment in idiopathic dilated cardiomyopathy. Am J Med 1996;101:461–7.
132. Malik FS, Mehra MR, Uber PA, et al. Intravenous thyroid hormone supplementation in heart failure with cardiogenic shock. J Card Fail 1999;5:31–7.
133. Pingitore A, Galli E, Barison A, et al. Acute effects of triiodothyronine (T3) replacement therapy in patients with chronic heart failure and low-T3 syndrome: a randomized, placebo-controlled study. J Clin Endocrinol Metab 2008;93:1351–8.
134. Salzano A, D'Assante R, Lander M, et al. Hormonal replacement therapy in heart failure: focus on growth hormone and testosterone. Heart Fail Clin 2019;15:377–91.
135. Salzano A, Cittadini A, Bossone E, et al. Multiple hormone deficiency syndrome: a novel topic in chronic heart failure. Future Sci OA 2018;4:FSO311.
136. Salzano A, Marra AM, D'Assante R, et al. Growth hormone therapy in heart failure. Heart Fail Clin 2018;14:501–15.
137. Bossone E, Arcopinto M, Iacoviello M, et al. Multiple hormonal and metabolic deficiency syndrome in chronic heart failure: rationale, design, and demographic characteristics of the T.O.S.CA. Registry. Intern Emerg Med 2018;13:661–71.

The Gut Axis Involvement in Heart Failure
Focus on Trimethylamine *N*-oxide

Andrea Salzano, MD, MRCP[a,1], Shabana Cassambai, PhD[b,1],
Yoshiyuki Yazaki, MD[b], Muhammad Zubair Israr, PhD[b],
Dennis Bernieh, PhD[b], Max Wong, PhD[b], Toru Suzuki, MD, PhD, FRCP[b,*]

KEYWORDS

- Heart failure • Cardiovascular disease • TMAO • Gut • Prognosis • Risk stratification

KEY POINTS

- A key model of interest and one of recent attention is the association between heart failure (HF) and the gastrointestinal system, the so-called gut hypothesis.
- Growing evidence suggests that one of the more prominent molecules associated with the link between HF and the gut is the choline and carnitine metabolic by-product, trimethylamine *N*-oxide (TMAO).
- TMAO levels are increased in HF populations compared with healthy subjects. Higher TMAO levels are associated with poor prognosis, whereas low TMAO levels either at baseline or follow-up confer better prognosis.
- TMAO could represent a novel and independent therapeutic target for HF.

INTRODUCTION

Heart failure (HF) is the only cardiovascular disease that has maintained high levels of mortality in the past decade.[1] With the aim of understanding and reducing the burden associated with HF, research has focused on pathophysiologic models to complete knowledge of the pathways involved and design appropriate trials to identify novel drug targets and interventions.[2]

A key model of interest and one of recent attention is the association between HF and the gastrointestinal system,[3] the so-called gut hypothesis.[4] In HF, it is well established that the presence of bowel hypoperfusion, derived from reduced cardiac output, leads to mucosal ischemia that can increase bowel wall permeability and bacterial translocation. This bacterial translocation, through endotoxin production, is considered an important stimulus for elevated cytokine levels,[5] which is associated with impaired cardiovascular performance and poor prognosis.[6] On the other hand, chronic bowel congestion causes edema of the gastrointestinal tract, affecting the functions of the intestinal mucosa[7]; furthermore, many other factors that may alter the gut flora (eg, acute changes of fluid balance, acid/base disturbance, gastrointestinal dysmotility, and nutrient deprivation) are common in HF and might result in bacterial overgrowth or translocation. In this context,

This article originally appeared in *Heart Failure Clinics*, Volume 16, Issue 1, January 2020.
Disclosure Statement: A. Salzano receives research grant support from Cardiopath, UNINA, and Compagnia di San Paolo in the frame of Programme STAR. The other authors have nothing to disclose.
[a] IRCCS SDN, Diagnostic and Nuclear Research Institute, Via E Gianturco, 80143, Naples, Italy; [b] Department of Cardiovascular Sciences, NIHR Leicester Cardiovascular Biomedical Research Centre, University of Leicester, Glenfield Hospital, Leicester LE3 9QP, UK
[1] Contributed equally to this article.
* Corresponding author.
E-mail address: tsuzuki@leicester.ac.uk

growing evidence suggests that one of the more prominent molecules associated with the link between HF and the gut is the choline and carnitine metabolic by-product, trimethylamine *N*-oxide (TMAO), produced by the gut microbiota from the precursor trimethylamine (TMA), with subsequent oxidation via the liver enzyme, flavin-containing monooxygenase 3 (FMO3).[8–10]

In recent years, TMAO has been shown to be a strong prognostic biomarker in both acute HF[11] and stable chronic HF (CHF).[12–16] Furthermore, the magnitude of cardiovascular impairment and poor prognosis has been associated with the circulating levels of TMAO.

This review provides an overview of the current understanding of the interplay between TMAO and HF.

ROLE OF TRIMETHYLAMINE *N*-OXIDE IN THE PATHOPHYSIOLOGY OF HEART FAILURE
Trimethylamine N-oxide Metabolism

TMAO, a gut microbiota–mediated metabolite, is derived from the metabolism of choline and carnitine into TMA. TMAO is thought to be the missing link between the consumption of a Western diet and cardiovascular disease risk.[17] Intestinal bacteria are implicated in the production of the precursor to TMAO, TMA, through the anaerobic metabolism of choline and ʟ-carnitine, derived largely from eggs and red meat as well as other sources (**Fig. 1**). TMA lyase is the bacterial enzyme responsible for the generation of TMA, via *cutC/cutD* and *cntA/cntB* genes for choline and ʟ-carnitine, respectively.[18] The oxidation of TMA to TMAO occurs via the human liver enzyme FMO3,[19] which is involved in the detoxification of xenobiotics.[20] In healthy humans, TMAO is cleared rapidly from the body via urine[21] and is largely considered a waste product of choline metabolism.[22] Therefore, renal function can affect TMAO levels significantly. Individuals with FMO3 deficiency, however, have an accumulation of the toxic TMA, which is associated with a characteristic fishy body odor, known as trimethylaminuria. Consequently, trimethlyaminuria sufferers are advised to limit the choline, lecithin, and carnitine consumption in their diet to ensure reduced levels of TMA production.[23]

TMAO itself has a protective functional role in antagonizing the destabilizing effect of urea on proteins,[24] particularly in saltwater fish and crustaceans.[23] Although TMAO is excreted mainly through urine in humans, a study investigating

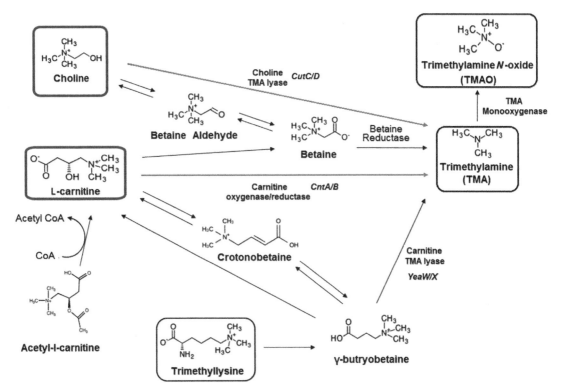

Fig. 1. A schematic depicting the multiple pathways and metabolites associated with the production of TMAO in humans. Orange boxes—sources of TMAO; blue arrows—key pathways of TMAO metabolism; black boxes—metabolites with associated cardiovascular or noxious properties.

the direct effects of TMAO on pathologic protein folding found a stabilizing chaperone effect whereby mutant protein folding, such as with the cystic fibrosis transmembrane conductance regulatory (CFTR) protein, was rescued.[25,26] Although the protein-stabilizing effects associated with TMAO are well known, TMAO has been shown to have a direct impact on atherosclerotic plaque formation, reduce ventricular function in HF, and induce renal fibrosis within in vivo and in vitro models.[17,27] These observations have been linked to an association with increased cardiovascular risk; population-based studies within acute HF and acute myocardial infarction patients[11,28] have found elevated circulating levels of TMAO to be correlated with death and hospitalization.

Literature regarding the association of TMAO with cardiovascular disease is widely debated. Certain fish are known to have high levels of TMAO, yet the consumption of fish has been linked to cardioprotective effects due to omega-3 fatty acids,[29,30] with no mention of the involvement of TMAO. Studies also have shown that the most significant increase in plasma TMAO levels is observed after the consumption of fish compared with other sources of protein.[31] These studies highlight the discrepancies regarding the effect of TMAO in situ, yet studies focusing on mechanistic investigations have previously shown that TMAO is causal of atherosclerosis, platelet hyper-reactivity, and cardiac fibrosis in a murine model of CHF,[32] therefore suggesting a direct link between TMAO and the propagation of cardiovascular risk factors.

Trimethylamine N-oxide and Diet

Plasma TMAO levels are determined by factors, including diet. Excessive consumption of dietary sugars and saturated fats, known as the Western diet, has been linked with obesity, metabolic syndrome, and impairment in cardiac function. The consumption of a Western diet has been shown to alter the gut microbiota composition, with decreased levels of *Bacteroidetes* and *Bifidobacteria* and increased levels of *Firmicutes* and *Proteobacteria*; the altered composition is thought to influence TMAO synthesis.[33] Studies have demonstrated the consumption of a Western diet leads to increased circulating TMAO levels in the blood[34] and cardiovascular disease risk.[17] A recent study showed Western diet–induced obese mice displayed impaired cardiac systolic and diastolic dysfunction, which, after voluntary exercise, resulted in slight decreases in weight gain and metabolic disorders but completely prevented cardiac dysfunction. The results from this study suggest the cardioprotective effects of voluntary exercise in Western diet–induced obesity can be terminated via TMAO supplementation.[35]

Protein-rich diets seem to have a positive correlation with TMAO excretion in the urine.[36] Large amounts of nondigestible carbohydrates can reduce TMAO formation by remodeling the gut microbiota; however, studies also have shown that TMAO levels increase in the short term.[37,38] Nonetheless, the Western diet, rich of eggs and red meat, is considered the major influence between TMAO levels and cardiovascular disease risk.[39]

Trimethylamine N-oxide in Preclinical Models of Heart Failure

The recent interest in the intestinal microbiota has sparked the discussion of novel approaches to therapeutic medicine; dysbiosis of the gut microbiota has been associated with diseases, such as obesity and atherosclerosis,[40,41] implicating the gut microbiota as a potential therapeutic target. Studies in humans and animal models have shown the correlation of cardiovascular disease adverse events and increased levels of TMAO.[11,17,27,28,42,43] Despite the debated role of TMAO, it is clear from clinical and preclinical studies that the gut microbiota is involved in facilitating the changes associated with diseases, such as HF. Animal models of diet-induced obesity and pressure overload–induced HF have demonstrated a role for TMAO in accelerating cardiovascular risk, such as renal dysfunction or atherosclerotic lesions.[42,44] Moreover, studies that have used animal models of myocardial infarction and a humanized microbiome have demonstrated that targeting the gut microbiota leads to attenuation of myocardial hypertrophy and HF[45] as well as reduced TMAO levels.[46]

Several methods of targeting TMAO have been explored in a bid to identify the role of TMAO in cardiovascular disease risk, including inhibition of TMA lyases[18] and the use of fecal transplantation and probiotics to repopulate the intestinal flora.[34,46] These interventions, however, have shown mixed results with animal models extrapolated into clinical settings or healthy volunteers. Additionally, there have been no studies to date that show that lowering TMAO has any beneficial effect on heart health. Although many studies indicate a correlative relationship, there are few studies that look at the mechanistic approach for interventions in cases of TMAO and cardiovascular risk. This leaves the mechanistic implications of pathogenesis largely unclear,[47] which also limits successful intervention. Several studies have failed to show an intervention consistently capable of lowering TMAO.[34,48] In addition, although some methods to reduce TMAO, such as fecal transplantation, show promise in animals and in vitro models, these have not been translated into humans successfully, highlighting the challenges that present when extrapolating experimental studies. There is, however, a role for the gut microbiota in heart health, which can be exploited for therapeutic purposes; therefore, ongoing research is necessary to determine how the modulation of the gut microbiome may lead to improved cardiovascular health, with more research necessary in clinical settings.

TRIMETHYLAMINE N-OXIDE IN HEART FAILURE
Acute Heart Failure

To date, only 1 study has investigated the role of TMAO in acute HF patients.[11] In 972 acute HF patients, the authors' group showed that individuals with higher TMAO levels were more likely to be older; have reduced renal function, decreased heart rate, blood pressure, and hemoglobin levels; have increased levels of N-terminal pro–B-type natriuretic peptide (NT-proBNP) and potassium; and have reduced left ventricular ejection fraction. With regard to comorbidities, more patients in the higher TMAO group had diabetes or previous HF and evidence of atrial fibrillation. The clinical status of these patients was the poorest, with more patients in New York Heart Association (NYHA) class IV in the higher TMAO group. When clinical parameters associated with TMAO levels were investigated, TMAO was significantly and positively correlated to age, blood urea nitrogen, serum creatinine, and NT-proBNP, whereas a negative correlation was found with estimated glomerular filtration rate (eGFR), systolic blood pressure, and heart rate. Age, blood urea nitrogen, and eGFR were the most significant independent predictors of TMAO levels, with a minor role for diabetes, smoking status, atrial fibrillation, and NYHA class.

With regard to prediction of outcomes, TMAO was a univariate predictor in a composite of death and hospitalization due to HF at 1 year and of death at 1 year. In particular, TMAO was predictive in a multivariate model with predictors, such as age, NT-proBNP, and NYHA class. For both endpoints, however, when renal function (eGFR and urea) were included, TMAO was no longer predictive of outcomes. With regard to in-hospital mortality, TMAO was able to improve the risk stratification in combination with clinical scores (ie, Acute Decompensated Heart Failure National Registry (ADHERE), Organized Program to Initiate

Lifesaving Treatment in Hospitalized Patients with Heart Failure (OPTIMIZE-HF), Get With The Guidelines-Heart Failure (GWTG-HF)), even when renal indices are included.

TMAO strengthened the prediction of the composite endpoint when combined with NT-proBNP. Patients with both markers elevated were at the highest risk of death/HF. This is not surprising, given these markers reflect 2 different pathways, and further supports the hypothesis that a combination of biomarkers involved in different pathways could be the key point in the utilization and interpretation of biomarkers within cardiovascular disease.[49,50]

Chronic Heart Failure

CHF has been investigated more thoroughly in the context of TMAO. The first investigation of TMAO in CHF was performed a few years ago[15]; it demonstrated for the first time that TMAO levels were significantly higher in HF than in healthy subjects. In a cohort of 720 stable CHF patients, the investigators demonstrated an association between elevated TMAO levels and poor outcome in HF. In particular, patients with higher TMAO levels tended to be older, with a greater prevalence of diabetes mellitus (DM) and renal insufficiency. Furthermore, brain natriuretic peptide (BNP) values were higher in this category of patients and TMAO levels were significantly correlated with BNP levels and eGFR. With regard to mortality, TMAO stratified by quartiles showed a graded increase in mortality risk at 5 years. No differences were found when patients were stratified with regard to etiology of HF, age, presence of DM, sex, or smoking habits. Finally, even when corrected for eGFR, high-sensitivity C-reactive protein (CRP), and BNP levels, patients in the highest TMAO quartile remained at a significantly higher risk of mortality.

In a second study performed by the same group,[13] high TMAO as well as choline and betaine (2 substrates in the formation of TMAO [see **Fig. 1**]) were associated with higher NT-proBNP levels and more advanced left ventricular diastolic dysfunction. Levels of these metabolites were not related to systolic function or inflammatory or endothelial damage injury biomarkers. Despite the association of all 3 metabolites with increased risk for 5-year adverse clinical events (death/transplantation), only TMAO remained independently associated when corrected for age, renal function, NT-proBNP levels, and echocardiographic parameters of diastolic dysfunction. Therefore, TMAO demonstrated a stronger prognostic value compared with choline and betaine.

Another investigation conducted on TMAO, choline, and betaine, in a cohort of 155 patients with HF, 100 patients with coronary artery disease (CAD), and 33 healthy matched individuals,[12] showed HF patients with the highest levels of these metabolites compared with the other groups. All 3 markers were associated with NYHA class and NT-proBNP and inversely associated with eGFR and were significantly related to pulmonary pressure (estimated with right-sized catheterization). Furthermore, TMAO was associated with previous diagnosis of ischemic disease and with age. Among the HF patients, TMAO levels tended to be higher in patients with a diagnosis of CAD, independent of several confounding factors (eg, age, eGFR, CRP, and NT-proBNP). The association of TMAO levels with echocardiographic markers of diastolic dysfunction was not confirmed in this study. For mortality, TMAO levels but not choline or betaine were associated with poor prognosis, with approximately half of the cases in the upper tertile resulting in death or heart transplantation. When adjusted for multiple confounders (eg, eGFR, CRP, and NT-proBNP), however, this association no longer was significant.

Recently, the authors' group has demonstrated, using the BIOSTAT-CHF (Biology Study to Tailored Treatment in Chronic Heart Failure) cohort,[51,52] that TMAO levels are associated with adverse outcome (mortality and mortality/HF).[16] For the first time, the response of circulating TMAO levels to treatment and its associations with outcome were investigated. The authors found that contrary to natriuretic peptides, TMAO levels did not respond to guideline treatment. In addition, patients with sustained elevated levels of TMAO had the worst outcome. In particular, low TMAO levels at baseline and/or follow-up were associated with better prognosis. TMAO levels remained associated with outcomes even when adjusted for BIOSTAT-CHF risk models, which includes age, blood urea nitrogen, BNP, and other biochemical biomarkers and comorbidities. Notably, a post-hoc analysis performed on this cohort showed that, when grouped using a diet-based categorization by country of enrollment, TMAO levels differed by geographical location, displaying a different association with outcome by region (i.e. mortality risk of patients with elevated TMAO was higher in patients enrolled in Center-East Europe than in patients enrolled in Northern, Western and Southern countries, regardless of main confounders and gene variants).[53]

In the Ludwigshafen Risk and Cardiovascular Health Study study, TMAO levels and association with outcome were compared between HF with reduced ejection fraction (HFrEF) and HF with preserved ejection fraction (HFpEF).[14] In particular, TMAO was significantly associated with outcome in HFrEF but not in HFpEF when adjusted for several factors, including age, sex, eGFR, and DM. TMAO was more predictive in patients without DM and in patients with the lowest tertile of eGFR. In addition, TMAO showed a predictive value above and beyond NT-proBNP within this cohort, because NT-proBNP levels lose significance when adjusted for CRP. With regard to HFpEF, recently it has been demonstrated that TMAO levels were elevated to a similar extent in HFpEF and HFrEF patients when compared to cardiovascular disease free subject; further, TMAO levels showed an association with short-term and long-term events, in particular when used as a dichotomised variable (cut-off of 5 mmol/l, derived from the upper quartile of the control healthy population). In addition, when patients have been stratified with regard to TMAO and BNP levels, the combined use of these two biomarkers may be useful in risk stratification of HFpEF patients, in particular in those in which BNP is less elevated.[54]

Finally, in a small single-center study, TMAO levels were assessed for the first time in a japanese cohort, confirming that TMAO levels were elevated in HF patients compared with controls subjects.[55] Additionally, TMAO levels were related to the gut microbiome composition, in particular with the abundance of the *Escherichia/Shigella* genus.

CLINICAL CONTEXT AND FUTURE PERSPECTIVES

Overall, the data from published studies show a positive association between TMAO levels and prognosis in HF (**Table 1**), as explicated in a recent meta-analysis.[56] This observation is not surprising, given that high concentrations of TMAO are associated with increased risk of cardiovascular events and all-cause mortality, with a dose-dependent relationship.[56] In particular, the association of TMAO with outcomes are strongest in patients with CAD, and this could be linked with the proposed proatherogenic role of TMAO.

Some points, however, remain a matter of debate. To date, it is not possible to conclude whether high TMAO levels are causative of the increased risk of poor outcome in HF patients or if the HF causes the increase in TMAO levels and this is associated with poor prognosis. Although these effects are correlative, several studies have suggested a mechanistic link

Table 1
Previous reports for associations between TMAO and outcome in heart failure patients

Authors	Year Journal	Location	Study Population	Follow-Up Length	Outcomes	TMAO Levels (μmol/L)
Tang et al,[15]	2014 J Am Coll Cardiol	USA	CHF n = 720	5 y	All-cause mortality	5.0 [3.0–8.5]
Tang et al,[13]	2015 J Cardiac Fail	USA	CHF n = 112	5 y	All-cause mortality and heart transplantation	5.8 [3.6–12.1]
Troseid et al,[12]	2015 J Intern Med	Norway	CHF n = 155	5.2 y	All-cause mortality and heart transplantation	13.5 ± 18.5 (CAD) 7.1 ± 5.6 (DCM)
Suzuki et al,[11]	2016 Heart	UK	AHF n = 972	1 y	All-cause mortality and a composite of mortality/ rehospitalisation	5.6 [3.4–10.5]
Shuett et al,[14]	2017 J Am Coll Cardiol	Germany	CHF (HFpEF and HFrEF) n = 823	9.7 y	All-cause mortality and cardiovascular mortality	4.7 [3.4–6.8] (HFrEF) 4.7 [3.2–6.9] (HFpEF)
Suzuki et al,[16]	2018 Eur J Heart Fail	11 European countries	Worsening or new-onset HF n = 2234	3 y	All-cause mortality and a composite of mortality/ rehospitalisation	5.9 [3.6–10.8]
Yazaki et al,[53]	2019 Eur J Heart Fail	11 European countries	Worsening or new-onset HF grouped by region n = 2234	3 y	All-cause mortality and a composite of mortality/ rehospitalisation	7.4 [4.1–13.6] NW 4.6 [2.9–7.5] CE 6.2 [3.6–11.5] S
Salzano et al,[54]	2019 Eur J Prev Cardiol	UK	CHF (HFpEF and HFrEF) n = 156	5 y	Composite endpoint of all-cause mortality/ hospitalisation for HF at 18 mo (short-term) and at 60 mo (long-term)	8.4 [3.7–13.8] HFrEF 6.6 [4.3–12.3] HFpEF
Hayashi et al,[55]	2018 Circ J	Japan	Decompensated HF n = 22	Cross-sectional	TMAO levels (during de-compensation and during compensation phases) and gut microbioma composition were altered when compared to control subjects	17.3 ± 11.7 (Decomp) 17.7 ± 12.6 (Comp)

Abbreviations: AHF, acute heart failure; CAD, coronary artery disease; CE, central/eastern region; CHF, chronic heart failure; Comp, compensated; DCM, dilated cardiomyopathy; Decomp, decompensated; HFpEF, heart failure with preserved ejection fraction; HFrEF, heart failure with reduced ejection fraction; NW, northern/western region; S, southern region; TMAO, trimethylamine N-oxide.

between myocardial function and altered intestinal microbiota,[3,4] which may underlie the association with poor outcome. The relationship between TMAO and left ventricular systolic function is unknown; however, diastolic dysfunction has been observed,[13] suggesting a stronger link with cardiac congestion rather than with impaired perfusion. This association may be explained by the intestinal congestion observed within patients with more severe HF, resulting in alterations of the microbiota composition, with subsequent impact on TMAO levels. Another issue not yet clarified is whether TMAO has the same role in HFrEF and in HFpEF. Only two studies have tested the association of TMAO in HFrEF and HFpEF,[14] and further research is needed to clarify the association of TMAO in these conditions.

The role of diet and kidney function is also highly debated regarding the association of TMAO with HF. Some reports showed attenuated association of TMAO levels with outcomes after adjustment for confounders.[11,12] In contrast, in other HF populations, TMAO levels were reported to be associated with mortality even after adjustment for renal function.[13,15,16] With this regard, a recent meta-analysis demonstrated significant differences in the relationship between TMAO and all-cause mortality in patients with and without chronic kidney disease,[56] showing no significant difference between the 2 groups.

In addition, considering that TMAO levels were shown not to be affected by traditional guideline-recommended HF treatment,[16] this presents a novel field of research for investigation, whereby modification of the gut microbiota could be a novel therapeutic approach, and to date there are no large-scale trials that have been conducted to test this hypothesis.

Trimethylamine N-oxide and Heart Failure: Unmet Needs

On the basis of data present in the literature, there are several limitations with regard to knowledge about TMAO in HF. In brief,

- Largely, the data obtained from these studies represent single ethnic groups, mainly white patients. Few studies are representative of other ethnic groups, and, therefore, drawing generalized conclusions based on a single ethnicity is misrepresentative.
- To date, it is not clearly understood whether HF affects TMAO levels or if TMAO is involved in the pathophysiology of HF.
- The role of confounding factors does not have a consensus in the literature and

studies presented; therefore, the interplay of several factors, such as eGFR, age, and sex, needs to be clearly addressed concerning TMAO.

- All observations deriving from HF studies have limited or no data about the dietary condition of patients.
- There are no studies investigating pharmacologic intervention on TMAO levels in HF.
- There is no clear evidence to suggest that lowering TMAO levels in patients shows better prognosis.
- It is not clear whether TMAO has an association with mortality in HFpEF.

In the authors' opinion, these points need to be addressed in future research, in order to gain a full understanding of the role of TMAO in HF.

SUMMARY

In conclusion, TMAO levels are increased in HF populations compared with healthy subjects. Higher TMAO levels are associated with poor prognosis, whereas low TMAO levels either at baseline or follow-up confer better prognosis. In order to draw appropriate conclusions regarding the role of TMAO in HF, additional studies are needed to address the current limitations highlighted. The finding that TMAO levels seem to be not affected by guideline-HF treatment may shed light on TMAO as a novel and independent therapeutic target for HF that requires specific treatment.

REFERENCES

1. Braunwald E. Heart failure. JACC Heart Fail 2013;1: 1–20.
2. Ponikowski P, Voors AA, Anker SD, et al. 2016 ESC guidelines for the diagnosis and treatment of acute and chronic heart failure: the Task Force for the diagnosis and treatment of acute and chronic heart failure of the European Society of Cardiology (ESC). Developed with the special contribution of the Heart Failure Association (HFA) of the ESC. Eur J Heart Fail 2016;18: 891–975.
3. Krack A, Sharma R, Figulla HR, et al. The importance of the gastrointestinal system in the pathogenesis of heart failure. Eur Heart J 2005;26: 2368–74.
4. Nagatomo Y, Tang WH. Intersections between microbiome and heart failure: revisiting the gut hypothesis. J Card Fail 2015;21:973–80.
5. Sandek A, Bjarnason I, Volk HD, et al. Studies on bacterial endotoxin and intestinal absorption

function in patients with chronic heart failure. Int J Cardiol 2012;157:80–5.

6. Marra AM, Arcopinto M, Salzano A, et al. Detectable interleukin-9 plasma levels are associated with impaired cardiopulmonary functional capacity and all-cause mortality in patients with chronic heart failure. Int J Cardiol 2016;209: 114–7.

7. Pasini E, Aquilani R, Testa C, et al. Pathogenic gut flora in patients with chronic heart failure. JACC Heart Fail 2016;4:220–7.

8. Baker JR, Chaykin S. The biosynthesis of trimethylamine-N-oxide. J Biol Chem 1962;237:1309–13.

9. Cassambai S, Salzano A, Yazaki Y, et al. Impact of acute choline loading on circulating trimethylamine N-oxide levels. Eur J Prev Cardiol 2019. https://doi.org/10.1177/2047487319831372. 204748 7319831372.

10. Albert CL, Tang WHW. Metabolic biomarkers in heart failure. Heart Fail Clin 2018;14:109–18.

11. Suzuki T, Heaney LM, Bhandari SS, et al. Trimethylamine N-oxide and prognosis in acute heart failure. Heart 2016;102:841–8.

12. Troseid M, Ueland T, Hov JR, et al. Microbiota-dependent metabolite trimethylamine-N-oxide is associated with disease severity and survival of patients with chronic heart failure. J Intern Med 2015; 277:717–26.

13. Tang WH, Wang Z, Shrestha K, et al. Intestinal microbiota-dependent phosphatidylcholine metabolites, diastolic dysfunction, and adverse clinical outcomes in chronic systolic heart failure. J Card Fail 2015;21:91–6.

14. Schuett K, Kleber ME, Scharnagl H, et al. Trimethylamine-N-oxide and heart failure with reduced versus preserved ejection fraction. J Am Coll Cardiol 2017; 70:3202–4.

15. Tang WH, Wang Z, Fan Y, et al. Prognostic value of elevated levels of intestinal microbe-generated metabolite trimethylamine-N-oxide in patients with heart failure: refining the gut hypothesis. J Am Coll Cardiol 2014;64:1908–14.

16. Suzuki T, Yazaki Y, Voors AA, et al. Association with outcomes and response to treatment of trimethylamine N-oxide in heart failure (from BIOSTAT-CHF). Eur J Heart Fail 2019;21(7):877–86.

17. Koeth RA, Wang Z, Levison BS, et al. Intestinal microbiota metabolism of L-carnitine, a nutrient in red meat, promotes atherosclerosis. Nat Med 2013;19: 576–85.

18. Wang Z, Roberts AB, Buffa JA, et al. Non-lethal Inhibition of gut microbial trimethylamine production for the treatment of atherosclerosis. Cell 2015;163: 1585–95.

19. Bennett BJ, de Aguiar Vallim TQ, Wang Z, et al. Trimethylamine-N-oxide, a metabolite associated with atherosclerosis, exhibits complex genetic and dietary regulation. Cell Metab 2013;17: 49–60.

20. Mayatepek E, Flock B, Zschocke J. Benzydamine metabolism in vivo is impaired in patients with deficiency of flavin-containing monooxygenase 3. Pharmacogenetics 2004;14:775–7.

21. Fennema D, Phillips IR, Shephard EA. Trimethylamine and trimethylamine N-Oxide, a flavin-containing monooxygenase 3 (FMO3)-mediated host-microbiome metabolic axis implicated in health and disease. Drug Metab Dispos 2016;44: 1839–50.

22. Ufnal M, Zadlo A, Ostaszewski R. TMAO: a small molecule of great expectations. Nutrition 2015;31: 1317–23.

23. Christodoulou J. Trimethylaminuria: an under-recognised and socially debilitating metabolic disorder. J Paediatr Child Health 2012;48:E153–5.

24. Zou Q, Bennion BJ, Daggett V, et al. The molecular mechanism of stabilization of proteins by TMAO and its ability to counteract the effects of urea. J Am Chem Soc 2002;124:1192–202.

25. Welch WJ. Role of quality control pathways in human diseases involving protein misfolding. Semin Cell Dev Biol 2004;15:31–8.

26. Leandro P, Gomes CM. Protein misfolding in conformational disorders: rescue of folding defects and chemical chaperoning. Mini Rev Med Chem 2008; 8:901–11.

27. Wang Z, Klipfell E, Bennett BJ, et al. Gut flora metabolism of phosphatidylcholine promotes cardiovascular disease. Nature 2011;472:57–63.

28. Suzuki T, Heaney LM, Jones DJ, et al. Trimethylamine N-oxide and risk stratification after acute myocardial infarction. Clin Chem 2017;63:420–8.

29. Sala-Vila A, Guasch-Ferre M, Hu FB, et al. Dietary alpha-Linolenic acid, marine omega-3 fatty acids, and mortality in a population with high fish consumption: findings from the PREvencion con DIeta MEDiterranea (PREDIMED) Study. J Am Heart Assoc 2016;5 [pii:e002543].

30. Albert CM, Campos H, Stampfer MJ, et al. Blood levels of long-chain n-3 fatty acids and the risk of sudden death. N Engl J Med 2002;346:1113–8.

31. Cheung W, Keski-Rahkonen P, Assi N, et al. A metabolomic study of biomarkers of meat and fish intake. Am J Clin Nutr 2017;105:600–8.

32. Zhu W, Gregory JC, Org E, et al. Gut microbial metabolite TMAO enhances platelet hyperreactivity and thrombosis risk. Cell 2016;165:111–24.

33. Chen K, Zheng X, Feng M, et al. Gut microbiota-dependent metabolite trimethylamine N-oxide contributes to cardiac dysfunction in western diet-induced obese mice. Front Physiol 2017;8:139.

34. Boutagy NE, Neilson AP, Osterberg KL, et al. Probiotic supplementation and trimethylamine-N-oxide

production following a high-fat diet. Obesity (Silver Spring) 2015;23:2357–63.

35. Zhang H, Meng J, Yu H. Trimethylamine N-oxide supplementation abolishes the cardioprotective effects of voluntary exercise in mice fed a western diet. Front Physiol 2017;8:944.

36. Rasmussen LG, Winning H, Savorani F, et al. Assessment of the effect of high or low protein diet on the human urine metabolome as measured by NMR. Nutrients 2012;4:112–31.

37. Bergeron N, Williams PT, Lamendella R, et al. Diets high in resistant starch increase plasma levels of trimethylamine-N-oxide, a gut microbiome metabolite associated with CVD risk. Br J Nutr 2016;116: 2020–9.

38. Janeiro M, Ramírez M, Milagro F, et al. Implication of trimethylamine N-oxide (TMAO) in disease: potential biomarker or new therapeutic target. Nutrients 2018; 10:1398.

39. Wang Z, Bergeron N, Levison BS, et al. Impact of chronic dietary red meat, white meat, or non-meat protein on trimethylamine N-oxide metabolism and renal excretion in healthy men and women. Eur Heart J 2019;40(7):583–94.

40. Carding S, Verbeke K, Vipond DT, et al. Dysbiosis of the gut microbiota in disease. Microb Ecol Health Dis 2015;26:26191.

41. Yin J, Liao SX, He Y, et al. Dysbiosis of gut microbiota with reduced trimethylamine-N-oxide level in patients with large-artery atherosclerotic stroke or transient ischemic attack. J Am Heart Assoc 2015; 4 [pii:e002699].

42. Organ CL, Otsuka H, Bhushan S, et al. Choline diet and its gut microbe-derived metabolite, trimethylamine N-oxide, exacerbate pressure overload-induced heart failure. Circ Heart Fail 2016;9: e002314.

43. Randrianarisoa E, Lehn-Stefan A, Wang X, et al. Relationship of serum trimethylamine N-oxide (TMAO) levels with early atherosclerosis in humans. Sci Rep 2016;6:26745.

44. Sun G, Yin Z, Liu N, et al. Gut microbial metabolite TMAO contributes to renal dysfunction in a mouse model of diet-induced obesity. Biochem Biophys Res Commun 2017;493:964–70.

45. Gan XT, Ettinger G, Huang CX, et al. Probiotic administration attenuates myocardial hypertrophy and heart failure after myocardial infarction in the rat. Circ Heart Fail 2014;7:491–9.

46. Martin FP, Wang Y, Sprenger N, et al. Probiotic modulation of symbiotic gut microbial-host metabolic interactions in a humanized microbiome mouse model. Mol Syst Biol 2008;4:157.

47. Savi M, Bocchi L, Bresciani L, et al. Trimethylamine-N-oxide (TMAO)-induced impairment of cardiomyocyte function and the protective role of urolithin B-glucuronide. Molecules 2018;23 [pii:E549].

48. Borges NA, Stenvinkel P, Bergman P, et al. Effects of probiotic supplementation on trimethylamine-N-oxide plasma levels in hemodialysis patients: a pilot study. Probiotics Antimicrob Proteins 2019;11(2): 648–54.

49. Salzano A, Marra AM, Proietti M, et al. Biomarkers in heart failure and associated diseases. Dis Markers 2019;2019:8768624.

50. Salzano A, Marra AM, D'Assante R, et al. Biomarkers and imaging: complementary or subtractive? Heart Fail Clin 2019;15:321–31.

51. Voors AA, Anker SD, Cleland JG, et al. A systems BIOlogy Study to TAilored Treatment in Chronic Heart Failure: rationale, design, and baseline characteristics of BIOSTAT-CHF. Eur J Heart Fail 2016; 18:716–26.

52. Streng KW, Nauta JF, Hillege HL, et al. Non-cardiac comorbidities in heart failure with reduced, mid-range and preserved ejection fraction. Int J Cardiol 2018;271:132–9.

53. Yazaki Y, Salzano A, Nelson CP, et al. Geographical location affects the levels and association of trimethylamine N-oxide with heart failure mortality in BIOSTAT-CHF: a post-hoc analysis. Eur J Heart Fail 2019 Jul 28. https://doi.org/10.1002/ejhf.1550. [Epub ahead of print].

54. Salzano A, Israr MZ, Yazaki Y, et al. Combined use of trimethylamine N-oxide with BNP for risk stratification in heart failure with preserved ejection fraction: findings from the DIAMONDHFpEF study. Eur J Prev Cardiol 2019 Aug 14. https://doi.org/10.1177/ 2047487319870355. 2047487319870355. [Epub ahead of print].

55. Hayashi T, Yamashita T, Watanabe H, et al. Gut microbiome and plasma microbiome-related metabolites in patients with decompensated and compensated heart failure. Circ J 2018;83: 182–92.

56. Schiattarella GG, Sannino A, Toscano E, et al. Gut microbe-generated metabolite trimethylamine-N-oxide as cardiovascular risk biomarker: a systematic review and dose-response meta-analysis. Eur Heart J 2017;38:2948–56.

Chronic Obstructive Pulmonary Disease and Heart Failure: A Breathless Conspiracy

Pierpaolo Pellicori, MD, FESC[a],*, John G.F. Cleland, MD, FRCP, FESC[a],
Andrew L. Clark, MA, MD, FRCP[b]

KEYWORDS

- COPD • Heart failure • Natriuretic peptides • Diagnosis • Review • Therapy

KEY POINTS

- COPD and heart failure are both common and share many risk factors.
- Heart failure and COPD frequently coexist, and such patients have a poor prognosis.
- Determining whether breathlessness is due predominantly to lung or heart disease can be difficult; missed diagnoses are common.
- The combined effect of treatments for HFrEF on outcome is large and therefore the diagnosis should not be missed.
- COPD may deter the introduction or up-titration of β-blockers, a key treatment of HFrEF.
- Treatments do not substantially alter outcomes for COPD or HFpEF.

INTRODUCTION

Heart failure (HF) and chronic obstructive pulmonary disease (COPD) are increasingly common and often coexist. Together they probably cause or complicate about 10% of all hospital admissions. However, perhaps fewer than half of patients who have these conditions have appropriate investigation and diagnosis. Furthermore, the diagnosis of one condition may obscure the presence of the other.[1,2] HF and COPD have much in common, including risk factors (for instance, a lifelong history of smoking and obesity), symptoms (breathlessness and cough), and clinical signs (lung crackles and peripheral edema). Differentiating between the 2 conditions is a diagnostic challenge, but their correct identification is essential: the correct treatment will improve the long-term outcome of many patients with HF, whereas there is little treatment that has a profound impact on outcome for COPD.[3,4]

This review discusses the diagnostic challenges in distinguishing COPD from chronic HF in patients with exertional dyspnea. Also discussed are the prevalence, clinical relevance, and therapeutic implications associated with a concurrent diagnosis of COPD and HF.

CHRONIC OBSTRUCTIVE PULMONARY DISEASE AND HEART FAILURE: A DIAGNOSTIC CHALLENGE
Clinical History and Physical Examination

An accurate clinical history usually leaves more doubts than certainties in a breathlessness patient because signs and symptoms are not specific for either condition. Advanced age increases the risk of having both COPD and HF. Many of those who report dyspnea on exercise

This article originally appeared in *Heart Failure Clinics*, Volume 16, Issue 1, January 2020.

Disclosure: The authors have nothing to disclose.

[a] Robertson Institute of Biostatistics and Clinical Trials Unit, University of Glasgow, University Avenue, Glasgow G12 8QQ, UK; [b] Department of Cardiology, Castle Hill Hospital, Hull York Medical School, University of Hull, Kingston upon Hull HU16 5JQ, UK

* Corresponding author.

E-mail address: pierpaolo.pellicori@glasgow.ac.uk

are or have been smokers, many are obese, and many have coronary artery disease. Cough is frequent, and can be due to COPD, HF, or use of angiotensin-converting enzyme inhibitors (ACE-I). Clinical signs of air-flow limitation (such as wheeze) or high cardiac filling pressure (such as lung crackles or raised jugular vein pressure) lack specificity and are common only when disease is severe.[5,6] Nonintentional weight loss, malnutrition, and cachexia are also common in the more advanced stages of either COPD or HF.[7,8]

Chest Radiography and Other Radiological Findings

A normal chest radiograph does not rule out a diagnosis of COPD or chronic HF.[9] Abnormal findings are nonspecific except, perhaps, when there is frank pulmonary edema. However, other causes of cough and exertional breathlessness can be diagnosed on a chest radiograph, such as lung cancer, tuberculosis, and pulmonary fibrosis. A plain radiograph should always be considered.

Electrocardiography

A normal electrocardiogram (ECG) excludes HF for practical purposes, but not COPD.[10] Although many subtle ECG changes have been reported in patients with COPD, their clinical relevance has not been demonstrated.[11] Prompt identification of atrial fibrillation, a common ECG finding in both conditions, is important because anticoagulation is usually indicated to prevent stroke.

Spirometry

A ratio of forced expiratory volume in the first second (FEV_1) to forced vital capacity (FVC) of less than 70% after administration of a bronchodilator is the key diagnostic criterion for COPD.[12] This definition seems straightforward, but spirometry can be easily misinterpreted, leading to inappropriate diagnosis and treatment.[13] Up to 25% of patients who meet the spirometric criterion for COPD will have a result within the normal range on repeat testing without receiving any treatment that could explain the difference.[14,15] By contrast, a substantial proportion of current, or past, smokers with respiratory symptoms, apparent exacerbations, and exercise limitation has evidence of airway disease on computed tomography scans, despite normal spirometry.[16] The FEV_1/FVC ratio also declines with age, and HF may cause further reductions.

Biomarkers

With rare exceptions (such as constrictive pericarditis), when intracardiac pressures increase or renal water and salt retention occurs leading to fluid overload, the heart produces natriuretic peptides (NPs) as a counter-regulatory strategy designed to cause natriuresis and vasodilation. Increasing plasma concentrations of NPs are the single most powerful predictor of adverse outcome in patients with HF, regardless of left ventricular ejection fraction.[17,18] A normal plasma concentration of NPs rules out serious cardiac dysfunction (in constrictive pericarditis, plasma concentrations of NPs are lower than expected from the clinical picture, but rarely normal). The diagnostic utility of NPs is currently recognized by all international guidelines on HF, including the National Institute for Health and Care Excellence and the European Society for Cardiology, to rule out important cardiac dysfunction in patients with suspected HF, acute or chronic.[3]

Screening studies suggest that up to 50% of patients with COPD have increased plasma concentrations of NPs, although no large definitive study exists (**Table 1**).[19–22] Raised plasma NP levels in patients with COPD predict a higher mortality, whether or not they have received a diagnosis of HF.[23,24] For patients with COPD, increased plasma concentrations of high-sensitivity troponin-I, suggesting ongoing myocardial damage, are also associated with high rates of cardiovascular events, but not with exacerbations of COPD.[25] No blood biomarkers are currently recommended for the identification of persons with COPD. Patients with an elevated plasma concentration of NP should be investigated further, usually by echocardiography.

Echocardiography

Cardiac imaging (most commonly echocardiography) is an essential investigation for breathless patients who have an elevated plasma NP or in whom a cardiac contribution to breathlessness is suspected or needs to be excluded. It is important not to miss patients with a reduced left ventricular ejection fraction or severe valve disease, for which highly effective treatments exist. If these abnormalities are excluded, a dilated left atrium implies that the patient has abnormal left ventricular diastolic function and suggests the diagnosis of HF with preserved left ventricular ejection fraction (HFpEF). An echocardiogram should be considered in patients with an exacerbation of COPD, as approximately 25% of patients will have an important, potentially treatable, underlying heart problem.[26,27]

Table 1
Screening by natriuretic peptides (NPs) in patients with chronic obstructive pulmonary disease (COPD; only studies with >100 patients)

Study	Year	N	Age (y)	Men (%)	COPD Diagnosis	HF (%)	Diuretic (%)	Edema (%)	Current Smoker (%)	IHD (%)	AF (&)	Creatinine	Abnormal NPs (%)	Criteria Used to Diagnose HF and Prevalence
Cross-sectional[19]	2001–2003	200	73	58	Clinical or GOLD (59%)	0	22	19	NR	34	9	90 μmol/L	~50	ESC criteria: 26% (15% HFrEF)
Cross-sectional[20]	2006	170	64	75	GOLD	Excl.	NR	Excl.	42	NR	NR	NR	23	Echocardiography: 3% had LVEF ≤50%
Prospective, observational[21]	2004–2008	140	67	46	GOLD	NR	27	19	82	NR	9	92 μmol/L	>50	Echocardiography: 11% had LVEF <45%
Prospective, observational[22]	NR	218	70	76	GOLD	0	22	19	24	17	NR	5% CKD	>50	Echocardiography: 14% HFrEF

Abnormal NPs includes NT-proBNP greater than 125 ng/L or BNP greater than 35 ng/L.

Abbreviations: AF, atrial fibrillation; BNP, B-type natriuretic peptide; CKD, chronic kidney disease; ESC, European Society of Cardiology; Excl., excluded; GOLD, Global Initiative for Chronic Obstructive Lung Disease criteria; HF, heart failure; HFrEF, heart failure with reduced left ventricular ejection fraction; IHD, ischemic heart disease; LVEF, left ventricular ejection fraction; N, number of patients; NR, not reported; NT-proBNP, N-terminal prohormone B-type natriuretic peptide.

HOW COMMON ARE CHRONIC OBSTRUCTIVE PULMONARY DISEASE AND HEART FAILURE?

Everyone gets breathless with sufficient exertion. Breathlessness precipitated by modest levels of exertion that a healthy young person can easily manage is very common, but is frequently not reported or investigated. Many subjects, or sometimes their doctors, attribute exertional dyspnea to simply "getting older" or "being unfit or fat." Consequently, many cases of HF and/or COPD are not diagnosed until symptoms or signs become severe enough to require a hospital admission. Use of a loop diuretic, also common in primary care as treatment of exertional dyspnea or ankle swelling, might temporarily mask symptoms of HF. Initiation of loop diuretics should prompt further investigation of cardiac function.[28] Robust, objective criteria to identify, or rule out, cardiac or lung disease as a cause of breathlessness are, with the exception of NPs, lacking. Thus, the reported prevalence of COPD and HF varies substantially, depending on the characteristics of the population studied, the context and period of time during which data were collected, the geographic area and exposure to different environmental risk factors, and, most importantly, the diagnostic criteria used to define HF and COPD.

At least 5% of the adult population is said to have COPD while the prevalence of HF is perhaps 1% to 2%. Many reports suggest that a large proportion of breathlessness patients have both conditions (**Tables 2**[26,29–36] **and 3**[37–48]). It is worth noting that the diagnosis of "heart failure" includes those with either a reduced (HFrEF) or preserved (HFpEF) left ventricular ejection fraction on imaging, which have a similar prevalence.

PREVALENCE AND PROGNOSTIC RELEVANCE OF HEART FAILURE IN PEOPLE WITH CHRONIC OBSTRUCTIVE PULMONARY DISEASE

In surveys of COPD, HF is usually reported in less than 20% of patients (see **Table 2**). Despite the high prevalence of ischemic heart disease, smoking, and echocardiographic abnormalities in patients with COPD, COPD itself is, surprisingly, not strongly associated with HF in epidemiologic studies. Perhaps once a diagnosis of COPD is made, clinicians do not look for other problems to explain symptoms. However, missing a diagnosis of HF may have important consequences. In a cohort of 404 patients older than 65 years with COPD diagnosed in primary care, a detailed cardiovascular examination identified previously undiagnosed HF in 21%, of whom about 50% had HFpEF and 50% HFrEF.[35] A diagnosis of HF approximately doubled the risk of mortality in models adjusted for age and other comorbidities. Of those with COPD who were thought not to have HF, 22% were treated with a diuretic, and about one-third had an NT-proBNP (N-terminal prohormone B-type natriuretic peptide) level greater than 125 ng/L, suggesting that many of these patients also had HF.

Among 1664 ambulatory patients with COPD enrolled in a multicenter registry in Spain and the United States (BODE), the prevalence of self-reported HF, supported by review of medical records, was ~16%, which was associated with a 33% increase in mortality.[29] A recent analysis of electronic health records from Sweden, which included data from primary and secondary care on ~90,000 patients aged ≥35 years, showed that, compared with those with COPD alone (n = 885, 1%), those who had HF as a coded codiagnosis (n = 99, 10%) had 7-fold higher mortality.[36]

PREVALENCE AND PROGNOSTIC RELEVANCE OF CHRONIC OBSTRUCTIVE PULMONARY DISEASE IN PEOPLE WITH HEART FAILURE

The prevalence of COPD among patients with HF ranges from 10% to 20% in large trials and registries where COPD was either self-reported by patients or based on the opinion (nonstandardized) of researchers (see **Table 3**). In smaller studies that used lung function tests to evaluate air-flow obstruction objectively, up to 50% of patients with HF had abnormal spirometry. This wide discrepancy might suggest that the diagnosis of COPD is often missed, perhaps because cardiologists pay little attention to airway disease in the presence of a more deadly, but treatable, condition. However, it is also possible that HF has effects on the lung that mimic the effects of COPD, leading to overdiagnosis. Interstitial lung edema can compress alveoli and distal airways; cardiomegaly or pleural effusion can reduce the intrathoracic space and compress lung volumes; decreased respiratory muscle strength can reduce inspiratory and expiratory forces; and frailty may impair the ability to perform spirometry accurately and normal values in those older than 80 years are not well defined, which might lead to overdiagnosis by spirometry.[49] Moreover, effective treatment of HF can normalize spirometry and reduce hospitalizations for respiratory infection.[50,51] Interpreting spirometric data in a patient with poorly controlled HF can be difficult.

Table 2
Prevalence of heart failure in patients with chronic obstructive pulmonary disease

First Author,[Ref.] Year	Sample (N)	Year	Country	COPD Population and Definition	HF Definition	Prevalence of HF (%)	CV Therapies in Patients with COPD	Outcome Findings
Divo et al,[29] 2012	1664	1997–2009	USA and Spain	Ambulatory, GOLD (≥3: 56%)	Self-reported/ medical records	16	NR	HF increased risk of death (HR: 1.33; 95% CI: 1.06–1.68; P = .02)
Cazzola et al,[30] 2010	341,329	2006	Italy	Primary care; ICD-9	ICD-9	8	NR	NR
Curkendall et al,[31] 2006	11,493	1997–2000	Canada	Government database; ICD-9 and prescribed inhaler	ICD-9	19	Diuretics: 57% Digoxin: 17% BB: 10% ACE-I: 34%	Patients diagnosed and treated with COPD are at high risk for CV morbidity and mortality
Holguin et al,[32] 2005	~47 million	1979–2001	USA	Hospital discharge; ICD-9	ICD-9	10	NR	Compared with those without COPD, in-hospital mortality for HF is higher in patients with COPD
McCullough et al,[33] 2003	417	1999–2000	USA/ Europe	Emergency department (dyspnea); self-reported	Framingham and NHANES criteria	21	HF: Diuretic: 53% Digoxin: 35% ACE-I: 37% BB: 21% No HF: Diuretic: 25% Digoxin: 6% ACE-I: 19% BB: 7%	The emergency physician identified only 37% of HF cases Patients with HF had higher BNP (mean 587 pg/mL) than those without (108 pg/mL)

(continued on next page)

Table 2
(continued)

First Author,[Ref.] Year	Sample (N)	Year	Country	COPD Population and Definition	HF Definition	Prevalence of HF (%)	CV Therapies in Patients with COPD	Outcome Findings
Freixa et al,[26] 2013	342	2004–06	Spain	First COPD admission; ATS/ERS criteria	Self-reported + echocardiography 3 mo after discharge	13 LVSD (9 unknown) 14 DD ≥grade 3 (10 unknown)	NR	NR
Spece et al,[34] 2018	2391	2005–11	USA	Hospital discharge; ICD-9	ICD-9	23	NR	CV causes are common reasons for readmission
Boudestein et al,[35] 2009	404	2001–03	Netherlands	Primary care, clinically diagnosed	ESC criteria	21 (previously undiagnosed; 50 had HFpEF)	HF and COPD: Diuretic: 34% ACE-I/ARB: 35% BB: 16% / COPD only: Diuretic: 22% ACE-I/ARB: 22% BB: 11%	Newly diagnosed HF was independent predictor of mortality (HR 2.1; 95% CI 1.2–3.6; *P* = .01)
Kaszuba et al,[36] 2018	984 (~3%)	2007	Sweden	Primary and secondary care; ICD-10	ICD-10	10	NR	In univariate analysis, mortality in patients with COPD and coexisting HF was 7 times higher than in those with COPD alone

Abbreviations: ACE-I, angiotensin-converting enzyme inhibitor; ARB, angiotensin II receptor blocker; ATS, American Thoracic Society; BB, β-blockers; CV, cardiovascular; ESC, European Society of Cardiology; ERS, European Respiratory Society; HFpEF, heart failure with preserved LVEF; HFrEF, heart failure with reduced LVEF; ICD, International Classification of Diseases; LVEF, left ventricular ejection fraction; LVSD, left ventricular systolic dysfunction; N, number of patients.

Table 3

Prevalence and clinical relevance of chronic obstructive pulmonary disease in patients with heart failure in selected recent registries and clinical trials

First Author,Ref. Year	Prevalence of COPD (%)	Sample (N)	Year	Country	HF Population/ Diagnosis	Treatment for Heart Failure			Outcome
						BB (COPD vs no COPD)	ACE-i/ARB (COPD vs no COPD)	Diuretic (COPD vs no COPD)	
COPD adjudicated by clinical notes/clinical evidence/medical history/therapy for COPD									
De Blois et al,[37] 2010	17	4132	2000–2008	Norway	Mixed, >80% HFrEF/ ESC guidelines	74% vs 84% (P<.001)	Similar: ~90%	90% vs 86% (P = .002)	COPD independently predicted death (HR 1.19; 95% CI 1.02–1.39; P = .03)
Mentz et al,[38] 2012	10	4133	2003–2006	USA, Europe, South Africa	Acute/LVEF ≤40%	63% vs 71% (P = .001)	80% vs 85% (P = .01)	Similar: ~97%	COPD was associated with ACM and CV death/HFH only in univariable analysis
Canepa et al,[39] 2018	19 AHF 14 CHF	16,329	2011–2013	Europe	Mixed, ~70% HFrEF/IV therapy for AHF	CHF: 77% vs 85% (P<.001) AHF:51% vs 56% (P<.001)	CHF: ~85%, similar AHF: 64%, similar	CHF: 88% vs 78% (P<.001) AHF: 73% vs 62% (P<.001)	Greater in-hospital mortality in those with COPD (8% vs 5%) COPD was not independent predictor of ACM, but predicted HFH
Canepa et al,[40] 2017	22	6975	2002–2005	Italy	Chronic, ~90% HFrEF/ LVEF <40% or HFH in previous 12 mo	44% vs 71% (P<.001)	91% vs 94% (P<.0001)	93% vs 89% (P<.001)	COPD was an independent predictor of ACM (HR 1.28, 95% CI 1.15–1.43, P<.0001) and hospitalizations
Tavazzi et al,[41] 2013	11	6505	2006–2009	37 Countries	Chronic, HFrEF/LVEF <35%, SR and HFH in prior 12 mo	69% vs 92% (P<.001)	ACE-i: similar (~79%)	89% vs 82% (P<.001)	The primary end point (CV death or HHF), but not ACM, was more frequent in patients with COPD

(continued on next page)

Table 3
(continued)

First Author,[Ref.] Year	Prevalence of COPD (%)	Sample (N)	Year	Country	HF Population/ Diagnosis	Treatment for Heart Failure			Outcome
						BB (COPD vs no COPD)	ACE-i/ARB (COPD vs no COPD)	Diuretic (COPD vs no COPD)	
Parissis et al,[42] 2014	25	4953	2006–2007	9 Countries	Acute, >50% HFrEF/ ESC guidelines	21% vs 24% (*P* = .055)	ACE-I: 34% vs 31% (*P* = .042) ARB: 26% vs 28% (ns)	35% vs 31% (*P* = .006)	Similar in-hospital mortality (~10%)
Mentz et al,[43] 2012	25	20,118	2003–2004	USA	Acute, HFrEF/LVSD at admission	52% vs 57% (*P*<.001)	Similar (54%)	LD: 69% vs 61% (*P*<.001)	COPD increased in-hospital non-CV mortality, but not post-discharge mortality
COPD diagnosed by spirometry									
Cuthbert et al,[44] 2019	50%	3514	2000–2016	UK	Chronic at first visit, ~25% HFpEF/ reduced LVEF or NT-proBNP >400 ng/L	54% vs 62%	Similar: 71% vs 72%	LD: Similar: 72% vs 70%	COPD weakly associated with ACM in HFrEF, but not HFpEF
Jacob et al,[45] 2017	26%	8099	2009–2012	Spain	Acute, 38% HFrEF/ clinical and radiological	Admission: 30% vs 45% (*P*<.001)	Admission: similar (~56%)	LD: 75% vs 68% (*P*<.001)	COPD only associated with readmissions at 30 d
Iversen et al,[46] 2010	35% (vs 22% self-reported)	532	2001–2004	Denmark	Acute, 42% HFpEF/ requiring IV diuretic	17% vs 32% (*P* = .002)	Similar (~35%)	71% vs 64% (*P* = .18).	PFTs provide prognostic information in HF
Plesner et al,[47] 2017	39%	573	2009–2011	Denmark	Chronic at first visit/ LVEF <45%	Similar: 75% vs 78%	88% vs 94% (*P* = .03)	LD: 64% vs 48% (*P*<.01)	Abnormal spirometry predicted ACM
Yoshihisa et al,[48] 2014	28%	378	2009–2012	Japan	Acute, ~50% HFpEF/ Framingham criteria	67% vs 79% (*P* = .014)	Similar (87%)	NR	PFTs provide prognostic information in HF

Abbreviations: ACE-I, angiotensin-converting enzyme inhibitor; ACM, all-cause mortality; ARB, angiotensin II receptor blocker; BB, β-blockers; BNP, B-type natriuretic peptide; CV, cardiovascular; HFH, heart failure hospitalizations; HFpEF, heart failure with preserved LVEF; HFrEF, heart failure with reduced LVEF; IV, intravenous; LD, loop diuretic; LVEF, left ventricular ejection fraction; NR, not recorded; ns, not significant; NT-proBNP, N-terminal prohormone B-type natriuretic peptide; PFTs, pulmonary function tests.

In contrast to the clear increase in mortality associated with a diagnosis of HF in patients with COPD, the implications of an additional diagnosis of COPD for patients with HF are less clear. In a cohort of nearly 5000 patients referred between 2000 and 2016 to a single outpatient clinic with suspected HF in the United Kingdom who underwent comprehensive evaluation by echocardiography, NPs, and spirometry, a diagnosis of COPD, defined as FEV_1/FVC less than 0.7, was only weakly, and not independently, associated with an increased risk of death among patients with HFrEF, and not at all in those with HFpEF.[44] Using anonymized electronic records from more than 50,000 patients with incident HF in primary care in the United Kingdom, Lawson and colleagues[52] found that COPD was only associated with an increased risk of death and/or hospitalizations in the most severe cases, with the risk increasing progressively with the use of triple inhaler therapy, the need for oral steroids, and the use of long-term home oxygen.

Recent data from the European Society of Cardiology Heart Failure Long-Term Registry, which enrolled more than 16,000 patients with HF across 211 centers in Europe over a period of 24 months, suggest that COPD increases the risk of cardiovascular mortality (but not all-cause mortality) and readmissions, particularly because of worsening HF, over the following 12 months.[39] Similar results were reported in an analysis of the Systolic Heart failure treatment with the I_f Inhibitor ivabradine Trial (SHIFT). The composite of cardiovascular deaths or HF hospitalizations occurred more often in patients with both HF and COPD, rather than HF alone, but no difference in mortality was observed.[41] Whether these associations are related to COPD itself (which might predispose to frequent respiratory infections or arrhythmias, leading to HF admissions) or other factors (such as a lower use of HF medications in patients with concurrent COPD and HFrEF) is not clear.[53–55]

THERAPEUTIC CONCERNS

β-Blockers improve the long-term prognosis of patients with HF caused by left ventricular systolic dysfunction.[3,56] However, concerns about the potential for β-blockers to cause bronchoconstriction and block the effect of sympathomimetic bronchodilators dissuades many from giving these agents in adequate doses, if at all, to patients with concomitant HF and COPD (see **Table 3**). However, the available clinical evidence suggests that these fears are unfounded. Small randomized trials show that any decline in FEV_1 associated with β-blockers does not translate into worsening symptoms or quality of life in patients with HF and COPD.[57,58] The use of a cardioselective β-blocker, such as bisoprolol or nebivolol, might be preferred, at least theoretically, when there is concern about tolerability.[59,60]

Perhaps surprisingly, there is accumulating evidence from observational studies and subanalyses from randomized trials conducted in patients with COPD suggesting that a higher heart rate is associated with an increase in mortality and that β-blockers might reduce exacerbations of COPD and prolong survival.[61–63] Some of this apparent benefit might reflect inadvertent, "accidental" treatment of undiagnosed HF. A multicenter, prospective, randomized, double-blind, placebo-controlled trial is currently ongoing to test whether metoprolol reduces time to first exacerbation of COPD and of cardiovascular events in patients with moderate to severe COPD (ClinicalTrials.gov Identifier: NCT02587351).[64]

There is no evidence that treatment of COPD substantially improves long-term survival. β-Agonists can improve lung function tests in patients with COPD, but might worsen cardiovascular and HF outcomes, especially for patients with HFrEF who are not protected by β-blockers.[65–67] Inhaled steroids may increase the risk of pneumonia.[68] Oral steroids may increase sodium and water retention.[69] Certainly, a large proportion of patients with COPD can tolerate de-escalation of respiratory therapies, particularly those at low risk of exacerbations. Attempts to identify patients in whom treatments for COPD can be discontinued should be encouraged.[70,71]

SUMMARY

Neither COPD nor HF has a robust definition, creating uncertainty about the true prevalence of either condition. Missed diagnoses are common, especially when one or other condition provides a seemingly adequate explanation for a patient's symptoms. However, there is no doubt that these two conditions commonly coexist.

For patients with COPD no specific treatment improves survival, but they encounter high rates of cardiovascular events and often die of the consequences. Greater focus on cardiovascular rather than respiratory disease in patients with COPD might improve outcomes. However, there is no doubt that appropriate treatment reduces the morbidity and mortality of patients with HFrEF, with or without coexisting COPD.

REFERENCES

1. Peña VS, Miravitlles M, Gabriel R, et al. Geographic variations in prevalence and underdiagnosis of COPD: results of the IBERPOC multicentre epidemiological study. Chest 2000;118:981–9.

2. van Riet EE, Hoes AW, Limburg A, et al. Prevalence of unrecognized heart failure in older persons with shortness of breath on exertion. Eur J Heart Fail 2014;16:772–7.

3. Ponikowski P, Voors AA, Anker SD, et al. 2016 ESC Guidelines for the diagnosis and treatment of acute and chronic heart failure: the task force for the diagnosis and treatment of acute and chronic heart failure of the European Society of Cardiology (ESC). Developed with the special contribution of the Heart Failure Association (HFA) of the ESC. Eur J Heart Fail 2016;18:891–975.

4. Calzetta L, Rogliani P, Matera MG, et al. A systematic review with meta-analysis of dual bronchodilation with LAMA/LABA for the treatment of stable COPD. Chest 2016;149:1181–96.

5. Holleman DR Jr, Simel DL. Does the clinical examination predict airflow limitation? JAMA 1995;273: 313–9.

6. Pellicori P, Shah P, Cuthbert J, et al. Prevalence, pattern and clinical relevance of ultrasound indices of congestion in outpatients with heart failure. Eur J Heart Fail 2019. https://doi.org/10.1002/ejhf.1383.

7. Sze S, Pellicori P, Kamzi S, et al. Effect of beta-adrenergic blockade on weight changes in patients with chronic heart failure. Int J Cardiol 2018;264: 104–12.

8. Sze S, Pellicori P, Kazmi S, et al. Prevalence and prognostic significance of malnutrition using 3 scoring systems among outpatients with heart failure: a comparison with body mass index. JACC Heart Fail 2018;6:476–86.

9. Clark AL, Coats AJ. Unreliability of cardiothoracic ratio as a marker of left ventricular impairment: comparison with radionuclide ventriculography and echocardiography. Postgrad Med J 2000;76(895): 289–91.

10. Davie AP, Francis CM, Love MP, et al. Value of the electrocardiogram in identifying heart failure due to left ventricular systolic dysfunction. BMJ 1996;312: 222.

11. Larssen MS, Steine K, Hilde JM, et al. Mechanisms of ECG signs in chronic obstructive pulmonary disease. Open Heart 2017;4:e000552.

12. Vogelmeier CF, Criner GJ, Martinez FJ, et al. Global strategy for the diagnosis, management, and prevention of chronic obstructive lung disease 2017 report. GOLD Executive Summary. Am J Respir Crit Care Med 2017;195:557–82.

13. Woodruff PG, Barr RG, Bleecker E, et al, SPIROMICS Research Group. Clinical significance of symptoms in smokers with preserved pulmonary function. N Engl J Med 2016;374:1811–21.

14. Aaron SD, Tan WC, Bourbeau J, et al, Canadian Respiratory Research Network. Diagnostic instability and reversals of chronic obstructive pulmonary disease diagnosis in individuals with mild to moderate airflow obstruction. Am J Respir Crit Care Med 2017;196:306–14.

15. Perez-Padilla R, Wehrmeister FC, Montes de Oca M, et al, PLATINO group. Instability in the COPD diagnosis upon repeat testing vary with the definition of COPD. PLoS One 2015;10:e0121832.

16. Regan EA, Lynch DA, Curran-Everett D, et al, Genetic Epidemiology of COPD (COPDGene) Investigators. Clinical and radiologic disease in smokers with normal spirometry. JAMA Intern Med 2015; 175:1539–49.

17. Zhang J, Pellicori P, Pan D, et al. Dynamic risk stratification using serial measurements of plasma concentrations of natriuretic peptides in patients with heart failure. Int J Cardiol 2018;269:196–200.

18. Cleland JG, Pellicori P. Defining diastolic heart failure and identifying effective therapies. JAMA 2013; 309:825–6.

19. Rutten FH, Cramer MJ, Zuithoff NP, et al. Comparison of B-type natriuretic peptide assays for identifying heart failure in stable elderly patients with a clinical diagnosis of chronic obstructive pulmonary disease. Eur J Heart Fail 2007;9:651–9.

20. Watz H, Waschki B, Boehme C, et al. Extrapulmonary effects of chronic obstructive pulmonary disease on physical activity: a cross-sectional study. Am J Respir Crit Care Med 2008;177: 743–51.

21. Gale CP, White JE, Hunter A, et al. Predicting mortality and hospital admission in patients with COPD: significance of NT pro-BNP, clinical and echocardiographic assessment. J Cardiovasc Med (Hagerstown) 2011;12:613–8.

22. Macchia A, Rodriguez Moncalvo JJ, Kleinert M, et al. Unrecognised ventricular dysfunction in COPD. Eur Respir J 2012;39:51–8.

23. Pavasini R, Tavazzi G, Biscaglia S, et al. Amino terminal pro brain natriuretic peptide predicts all-cause mortality in patients with chronic obstructive pulmonary disease: Systematic review and meta-analysis. Chron Respir Dis 2017;14:117–26.

24. Hawkins NM, Khosla A, Virani SA, et al. B-type natriuretic peptides in chronic obstructive pulmonary disease: a systematic review. BMC Pulm Med 2017;17:11.

25. Adamson PD, Anderson JA, Brook RD, et al. Cardiac troponin I and cardiovascular risk in patients with chronic obstructive pulmonary disease. J Am Coll Cardiol 2018;72:1126–37.

26. Freixa X, Portillo K, Paré C, et al, PAC-COPD Study Investigators. Echocardiographic abnormalities in

patients with COPD at their first hospital admission. Eur Respir J 2013;41:784–91.

27. Houben-Wilke S, Spruit MA, Uszko-Lencer NHMK, et al. Echocardiographic abnormalities and their impact on health status in patients with COPD referred for pulmonary rehabilitation. Respirology 2017;22:928–34.

28. Pellicori P, Cleland JG, Zhang J, et al. Cardiac dysfunction, congestion and loop diuretics: their relationship to prognosis in heart failure. Cardiovasc Drugs Ther 2016;30:599–609.

29. Divo M, Cote C, de Torres JP, et al, BODE Collaborative Group. Comorbidities and risk of mortality in patients with chronic obstructive pulmonary disease. Am J Respir Crit Care Med 2012;186:155–61.

30. Cazzola M, Bettoncelli G, Sessa E, et al. Prevalence of comorbidities in patients with chronic obstructive pulmonary disease. Respiration 2010;80:112–9.

31. Curkendall SM, DeLuise C, Jones JK, et al. Cardiovascular disease in patients with chronic obstructive pulmonary disease, Saskatchewan Canada cardiovascular disease in COPD patients. Ann Epidemiol 2006;16:63–70.

32. Holguin F, Folch E, Redd SC, et al. Comorbidity and mortality in COPD-related hospitalizations in the United States, 1979 to 2001. Chest 2005;128:2005–11.

33. McCullough PA, Hollander JE, Nowak RM, et al, BNP Multinational Study Investigators. Uncovering heart failure in patients with a history of pulmonary disease: rationale for the early use of B-type natriuretic peptide in the emergency department. Acad Emerg Med 2003;10:198–204.

34. Spece LJ, Epler EM, Donovan LM, et al. Role of co-morbidities in treatment and outcomes after chronic obstructive pulmonary disease exacerbations. Ann Am Thorac Soc 2018;15:1033–8.

35. Boudestein LC, Rutten FH, Cramer MJ, et al. The impact of concurrent heart failure on prognosis in patients with chronic obstructive pulmonary disease. Eur J Heart Fail 2009;11:1182–8.

36. Kaszuba E, Odeberg H, Råstam L, et al. Impact of heart failure and other comorbidities on mortality in patients with chronic obstructive pulmonary disease: a register-based, prospective cohort study. BMC Fam Pract 2018;19:178.

37. De Blois J, Simard S, Atar D, et al, Norwegian Heart Failure Registry. COPD predicts mortality in HF: the Norwegian Heart Failure Registry. J Card Fail 2010;16:225–9.

38. Mentz RJ, Schmidt PH, Kwasny MJ, et al. The impact of chronic obstructive pulmonary disease in patients hospitalized for worsening heart failure with reduced ejection fraction: an analysis of the EVEREST Trial. J Card Fail 2012;18:515–23.

39. Canepa M, Straburzynska-Migaj E, Drozdz J, et al, ESC-HFA Heart Failure Long-Term Registry Investigators. Characteristics, treatments and 1-year prognosis of hospitalized and ambulatory heart failure patients with chronic obstructive pulmonary disease in the European Society of Cardiology Heart Failure Long-Term Registry. Eur J Heart Fail 2018;20:100–10.

40. Canepa M, Temporelli PL, Rossi A, et al, GISSI-HF Investigators. Prevalence and prognostic impact of chronic obstructive pulmonary disease in patients with chronic heart failure: data from the GISSI-HF Trial. Cardiology 2017;136:128–37.

41. Tavazzi L, Swedberg K, Komajda M, et al, SHIFT Investigators. Clinical profiles and outcomes in patients with chronic heart failure and chronic obstructive pulmonary disease: an efficacy and safety analysis of SHIFT study. Int J Cardiol 2013;170:182–8.

42. Parissis JT, Andreoli C, Kadoglou N, et al. Differences in clinical characteristics, management and short-term outcome between acute heart failure patients chronic obstructive pulmonary disease and those without this co-morbidity. Clin Res Cardiol 2014;103:733–41.

43. Mentz RJ, Fiuzat M, Wojdyla DM, et al. Clinical characteristics and outcomes of hospitalized heart failure patients with systolic dysfunction and chronic obstructive pulmonary disease: findings from OPTIMIZE-HF. Eur J Heart Fail 2012;14:395–403.

44. Cuthbert JJ, Kearsley JW, Kazmi S, et al. The impact of heart failure and chronic obstructive pulmonary disease on mortality in patients presenting with breathlessness. Clin Res Cardiol 2019;108:185–93.

45. Jacob J, Tost J, Miró Ò, et al, ICA-SEMES Research Group. Impact of chronic obstructive pulmonary disease on clinical course after an episode of acute heart failure. EAHFE-COPD study. Int J Cardiol 2017;227:450–6.

46. Iversen KK, Kjaergaard J, Akkan D, et al, ECHOS Lung Function Study Group. The prognostic importance of lung function in patients admitted with heart failure. Eur J Heart Fail 2010;12:685–91.

47. Plesner LL, Dalsgaard M, Schou M, et al. The prognostic significance of lung function in stable heart failure outpatients. Clin Cardiol 2017;40:1145–51.

48. Yoshihisa A, Takiguchi M, Shimizu T, et al. Cardiovascular function and prognosis of patients with heart failure coexistent with chronic obstructive pulmonary disease. J Cardiol 2014;64:256–64.

49. Pellicori P, Salekin D, Pan D, et al. This patient is not breathing properly: is this COPD, heart failure, or neither? Expert Rev Cardiovasc Ther 2017;15:389–96.

50. Brenner S, Güder G, Berliner D, et al. Airway obstruction in systolic heart failure—COPD or congestion? Int J Cardiol 2013;168:1910–6.

51. Krahnke JS, Abraham WT, Adamson PB, et al, Champion Trial Study Group. Heart failure and

respiratory hospitalizations are reduced in patients with heart failure and chronic obstructive pulmonary disease with the use of an implantable pulmonary artery pressure monitoring device. J Card Fail 2015; 21:240–9.

52. Lawson CA, Mamas MA, Jones PW, et al. Association of medication intensity and stages of airflow limitation with the risk of hospitalization or death in patients with heart failure and chronic obstructive pulmonary disease. JAMA Netw Open 2018;1: e185489.

53. Kapoor JR, Kapoor R, Ju C, et al. Precipitating clinical factors, heart failure characterization,and outcomes in patients hospitalized with heart failure with reduced, borderline, and preserved ejection fraction. JACC Heart Fail 2016;4:464–72.

54. Platz E, Jhund PS, Claggett BL, et al. Prevalence and prognostic importance of precipitating factors leading to heart failure hospitalization: recurrent hospitalizations and mortality. Eur J Heart Fail 2018;20: 295–303.

55. Arrigo M, Gayat E, Parenica J, et al, GREAT Network. Precipitating factors and 90-day outcome of acute heart failure: a report from the intercontinental GREAT registry. Eur J Heart Fail 2017;19: 201–8.

56. Cleland JGF, Bunting KV, Flather MD, et al, Beta-blockers in Heart Failure Collaborative Group. Beta-blockers for heart failure with reduced, mid-range, and preserved ejection fraction: an individual patient-level analysis of double-blind randomized trials. Eur Heart J 2018;39:26–35.

57. Hawkins NM, MacDonald MR, Petrie MC, et al. Bisoprolol in patients with heart failure and moderate to severe chronic obstructive pulmonary disease: a randomized controlled trial. Eur J Heart Fail 2009; 11:684–90.

58. Jabbour A, Macdonald PS, Keogh AM, et al. Differences between beta-blockers in patients with chronic heart failure and chronic obstructive pulmonary disease: a randomized crossover trial. J Am Coll Cardiol 2010;55:1780–7.

59. Düngen HD, Apostolovic S, Inkrot S, et al, CIBIS-ELD investigators and Project Multicentre Trials in the Competence Network Heart Failure. Titration to target dose of bisoprolol vs. carvedilol in elderly patients with heart failure: the CIBIS-ELD trial. Eur J Heart Fail 2011;13:670–80.

60. Sessa M, Mascolo A, Mortensen RN, et al. Relationship between heart failure, concurrent chronic obstructive pulmonary disease and beta-blocker use: a Danish nationwide cohort study. Eur J Heart Fail 2018;20:548–56.

61. Du Q, Sun Y, Ding N, et al. Beta-blockers reduced the risk of mortality and exacerbation in patients with COPD: a meta-analysis of observational studies. PLoS One 2014;9:e113048.

62. Bhatt SP, Wells JM, Kinney GL, et al, COPDGene Investigators. β-Blockers are associated with a reduction in COPD exacerbations. Thorax 2016;71:8–14.

63. Byrd JB, Newby DE, Anderson JA, et al, SUMMIT Investigators. Blood pressure, heart rate, and mortality in chronic obstructive pulmonary disease: the SUMMIT trial. Eur Heart J 2018;39:3128–34.

64. Bhatt SP, Connett JE, Voelker H, et al. β-Blockers for the prevention of acute exacerbations of chronic obstructive pulmonary disease (βLOCK COPD): a randomised controlled study protocol. BMJ Open 2016;6:e012292.

65. Salpeter SR, Ormiston TM, Salpeter EE. Cardiovascular effects of beta-agonists in patients with asthma and COPD: a meta-analysis. Chest 2004;125: 2309–21.

66. Gershon A, Croxford R, Calzavara A, et al. Cardiovascular safety of inhaled long-acting bronchodilators in individuals with chronic obstructive pulmonary disease. JAMA Intern Med 2013;173: 1175–85.

67. Bermingham M, O'Callaghan E, Dawkins I, et al. Are beta2 agonists responsible for increased mortality in heart failure? Eur J Heart Fail 2011;13:885–91.

68. Oba Y, Keeney E, Ghatehorde N, et al. Dual combination therapy versus long-acting bronchodilators alone for chronic obstructive pulmonary disease (COPD): a systematic review and network meta-analysis. Cochrane Database Syst Rev 2018;(12): CD012620.

69. Ericson-Nielsen W, Kaye AD. Steroids: pharmacology, complications, and practice delivery issues. Ochsner J 2014;14:203–7.

70. Magnussen H, Disse B, Rodriguez-Roisin R, et al, WISDOM Investigators. Withdrawal of inhaled glucocorticoids and exacerbations of COPD. N Engl J Med 2014;371:1285–94.

71. Chapman KR, Hurst JR, Frent SM, et al. Long-term triple therapy de-escalation to indacaterol/glycopyrronium in patients with chronic obstructive pulmonary disease (SUNSET): a randomized, double-blind, triple-dummy clinical trial. Am J Respir Crit Care Med 2018;198:329–39.

Sleep Breathing Disorders in Heart Failure

Amanda C. Coniglio, MD[a], Robert J. Mentz, MD[a,b],*

KEYWORDS

- Heart failure • Sleep-disordered breathing • Central sleep apnea • Obstructive sleep apnea
- Adaptive servoventilation • Phrenic nerve stimulation

KEY POINTS

- SDB is common in HF patients and often underdiagnosed because of a lack of consistent and/or distinguishing symptoms.
- CPAP treatment may improve sleep quality and daytime sleepiness in patients with obstructive sleep apnea and cardiovascular disease.
- ASV is currently not recommended for the treatment of SDB (with predominant central sleep apnea) in HFrEF patients; active research is under way to evaluate its safety and efficacy.
- SDB can be reduced in some HF patients with optimized medical therapy and with cardiac resynchronization therapy when appropriate.

EPIDEMIOLOGY AND DEFINITIONS

Sleep-disordered breathing (SDB) has become an increasingly recognized cause of morbidity and mortality in adults, and is largely underdiagnosed and undertreated. SDB is thought to affect approximately 10% of the adult population, although in patients with heart failure (HF) the prevalence may be as high as 50% to 75%.[1,2]

SDB is characterized by interruptions in breathing during sleep resulting in chemical, autonomic, mechanical, and inflammatory effects on the cardiovascular system. The severity of SDB is determined by the apnea-hypopnea index (AHI), the number of episodes per hour of sleep during which there is a reduction in airflow of at least greater than 50% for greater than 10 seconds (apnea) that is accompanied by an oxygen desaturation of greater than 3% to 4%.[3] Within SDB, there are several subtypes of sleep disturbances including obstructive sleep apnea (OSA), central sleep apnea (CSA) and Cheyne-Stokes respiration (CSR). OSA occurs when there is obstruction of the upper airway causing cessation of airflow during continued inspiratory effort, and is more prevalent in HF patients than in the general population.[4] The most common cause of OSA is obesity; other risks include upper airway edema, enlarged tonsils, variants in craniofacial structures, and upper airway muscle dysfunction.[5,6] Contrary to OSA, CSA occurs when the partial pressure of carbon dioxide falls below the apneic threshold, a level of carbon dioxide below which the nervous system fails to trigger breathing.[7,8] CSR is a distinct subset of CSA during which there are fluctuations in ventilation resulting in a crescendo-decrescendo pattern of breathing (**Fig. 1**).[9] This particular pattern is thought to be due to instability in the central respiratory control mechanism and is common in HF patients, particularly those with more advanced disease, occurring in 45% to 55% of patients.[10] It has even been reported to

This article originally appeared in *Heart Failure Clinics*, Volume 16, Issue 1, January 2020.

Disclosure: Dr R.J. Mentz has received research support from ResMed. Dr A.C. Coniglio has no relevant disclosures.

[a] Department of Medicine, Duke University School of Medicine, Durham, NC, USA; [b] Duke Clinical Research Institute, PO Box 17969, Durham, NC 27715, USA

* Corresponding author. Duke Clinical Research Institute, PO Box 17969, Durham, NC 27715.

E-mail address: robert.mentz@duke.edu

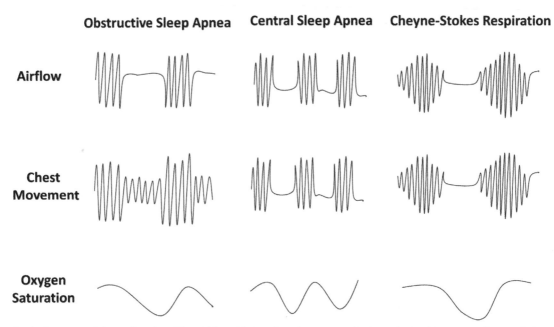

Fig. 1. Patterns of sleep-disordered breathing. Obstructive sleep apnea is characterized by upper airway obstruction with cessation of air movement despite continued chest wall movement, resulting in hypoxia and hypercapnia. Central sleep apnea differs in that there is an absence of centrally triggered breathing, resulting in cessation of chest wall movement and oxygen movement. Cheyne-Stokes respiration is a unique subtype of central sleep apnea marked by oscillations in speed and depth of breathing with periods of apnea.

occur in severe HF patients while awake or with exercise.[11] Pulmonary edema in HF may cause CSR by stimulating the pulmonary juxtacapillary receptors, leading to increased peripheral and central chemoreceptor responsiveness.[12,13]

OSA is associated with increased risk of hypertension, stroke, HF, atrial fibrillation, and coronary heart disease.[14] A prospective observational cohort study of patients with HF with reduced ejection fraction (HFrEF) admitted for HF exacerbations showed that 61% of patients had OSA and 21% had CSA.[15] When OSA or CSA is present in HF patients and untreated, mortality risk is doubled and thought to be due in large part to an increase in malignant ventricular arrhythmias.[16,17] In ischemic cardiomyopathy, untreated SDB portends an even worse outcome, with a threefold increase in mortality.[18]

PATHOPHYSIOLOGY

SDB causes a series of physiologic changes that negatively affect the cardiovascular system. In OSA, occlusion of airflow in the upper airway during active inspiration leads to a significant reduction in intrathoracic pressure. The changes in pressure result in increased venous blood return to the right heart and increased atrial and ventricular wall stress, while reducing blood

flow to the left side of the heart. There is increased right-sided afterload caused by hypoxia-mediated pulmonary vasoconstriction, and increased left-sided afterload resulting from the increased arterial wall stress with decreased intrathoracic pressure. With the increased afterload and decreased stroke volume, there is a decrease in arterial blood pressure generated.[19] Relative hypotension triggers baroreceptors to increase sympathetic tone, leading to vasoconstriction.[20] Meanwhile, the decrease in partial pressure of oxygen resulting from airway collapse and the subsequent increase in carbon dioxide levels further activates the sympathetic nervous system via peripheral and central chemoreceptors.[21] Over time, the chronic elevation in sympathetic tone promotes renal sodium retention and systemic congestion (**Fig. 2**).[22] Left untreated, the negative physiologic consequences of SDB promote left ventricular hypertrophy and increases oxidative stress, inflammation, endothelial dysfunction, and arrhythmias. However, with appropriate treatment of OSA, these negative consequences may be mitigated.[23,24]

Within the HF population overall, it is thought that patients have a higher ventilatory response and chemosensitivity to increased levels of carbon dioxide.[25] Furthermore, decreased cardiac output in HF patients creates a delay in the detection

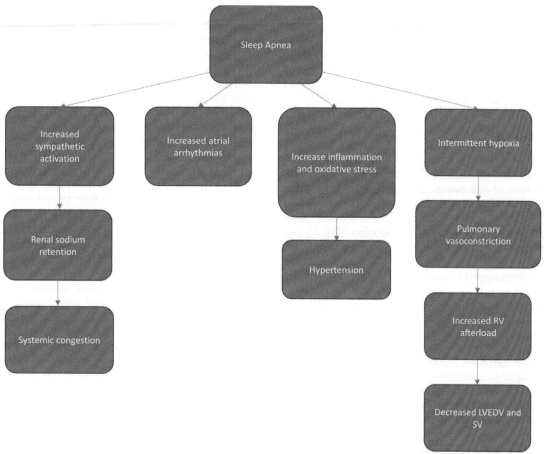

Fig. 2. Pathophysiologic consequences of sleep-disordered breathing. Sleep-disordered breathing leads to numerous maladaptive physiologic effects such as increased sympathetic activation, increased atrial arrhythmias, worsening daytime hypertension, and negative cardiac remodeling including left ventricular hypertrophy and decreased left ventricular ejection fraction.

of changes in oxygen and carbon dioxide levels, which exacerbates apnea/hyperventilation cycles.[26] CSA is thought to occur more commonly in HF patients if they are male, older than 60 years, have atrial fibrillation, or have hypocapnia while awake.[27] Given the strong link between HF and SDB, there has been much debate as to whether fluctuating apnea and hyperventilation is protective by preventing respiratory muscle fatigue and actually improving oxygen delivery during episodes of respiratory acidosis.[12,28]

DIAGNOSIS

The diagnosis of SDB is made when there are at least 5 AHI events per hour of sleep. The number of events per hour defines the severity of SDB, whereby 5 to 15 events per hour is mild, 15 to 30 events per hour is moderate, and greater than 30 events per hour is severe. Patients are defined as

having OSA or CSA if greater than 50% of their events are obstructive or central, respectively. The gold-standard test for SDB is nocturnal polysomnography (NPSG). This test occurs in a hospital or clinic setting and measures oral and nasal airflow, oxygen and carbon dioxide partial pressures, electrocardiograms, pulse oximetry, and abdominal and chest wall movements. Although this test is thought to be the most accurate, polysomnography is an acceptable alternative in patients with high pretest probability of SDB and can be carried out in a patient's home or in the hospital. Simple polysomnography has a sensitivity and specificity of 90% to 100% compared with NPSG.[29]

Although reports of daytime sleepiness, frequent nighttime wakening, and accounts of possible apnea certainly trigger concern for SDB, many HF patients do not report these symptoms despite the presence of SDB.[30] Therefore, the

American College of Cardiology/American Heart Association 2017 Focused Update recommends that all patients with New York Heart Association class II to IV HF should be formally screened for sleep apnea.[31] Studies are currently ongoing to determine whether pacemakers/defibrillators can be used as a screening tool to detect SDB.[32]

TREATMENT

All HF patients diagnosed with SDB should be on optimized HF medical therapy to help reduce their burden of AHI events. In appropriate candidates, cardiac resynchronization therapy (CRT) should also be recommended because there has been some benefit observed in reducing SDB.[33] Patients should avoid respiratory depressants such as narcotics, alcohol, and anxiolytics, and should be encouraged to exercise.

Continuous Positive Airway Pressure Therapy

Continuous positive airway pressure (CPAP) therapy has been a long-standing treatment for SDB. CPAP provides continued positive pressure via nasal or face mask to keep the airway patent during sleep and prevent obstruction. It is well established that CPAP reduces the number of AHI events and decreases daytime somnolence and blood pressure.[34]

In HF patients with OSA, CPAP decreased AHI events (from 30 events/h to 4 events/h), decreased systolic blood pressure, decreased heart rate, and increased left ventricular ejection fraction (LVEF) from 25% to 34% ($P<.001$).[35] The improvement in LVEF with CPAP treatment has been replicated in several additional studies.[36,37] A prospective cohort study has also demonstrated improved 20-year survival in HF patients treated with CPAP in comparison with those not treated ($P = .009$).[38]

The SAVE (Sleep Apnea Cardiovascular Endpoints) study is the largest randomized trial to date that evaluated CPAP in patients with moderate to severe OSA. In patients with pre-existing coronary artery disease or cerebrovascular disease, it found no significant decrease in cardiovascular events including stroke, heart attack, and death in patients who used CPAP.[39] However, the treatment group only used CPAP on average of 3.3 hours per night, indicating poor overall adherence to therapy. The study did show a lower risk of stroke with good CPAP adherence as well as improved snoring, daytime sleepiness, and quality of life.[40] Despite these results, several other studies have shown significant benefit in CPAP for other cardiovascular outcomes, particularly in patients with HF.[16,23,24]

In HF patients with CSA, research has shown benefit with CPAP therapy. The CANPAP (Canadian continuous positive airway pressure of central sleep apnea and heart failure) trial studied 258 patients with CSA and an average LVEF of 25% on optimal, contemporary medical HF therapy. Patients were randomized to receive CPAP therapy and were followed over a 2-year period. The treatment group had greater nocturnal oxygen saturation ($P<.001$), reduction in AHI events ($P<.001$), and increase in LVEF ($P = .016$) but showed no difference in transplant-free survival.[41] However, review of the data showed that 43% of the treatment group still had more than 15 AHI events per hour 3 months into the trial, suggesting poor compliance with CPAP therapy often attributed to discomfort with the mask, sensations of claustrophobia, and inability to sleep with the sound of the machine. When this was taken into account, secondary analysis of the data showed that CPAP was indeed associated with increased transplant-free survival ($P = .041$).[42] Investigators from the CANPAP trial have also reported an association of CPAP use in HFrEF patients with decrease in mitral regurgitation, improved quality of life, and reduced risk of death in subsequent trials.[43–45]

Adaptive Servoventilation Therapy

More recently, research has focused on the use of adaptive servoventilation (ASV) for the treatment of SDB. ASV administers continuous pressure to maintain upper airway patency similar to CPAP therapy; however, it is more advanced in its ability to sense apnea and hypopnea episodes and maintain either target tidal volumes or air flow via adjustments in pressure. The complexities of ASV therapies were developed as a means of better treating SDB, particularly CSA. The SERVE-HF (treatment of sleep-disordered breathing with predominant CSA by ASV in patients with heart failure) trial randomized 1325 HFrEF patients on contemporary, guideline-directed HF therapy with greater than 15 AHI events per hour to receive minute-ventilation-triggered ASV therapy for the treatment of CSA.[46] Treatment with ASV was found to be harmful with increased all-cause mortality (hazard ratio [HR] 1.28 [95% confidence interval 1.06–1.55]) predominantly attributable to increased cardiovascular events (HR 1.34 [1.09–1.65]) based on intention-to-treat analysis.[46] The results of this study led to discontinuation of other ongoing trials at that time examining ASV and led to a recommendation against the use of ASV in HF patients.[31] Further analysis of the data from SERVE-HF showed that the minute-ventilation-triggered ASV devices failed to control OSA and CSA.[46] Prior work has demonstrated that HF patients with pulmonary capillary wedge pressures less than 12 mm Hg have a reduction in cardiac output when exposed to positive pressure ventilation.[47] Given this result, it is hypothesized that the high default settings for inspiratory and expiratory pressure in the devices used in the SERVE-HF trial may have failed to correct obstruction, leading to worse outcomes in the treatment arm. More recent studies reported that treatment with ASV for suppression of CSA leads to increased periodic limb movements in sleep, which may also account for some of the morbidity seen in ASV treatment.[48]

ADVENT-HF (effect of adaptive servoventilation on survival and hospital admissions in heart failure) is a worldwide, multicenter, randomized trial that is currently ongoing to examine the effects of ASV on outcomes in HF patients with both OSA and CSA.[49] This study is using peak flow to trigger pressure support instead of the minute ventilation used to trigger pressure support in SERVE-HF, as this is thought to be a more benign way to treat SDB without the risk of cardiac output reduction. Initial analysis of the first 177 patients enrolled showed that peak-flow–targeted ASV is better tolerated and associated with higher compliance compared with other positive airway pressure devices.[50] Further results from this study are expected in 2020.

Alternative Therapies

In addition to CPAP and ASV, there have been several new strategies to improve SDB.

Given difficulties with CPAP compliance, phrenic nerve stimulation has recently been identified as a potential treatment strategy. Insertion of a transvenous neurostimulator to activate the phrenic nerve and trigger diaphragmatic contraction has been associated with a significant decrease in AHI events and is thought to be more physiologic than positive pressure ventilation.[51] In a small study of 96 patients with HF and CSA, phrenic nerve stimulation decreased HF hospitalizations and increased quality of life.[52] Phrenic nerve stimulation was approved by the Food and Drug Administration in October 2017 for the treatment of SDB but, thus far, there are no recommendations for the use of phrenic nerve stimulation in HF patients.

In those intolerant to other therapies, oxygen therapy alone has been shown to reduce desaturations in HF patients with CSA as well as to reduce AHI events.[53] Unfortunately, oxygen therapy alone does not improve LVEF or reduce the risk of arrhythmias.[54] The addition of acetazolamide has also been postulated to improve oxygenation and reduce AHI events, but further studies are currently needed to further elucidate its potential benefits.[55]

SUMMARY

SDB is more common in HF patients than in the general population, and is associated with increased morbidity and mortality. Numerous treatments are available including CPAP, ASV, and other more invasive strategies to reduce the number of AHI events nightly. Patients with HF and OSA should be treated with CPAP therapy (class IIb recommendation). ASV use is not recommended until further studies are conducted to ensure its safety in specific HF populations (class III recommendation).

Clinicians should optimize HF regimens, use CRT when appropriate, and avoid respiratory depressants to reduce the burden of nightly AHI events. All HF patients should be screened for SDB with polysomnography because they are often asymptomatic and benefit from diagnosis and treatment (class IIa recommendation). Patients with SDB should be treated with CPAP or phrenic nerve stimulation to prevent the detrimental effects of SDB including hypertension, worsening HF, ischemic disease, and arrhythmias.

REFERENCES

1. Young T, Peppard PE, Gottlieb DJ. Epidemiology of obstructive sleep apnea: a population health perspective. Am J Respir Crit Care Med 2002; 165(9):1217–39.
2. Franklin KA, Lindberg E. Obstructive sleep apnea is a common disorder in the population-a review on the epidemiology of sleep apnea. J Thorac Dis 2015; 7(8):1311–22.
3. Haruki N, Floras JS. Sleep-disordered breathing in heart failure- a therapeutic dilemma. Circ J 2017; 81(7):903–12.
4. Oldenburg O, Lamp B, Faber L, et al. Sleep-disordered breathing in patients with symptomatic heart failure: a contemporary study of prevalence in and characteristics of 700 patients. Eur J Heart Fail 2007;9(3):251–7.
5. Dempsey JA, Veasey SC, Morgan BJ, et al. Pathophysiology of sleep apnea. Physiol Rev 2010;90(1): 47–112.
6. Jordan AS, McSharry DG, Malhotra A. Adult obstructive sleep apnoea. Lancet 2014;383(9918): 736–47.
7. Javaheri S, Dempsey JA. Central sleep apnea. Compr Physiol 2013;3(1):141–63.

8. Lyons OD, Bradley TD. Heart failure and sleep apnea. Can J Cardiol 2015;31(7):898–908.

9. Perger E, Inami T, Lyons OD, et al. Distinct patterns of hyperpnea during Cheyne-Stokes respiration: implication for cardiac function in patients with heart failure. J Clin Sleep Med 2017;13(11):1235–41.

10. Vazir A, Hastings PC, Dayer M, et al. A high prevalence of sleep disordered breathing in men with mild symptomatic chronic heart failure due to left ventricular systolic dysfunction. Eur J Heart Fail 2007;9(3):243–50.

11. Arzt M, Harth M, Luchner A, et al. Enhanced ventilatory response to exercise in patients with chronic heart failure and central sleep apnea. Circulation 2003;107(15):1998–2003.

12. Naughton MT. Cheyne-Stokes respiration: friend or foe? Thorax 2012;67(4):357–60.

13. Sands SA, Owens RL. Congestive heart failure and central sleep apnea. Crit Care Clin 2015;31(3):473–95.

14. Peppard PE, Young T, Barnet JH, et al. Increased prevalence of sleep-disordered breathing in adults. Am J Epidemiol 2013;177(9):1006–14.

15. Khayat R, Abraham W, Patt B, et al. Central sleep apnea is a predictor of cardiac readmission in hospitalized patients with systolic heart failure. J Card Fail 2012;18(7):534–40.

16. Wang H, Parker JD, Newton GE, et al. Influence of obstructive sleep apnea on mortality in patients with heart failure. J Am Coll Cardiol 2007;49(15):1625–31.

17. Bitter T, Westerheide N, Prinz C, et al. Cheyne-Stokes respiration and obstructive sleep apnoea are independent risk factors for malignant ventricular arrhythmias requiring appropriate cardioverter-defibrillator therapies in patients with congestive heart failure. Eur Heart J 2011;32(1):61–74.

18. Yumino D, Wang H, Floras JS, et al. Relationship between sleep apnoea and mortality in patients with ischaemic heart failure. Heart 2009;95:819–24.

19. Yumino D, Kasai T, Kimmerly D, et al. Differing effects of obstructive and central sleep apneas on stroke volume in patients with heart failure. Am J Respir Crit Care Med 2013;187(4):433–8.

20. Bradley TD, Tkacova R, Hall MJ, et al. Augmented sympathetic neural response to simulated obstructive apnoea in human heart failure. Clin Sci (Lond) 2003;104(3):231–8.

21. Jouett NP, Watenpaugh DE, Dunlap ME, et al. Interactive effects of hypoxia, hypercapnia and lung volume on sympathetic nerve activity in humans. Exp Physiol 2015;100(9):1018–29.

22. Floras JS, Ponikowski P. The sympathetic/parasympathetic imbalance in heart failure with reduced ejection fraction. Eur Heart J 2015;36(30):1974–1982b.

23. Malone S, Liu PP, Holloway R, et al. Obstructive sleep apnoea in patients with dilated cardiomyopathy: effects of continuous positive airway pressure. Lancet 1991;338(8781):1480–4.

24. Kasai T, Narui K, Dohi T, et al. Prognosis of patients with heart failure and obstructive sleep apnea treated with continuous positive airway pressure. Chest 2008;133(3):690–6.

25. Javaheri S. A mechanism of central sleep apnea in patients with heart failure. N Engl J Med 1999;341(13):949–54.

26. Hall MJ, Xie A, Rutherford R, et al. Cycle length of periodic breathing in patients with and without heart failure. Am J Respir Crit Care Med 1996;154(2 Pt 1):376–81.

27. Sin DD, Fitzgerald F, Parker JD, et al. Risk factors for central and obstructive sleep apnea in 450 men and women with congestive heart failure. Am J Respir Crit Care Med 1999;160(4):1101–6.

28. Naghshin J, Rodriguez RH, Davis EM, et al. Chronic intermittent hypoxia exposure improves left ventricular contractility in transgenic mice with heart failure. J Appl Physiol (1985) 2012;113(5):791–8.

29. Pinna GD, Robbi E, Pizza F, et al. Can cardiorespiratory polygraphy replace portable polysomnography in the assessment of sleep-disordered breathing in heart failure patients? Sleep Breath 2014;18(3):475–82.

30. Vazir A, Sundaram V. Management of sleep apnea in heart failure. Heart Fail Clin 2018;14(4):635–42.

31. Yancy CW, Jessup M, Bozkurt B, et al. 2017 ACC/AHA/HFSA Focused Update of the 2013 ACCF/AHA Guideline for the Management of Heart Failure: A Report of the American College of Cardiology/American Heart Association Task Force on Clinical Practice Guidelines and the Heart Failure Society of America. J Card Fail 2017;23(8):628–51.

32. Gwag HB, Park Y, Lee SS, et al. Rationale, design, and endpoints of the 'DEvice-Detected CArdiac Tachyarrhythmic Events and Sleep-disordered Breathing (DEDiCATES)' study: Prospective multicenter observational study of device-detected tachyarrhythmia and sleep-disordered breathing. Int J Cardiol 2019;280:69–73.

33. Oldenburg O, Faber L, Vogt J, et al. Influence of cardiac resynchronisation therapy on different types of sleep disordered breathing. Eur J Heart Fail 2007;9(8):820–6.

34. Engleman HM, Martin SE, Deary IJ, et al. Effect of continuous positive airway pressure treatment on daytime function in sleep apnoea/hypopnoea syndrome. Lancet 1994;343(8897):572–5.

35. Kaneko Y, Floras JS, Usui K, et al. Cardiovascular effects of continuous positive airway pressure in patients with heart failure and obstructive sleep apnea. N Engl J Med 2003;348(13):1233–41.

36. Mansfield DR, Gollogly NC, Kaye DM, et al. Controlled trial of continuous positive airway pressure in obstructive sleep apnea and heart failure. Am J Respir Crit Care Med 2004;169(3):361–6.

37. Egea CJ, Aizpuru F, Pinto JA, et al. Cardiac function after CPAP therapy in patients with chronic heart failure and sleep apnea: a multicenter study. Sleep Med 2008;9(6):660–6.

38. Javaheri S, Caref EB, Chen E, et al. Sleep apnea testing and outcomes in a large cohort of Medicare beneficiaries with newly diagnosed heart failure. Am J Respir Crit Care Med 2011;183(4):539–46.

39. McEvoy RD, Antic NA, Heeley E, et al. CPAP for prevention of cardiovascular events in obstructive sleep apnea. N Engl J Med 2016;375(10):919–31.

40. Qiu ZH, Luo YM, McEvoy RD. The Sleep Apnea Cardiovascular Endpoints (SAVE) study: implications for health services and sleep research in China and elsewhere. J Thorac Dis 2017;9(8):2217–20.

41. Bradley TD, Logan AG, Kimoff RJ, et al. Continuous positive airway pressure for central sleep apnea and heart failure. N Engl J Med 2005;353(19):2025–33.

42. Arzt M, Floras JS, Logan AG, et al. Suppression of central sleep apnea by continuous positive airway pressure and transplant-free survival in heart failure: a post hoc analysis of the Canadian Continuous Positive Airway Pressure for Patients with Central Sleep Apnea and Heart Failure Trial (CANPAP). Circulation 2007;115(25):3173–80.

43. Tkacova R, Liu PP, Naughton MT, et al. Effect of continuous positive airway pressure on mitral regurgitant fraction and atrial natriuretic peptide in patients with heart failure. J Am Coll Cardiol 1997; 30(3):739–45.

44. Naughton MT, Benard DC, Liu PP, et al. Effects of nasal CPAP on sympathetic activity in patients with heart failure and central sleep apnea. Am J Respir Crit Care Med 1995;152(2):473–9.

45. Naughton MT, Liu PP, Bernard DC, et al. Treatment of congestive heart failure and Cheyne-Stokes respiration during sleep by continuous positive airway pressure. Am J Respir Crit Care Med 1995;151(1):92–7.

46. Cowie MR, Woehrle H, Wegscheider K, et al. Adaptive servo-ventilation for central sleep apnea in systolic heart failure. N Engl J Med 2015;373(12): 1095–105.

47. Bradley TD, Holloway RM, McLaughlin PR, et al. Cardiac output response to continuous positive airway pressure in congestive heart failure. Am Rev Respir Dis 1992;145(2 Pt 1):377–82.

48. Xie J, Covassin N, Chahal AA, et al. Effect of adaptive servo-ventilation on periodic limb movements in sleep in patients with heart failure. Am J Cardiol 2019;123(4):632–7.

49. Lyons OD, Floras JS, Logan AG, et al. Design of the effect of adaptive servo-ventilation on survival and cardiovascular hospital admissions in patients with heart failure and sleep apnoea: the ADVENT-HF trial. Eur J Heart Fail 2017;19(4):579–87.

50. Perger E, Lyons OD, Inami T, et al. Predictors of one year compliance with adaptive servo-ventilation in patients with heart failure and sleep- disordered breathing: preliminary data from the ADVENT-HF trial. Eur Respir J 2019;53(2) [pii:1801626].

51. Jagielski D, Ponikowski P, Augostini R, et al. Transvenous stimulation of the phrenic nerve for the treatment of central sleep apnoea: 12 months' experience with the remede((R)) System. Eur J Heart Fail 2016;18(11):1386–93.

52. Costanzo MR, Ponikowski P, Coats A, et al. Phrenic nerve stimulation to treat patients with central sleep apnoea and heart failure. Eur J Heart Fail 2018; 20(12):1746–54.

53. Nakao YM, Ueshima K, Yasuno S, et al. Effects of nocturnal oxygen therapy in patients with chronic heart failure and central sleep apnea: CHF-HOT study. Heart Vessels 2016;31(2):165–72.

54. Bordier P, Lataste A, Hofmann P, et al. Nocturnal oxygen therapy in patients with chronic heart failure and sleep apnea: a systematic review. Sleep Med 2016;17:149–57.

55. Javaheri S, Sands SA, Edwards BA. Acetazolamide attenuates Hunter-Cheyne-Stokes breathing but augments the hypercapnic ventilatory response in patients with heart failure. Ann Am Thorac Soc 2014;11(1):80–6.

When Pulmonary Hypertension Complicates Heart Failure

Alberto-Maria Marra, MD[a], Nicola Benjamin, MSc[b,c],
Antonio Cittadini, MD[d,e], Eduardo Bossone, MD, PhD[f],
Ekkehard Grünig, MD, PhD[b,c],*

KEYWORDS

- Pulmonary hypertension • Right ventricle • Chronic heart failure
- Heart failure with preserved ejection fraction

KEY POINTS

- Pulmonary hypertension often complicates chronic left-sided heart failure.
- The loss of left atrial function is the first step toward an increase in pulmonary vascular resistance.
- Right atrial dilatation is often the first sign of increased right heart afterload.
- Clinical trials with pulmonary arterial hypertension–targeted drugs led to conflicting results in pulmonary hypertension owing to chronic left-sided heart failure.

INTRODUCTION

Pulmonary hypertension (PH) is quite common in patients with chronic heart failure (CHF) and dramatically impacts their exercise capacity, quality of life, and prognosis.[1–3] The vast majority (almost 75%) of PH cases are caused by chronic left-sided CHF (PH-LHD).[2,4] According to the European guidelines,[5] CHF is divided into 3 phenotypes based on left ventricular ejection fraction (LVEF): (1) heart failure with reduced ejection fraction (HFrEF; LVEF <40%); (2) heart failure with preserved ejection fraction (HFpEF; LVEF ≥50%); and (3) heart failure with midrange ejection fraction (LVEF 41%–49%).[5] PH may occur in any kind of CHF phenotype, but most commonly affects patients with HFpEF, which in turn are older and typically display several cardiovascular and metabolic comorbidities.[6,7] Despite the frequency and impact of PH-LHD, apart from background therapy for CHF, today no targeted therapy is available for these patients.[8] Moreover, PH-LHD inexorably leads to right ventricular dysfunction, which has an additional detrimental effect on clinical status and outcomes.[1,7] A profound understanding of the mechanisms that may lead to the development of PH-LHD might be helpful to improve the management of these patients.[4]

This article originally appeared in *Heart Failure Clinics*, Volume 16, Issue 1, January 2020.
Disclosure Statement: Dr A.-M. Marra received an institutional grant from Italian Healthcare Ministry (Ricerca Finalizzata per Giovani Ricercatori. Progetto n. GR-2016-02364727). The other authors have nothing to disclose.
[a] IRCSS SDN, Via Gianturco 113, Naples I-80142, Italy; [b] Centre for Pulmonary Hypertension, Thoraxklinik at Heidelberg University Hospital, Röntgenstraße 1, Heidelberg D-69126, Germany; [c] Translational Lung Research Center Heidelberg (TLRC), Heidelberg, Germany; [d] Department of Translational Medical Sciences, Federico II University, Via Pansini 5, Naples I-80138, Italy; [e] Interdisciplinary Research Centre in Biomedical Materials (CRIB), Piazzale Tecchio 80, Naples I-80125, Italy; [f] Cardiology Division, A Cardarelli Hospital, Via Cardarelli 9, Naples I-80131, Italy
* Corresponding author. Centre for Pulmonary Hypertension, Thoraxklinik at Heidelberg University Hospital, Röntgenstraße 1, Heidelberg D-69126, Germany.
E-mail addresses: ekkehard_gruenig@t-online.de; ekkehard.gruenig@med.uni-heidelberg.de

Cardiol Clin 40 (2022) 191–198
https://doi.org/10.1016/j.ccl.2021.12.007

DEFINITION AND CLASSIFICATION OF PULMONARY HYPERTENSION IN CHRONIC LEFT-SIDED HEART FAILURE

According to current guidelines,[8] postcapillary PH is defined by the presence of a mean pulmonary arterial pressure (mPAP) $\geq$25 mm Hg and pulmonary arterial wedge pressure (PAWP) $\geq$15 mm Hg.[8] Postcapillary PH includes at greatest extent PH-LHD and some other rare forms of PH with unclear and/or multifactorial mechanisms (group 5). Within the last 10 years, growing evidence has suggested that healthy subjects showed mPAP values of 14 $\pm$ 5 mm Hg.[9] Several independent groups also reported that patients with an mPAP of 21 to 24 mm Hg are characterized by impaired exercise performance, right heart function at rest and during exercise, and impaired survival.[10–12] Consequently, during the 6th World Symposium of Pulmonary Hypertension, a lower cutoff (mPAP <20 mm Hg) and an elevated pulmonary vascular resistance (PVR) $\geq$3 wood units (WU) for diagnosis was proposed for all PH forms[13] and also included those associated with left-sided heart failure and PAWP of $\geq$15 mm Hg.[4]

PH owing to left-sided CHF is further divided into 2 phenotypes according to the diastolic pulmonary gradient (DPG), which specifically is the difference between diastolic pulmonary pressure and PAWP, and PVR, which is the ratio between the difference between mPAP and PAWP divided for the cardiac output (**Tables 1** and **2**). Isolated postcapillary PH (IpcPH) is present when DPG is less than 7 mm Hg and/or PVR $\leq$3 WU.[4,8] A combined postcapillary PH (CpcPH) is defined by a DPG $\geq$7 mm Hg and/or PVR >3 WU.[4,8]

The 2 phenotypes basically differentiate between backward transmission of increased left ventricular (LV) filling pressures and "reactive" PH with a precapillary component closer to pulmonary arterial hypertension (PAH).[4] Indeed, patients with CpcPH show reduced exercise capacity when compared with patients with IpcPH.[14] It has also been shown that the 2 conditions present with different genetic profiles.[15]

PATHOMECHANISMS AND THEIR CLINICAL MEANING IN PULMONARY HYPERTENSION-LEFT-SIDED CHRONIC HEART FAILURE

Left heart failure (LHF) is historically defined as a clinical syndrome caused by a structural and/or functional cardiac abnormality, resulting in a reduced cardiac output with elevated filling pressures at rest or during exercise or stress.[5]

The development of PH in CHF may be roughly divided into 6 stages, beginning with passive backward transmission of elevated LV filling pressures (first stage).[16] Left atrial (LA) dilation is often an early consequence of an increase in LV filling pressures. Functional mitral regurgitation has a further additive weight on the increase of LA pressure. The resulting increase in LA wall stress leads to chronic interstitial fibrosis, which results in impaired LA compliance, reduced LA contractility, and loss of the reservoir function of the LA.[17] In consequence, atrial fibrillation is a common finding in CHF.[18]

Regardless of the kind of LA remodeling (typically eccentric in HFrEF, increased stiffness in HFpEF) and magnitude of ejection fraction, LA dysfunction is associated with increased PVRs and right heart dysfunction.[18] In this regard, LA size has already been shown to be a strong and independent predictor of mortality in CHF.[19] Once the LA becomes no longer able to attenuate the burden of the increased LV-filling pressure (second stage), pulmonary circulation suffers from a long-lasting stress, characterized by damage of the alveolar-capillary barrier with increased leakage of fluids and cells into the alveolar lumen and interstitial edema.[20] On top of this process, inflammatory infiltrate and hypoxia-mediated vasoconstriction can aggravate PH in patients with CHF.[21]

All these stimuli are likely to drive structural remodeling of the pulmonary vessels, for example, by medial hypertrophy with intimal and adventitial fibrosis and luminal occlusion, especially in the presence of a precapillary component (third stage).[22–24] In contrast to PAH, histology of PH-LHD does not show plexiform lesions.[22,23]

Table 1
Hemodynamic definition of postcapillary pulmonary hypertension

	mPAP, mm Hg	PAWP, mm Hg	PVR		DPG, mm Hg
Postcapillary PH	$\geq$25	>15	Any		Any
IpcPH	$\geq$25	>15	$\leq$3 WU	*And/or*	<7
Combined postcapillary and precapillary PH	$\geq$25	>15	>3 WU	*And/or*	$\geq$7

Table 2
Typical features of pulmonary hypertension owing to left-sided heart disease

Past medical history	• Previous coronary heart disease • Previous cardiac surgery • Presence of multiple concomitant cardiovascular risk factors (diabetes, obesity, arterial hypertension, tobacco smoking, familial history of cardiovascular diseases)
Electrocardiogram	• Persistent atrial fibrillation • Left bundle branch block or left anterior hemiblock • Q waves • Atrial fibrillation
Echocardiography	• Markedly dilated left atrium • Severe LV hypertrophy • Severe diastolic dysfunction (E/E′ ratio >15) • Severe systolic dysfunction (ejection fraction <40%) • Severe aortic or mitral valve disease
Lung ultrasounds	• Kerley B lines • Pulmonary edema • Pleural effusion
Cardiopulmonary exercise test	• Exercise oscillatory ventilation • Normal up to mildly elevated minute ventilation/carbon dioxide production (VE/VCO$_2$) slope
Cardiac MRI	• LV strain pattern • LA/RA ratio >1

Pulmonary vascular remodeling has also been shown to be reversible in patients with PH-LHD, once LV is unloaded through implantation of LV assisted devices.[25,26]

Besides mPAP in CHF,[3] several other parameters of lung hemodynamics are independent predictors of poor outcome in CHF, such as PVR, PAWP, and pulmonary arterial compliance (PAC), which is the ratio between the stroke volume and the pulmonary pulse pressure.[15] The latter takes on great relevance because it is a surrogate index of the ventriculoarterial coupling, a compensatory mechanism whereby the right ventricle (RV) increases its contractility in order to contrast the higher pulmonary arterial load (fourth stage).[27] Interestingly, PAC is able to predict poorer outcomes at a greater extent than other parameters obtained by right heart catheterization (RHC).[14,28,29] The prognostic role of PAC is even maintained when PVR is not impaired,[28] suggesting that PAC is impaired early in the course of the disease. It may therefore enable an early identification of patients with impaired prognosis.[30]

The adaptation of right heart function crucially affects outcome in patients with PH-LHD and is even more important than the mere increase of pulmonary arterial pressures. Chronic pressure overload first leads to RV diastolic dysfunction, before RV systolic dysfunction appears.[31]

As a compensatory mechanism, the right atrium (RA) enhances its systolic function and its compliance in order to keep the flow through the pulmonary circulation (fifth stage).[31] Once the RA loses its compensatory function, the RV proceeds toward pathologic changes that include hypertrophy, chamber remodeling up to spherical shape, further increase in tricuspid regurgitation, and impairment of pump function.[32]

It has already been shown that exercise capacity and symptoms in CHF patients are determined by RV systolic function, regardless of LV performance[33,34] (sixth stage). Several large studies reported that RV pump dysfunction is associated with impaired survival rates regardless of the heart failure phenotype.[18,35,36]

RIGHT HEART CATHETERIZATION FOR DIFFERENTIAL DIAGNOSIS

Classification of patients is complicated by the common finding of an overlap phenotype in which characteristics of PH owing to left-sided heart failure and PAH are shared, also called "atypical PAH"[6] or "PAH with comorbidities."[37] In patients presenting an intermediate-risk profile, RHC might be indicated in order to assess the correct diagnosis, especially in those with risk factors for PAH (systemic sclerosis, portal hypertension, congenital heart disease, human immunodeficiency virus infection) or for chronic thromboembolic pulmonary hypertension (CTEPH) (previous lung embolism, hypercoagulability state).[4]

As mentioned above, the occurrence of a PAWP ≥15 mm Hg is mandatory to establish a diagnosis of PH owing to left-sided CHF, because the rise of PAWP mirrors LV end-diastolic pressure and generally is the consequence of elevated LV filling pressures.[8] Therefore, a correct PWAP assessment is of utmost importance in the context of PH diagnostic algorithm, and for this reason, attention should be paid regarding its measurement.[8]

According to guidelines, PAWP should be assessed at end-expiration at rest, with a proper "zero" point positioned at the midchest.[4] In case of atrial fibrillation, PAWP should be measured 130 to 160 milliseconds after the onset of the QRS complex. Typically, older patients with HFpEF may present artificially low values of PAWP because of dehydration.[2] For this reason, patients with borderline PAWP values (13–15 mm Hg) or patients with lower PAWP but echocardiographic signs of LV hypertrophy should undergo a provocative test to either confirm PAWP within normal range or eventually unmask increased LV filling pressures.[2] To date, 2 options can be suggested: either to perform an exercise RHC or perform a fluid challenge. Exercise RHC is a validated method that may also gather valid information about exercise capacity and functional status of the patients, especially when performed simultaneously with cardiopulmonary exercise test.[38] Patients with normal LV function very seldom exceed a PAWP ≥20 mm Hg during low-grade exercise (25 Watts). The main limitation of exercise RHC is that it requires specific equipment and should be performed in centers with high expertise. An alternative could be represented by fluid challenge test, which is easier to perform. However, it may lead to false interpretation because of its age dependency.[4]

PULMONARY ARTERIAL HYPERTENSION–TARGETED DRUGS IN PULMONARY HYPERTENSION OWING TO LEFT-SIDED HEART FAILURE

To date, no targeted therapy is available for patients who experienced right heart failure in the context of HFpEF or HFrEF. In the last decade, the relevance of PH and right heart failure in chronic LHF drove the conductance of several studies engaging PAH-targeted drugs in patients with HFpEF or HFrEF (**Table 3**).

A pilot monocentric study investigating the effect of sildenafil performed in Italy on patients with HFpEF led to encouraging preliminary results.[39] After 6 months of sildenafil (50 mg, 3 times a day), patients experienced a significant improvement in mPAP (−42.0% ± 13.0%) and RV function, as suggested by increased tricuspid annular plane systolic excursion (+69.0% ± 19.0%), RV ejection rate (+17.0% ± 8.3%), and reduced right atrial pressure (−54.0% ± 7.2%).[39] These results were not in line with those of Hoendermis and colleagues,[40] who tested the effects of 12 weeks of sildenafil on HFpEF patients on mPAP, without finding any difference between the active treatment group and placebo.

More recently, the "Sildenafil for improving outcomes after valvular correction" (SIOVAC) study reported worse clinical outcomes (death, hospital admission for heart failure, change in functional class, and patient global self-assessment) associated with sildenafil in patients affected by valvular heart diseases and increasedmPAPs who already received either surgical valve replacement or repair.[41] The largest study testing the effect of an endothelin receptor antagonist was the "Macitentan in subjects with combined prE- and post-capiLlary pulmOnary hypertension due to left ventricular Dysfunction" (MELODY-1) study.[42] The investigators of this trial reported negative results of macitentan treatment in patients with CHF, with almost 10% more fluid retention in the active treatment group. Several investigators speculated that these conflicting results are mainly due to the fact that increasing pulmonary blood flow may lead to increased LA filling, which might turn into lung edema in patients with particularly stiffened LA.[16]

A promising approach might be targeting guanylate cyclase with direct activation through riociguat, given the positive effects on right heart size and function associated with this drug in PAH and CTEPH.[43,44] Although the LEPHT study[45] reported no difference in mPAP in patients with HFrEF comparing patients who received riociguat to patients who received placebo, the secondary endpoints PVR ($P = .03$) and cardiac index (CI; $P = .0001$) showed a significant improvement. Moreover, a significant improvement in quality of life assessed with the Minnesota Living with Heart Failure questionnaire was registered.[45] More insights about the effects of riociguat in patients with PH owing to HFpEF will be gathered by the ongoing DYNAMIC study[46] (NCT02744339) or the PASSION-Study, which has started in 2019 (EudraCT n. 2017-003688-37).

Table 3
Randomized placebo-controlled clinical trials with pulmonary arterial hypertension–targeted drugs in pulmonary hypertension owing to left-sided heart failure

First Author, y (Study Acronym)	Drug	Sample Size (n)	Setting	Primary Endpoint	Main Results
Guazzi et al,[39] 2011 (no study acronym)	Sildenafil	44	HFpEF	Pulmonary hemodynamics, exercise capacity, and RV function	Improvement of pulmonary pressures and RV systolic function already after 6 mo
Bonderman et al,[45] 2013 (LEPHT)	Riociguat	201	HFrEF	Change in mPAP after 12 mo	No improvement of mPAP but improvement of secondary endpoints (PVR, CI)
Hoendermis et al,[40] 2015 (no study acronym)	Sildenafil	52	HFpEF	Change in mPAP after 12 mo	No effects on primary endpoints nor on secondary ones (PVR, CO, exercise capacity)
Vachiéry et al,[42] 2018 (MELODY-1)	Macitentan	48	LVEF ≥30% NYHA FC II-III 6MWD ≥150 m	Composite endpoint (death and HF hospitalization)	+10% fluid retention in patients treated with macitentan No effects on lung hemodynamics
Bermejo et al,[41] 2018 (SIOVAC)	Sildenafil	231	Patient with valvular heart disease after surgical correction	Composite clinical score combining death, hospital admission for HF, change in functional class, and patient global self-assessment	Worse clinical outcomes in patients treated with placebo

Abbreviations: 6MWD, 6-min walking distance; HF, heart failure; LEPHT, left ventricular systolic dysfunction associated with pulmonary hypertension riociguat trial.

CLINICAL MANAGEMENT OF RIGHT HEART FAILURE IN CHRONIC LEFT HEART FAILURE

The relevance of targeting pulmonary pressures in LHF has already been demonstrated by the CHAMPION trial that reported a significant improvement in terms of hospitalization because of acute decompensated LHF, when pulmonary pressures are used as a treatment target.[47,48]

Volume optimization is quite challenging in patients with right heart failure. Echocardiography is helpful for detecting signs of volume overload and venous congestion. An enlarged RA and an increased diameter of the vena cava inferior with low collapse are highly suggestive of volume overload.[49] Oral loop diuretics (in combination with thiazides and spironolactone) are therefore the basis of chronic LHF therapy. In severe acute right ventricular failure, intravenous diuretics are often able to provide volume optimization and symptom relief.[50]

In patients with HFrEF, the management of the functional mitral regurgitation, usually owing to the dilation of the LV, is an important treatment target. Functional mitral regurgitation is strongly associated with severe PH and dramatically impacts the patient's prognosis.[51] Transcatheter percutaneous mitral valve repair is sought to be a potential treatment for this condition, albeit conflicting results in 2 recently published large trials. The "Cardiovascular Outcomes Assessment of the MitraClip Percutaneous Therapy for Heart Failure Patients with Functional Mitral Regurgitation" (COAPT) resulted in a reduction of CHF-related hospitalization and all-cause mortality in patients treated with MitraClip on top of optimized medical therapy.[52] On the other hand, the "Percutaneous Repair with the Mitra Clip Device for Severe Functional/Secondary Mitral Regurgitation" (MITRA-FR) demonstrated no positive effects of this intervention.[53] Several investigators speculated that these conflicting results are mainly due to the fact that patients enrolled in the COAPT had higher New York Heart Association functional class (NYHA FC) than those of the MITRA-FR. The results of this trial led to the speculation that MitraClip may be beneficial in patients resistant to optimized pharmacologic as well as nonpharmacologic CHF therapy.[54]

For severe RV failure, vasopressors are needed in acute cases with severe hypotension. Noradrenaline (0.2–1.0 μg/kg*min) should be the first choice in patients with severe impairment of RV function, because it increases blood pressure and RV contractility.[55] Combination with levosimendan and phosphodiesterase III inhibitors with noradrenaline represents a reasonable second- and third-line strategy. Mechanical circulatory support[56,57] is needed for those patients who do not improve despite treatment with vasopressors and inotropes. Extracorporeal membrane oxygenation (ECMO) or life support rapidly supports RV systolic function.[58] Attention should be paid to typical complications of ECMO (infection or clot formation), which in turn may lead to death.[50]

Similarly to patients with PAH[59–63] also in HFpEF, exercise training is associated with exercise capacity improvement[64] and is currently recommended by CHF guidelines.[4]

SUMMARY AND FUTURE PERSPECTIVES

PH is a severe complication in patients affected by chronic left-sided heart failure. It dramatically impacts their exercise capacity, quality of life, and survival. PH in chronic left-sided heart failure is not merely caused by a backward transmission of pressures, but it is a complex process that involves atrial function, inflammation, and vasoconstriction. Once PVR increases and the impairment of PAC appears, the RA attempts to compensate the increased afterload. When this compensatory mechanism fails, RV dilatation and systolic dysfunction occur, leading to right heart failure and death. A correct assessment of PAWP is of utmost importance, and often the implementation of exercise RHC or fluid challenge might identify such cases with suspected "false-normal" PAWP (older people, diuretic therapy).

Multiple attempts were made in the last few years to test whether PAH-targeted drugs might be beneficial also for PH because of left-sided heart failure, leading to conflicting, and in some cases, negative results. Exercise training is likely to be a promising therapeutic strategy for patients affected by this condition.

REFERENCES

1. Guazzi M, Borlaug BA. Pulmonary hypertension due to left heart disease. Circulation 2012;126:975–90.
2. Rosenkranz S, Lang IM, Blindt R, et al. Pulmonary hypertension associated with left heart disease: updated recommendations of the Cologne Consensus Conference 2018. Int J Cardiol 2018;272:53–62.
3. Gerges C, Gerges M, Lang IM. Characterization of pulmonary hypertension in heart failure using the diastolic pressure gradient: the conundrum of high and low diastolic pulmonary gradient. JACC Heart Fail 2015;3:424–5.
4. Vachiéry J-L, Tedford RJ, Rosenkranz S, et al. Pulmonary hypertension due to left heart disease. Eur Respir J 2019;53:1801897.
5. Ponikowski P, Voors AA, Anker SD, et al. 2016 ESC guidelines for the diagnosis and treatment of acute and chronic heart failure. Eur Heart J 2016;37:2129–200.
6. Opitz CF, Hoeper MM, Gibbs JSR, et al. Pre-capillary, combined, and post-capillary pulmonary hypertension: a pathophysiological continuum. J Am Coll Cardiol 2016;68:368–78.
7. Gorter TM, van Veldhuisen DJ, Bauersachs J, et al. Right heart dysfunction and failure in heart failure with preserved ejection fraction: mechanisms and management. Position statement on behalf of the Heart Failure Association of the European Society of Cardiology. Eur J Heart Fail 2018;20:16–37.
8. Galiè N, Humbert M, Vachiery J-L, et al. 2015 ESC/ERS Guidelines for the diagnosis and treatment of pulmonary hypertension. Eur Heart J 2015;46:ehv317.
9. Kovacs G, Berghold A, Scheidl S, et al. Pulmonary arterial pressure during rest and exercise in healthy subjects: a systematic review. Eur Respir J 2009;34:888–94.
10. Coghlan JG, Wolf M, Distler O, et al. Incidence of pulmonary hypertension and determining factors in patients with systemic sclerosis. Eur Respir J 2018;51:1701197.
11. Nagel C, Marra AM, Benjamin N, et al. Reduced right ventricular output reserve in patients with systemic sclerosis and mildly elevated pulmonary artery pressures. Arthritis Rheumatol 2019;71(5):805–16.
12. Douschan P, Kovacs G, Avian A, et al. Mild elevation of pulmonary arterial pressure as a predictor of mortality. Am J Respir Crit Care Med 2018;197:509–16.
13. Simonneau G, Montani D, Celermajer DS, et al. Haemodynamic definitions and updated clinical classification of pulmonary hypertension. Eur Respir J 2019;53:1801913.

14. Dragu R, Rispler S, Habib M, et al. Pulmonary arterial capacitance in patients with heart failure and reactive pulmonary hypertension. Eur J Heart Fail 2015;17:74–80.

15. Miller WL, Grill DE, Borlaug BA. Clinical features, hemodynamics, and outcomes of pulmonary hypertension due to chronic heart failure with reduced ejection fraction: pulmonary hypertension and heart failure. JACC Heart Fail 2013;1:290–9.

16. Rosenkranz S, Gibbs JSR, Wachter R, et al. Left ventricular heart failure and pulmonary hypertension. Eur Heart J 2016;37:942–54.

17. Rossi A, Gheorghiade M, Triposkiadis F, et al. Left atrium in heart failure with preserved ejection fraction: structure, function, and significance. Circ Heart Fail 2014;7:1042–9.

18. Melenovsky V, Hwang S-J, Redfield MM, et al. Left atrial remodeling and function in advanced heart failure with preserved or reduced ejection fraction. Circ Heart Fail 2015;8:295–303.

19. Rossi A, Temporelli PL, Quintana M, et al, MeRGE Heart Failure Collaborators. Independent relationship of left atrial size and mortality in patients with heart failure: an individual patient meta-analysis of longitudinal data (MeRGE Heart Failure). Eur J Heart Fail 2009;11:929–36.

20. De Pasquale CG, Arnolda LF, Doyle IR, et al. Plasma surfactant protein-B: a novel biomarker in chronic heart failure. Circulation 2004;110:1091–6.

21. ten Freyhaus H, Dagnell M, Leuchs M, et al. Hypoxia enhances platelet-derived growth factor signaling in the pulmonary vasculature by down-regulation of protein tyrosine phosphatases. Am J Respir Crit Care Med 2011;183:1092–102.

22. Gerges C, Gerges M, Lang MB, et al. Diastolic pulmonary vascular pressure gradient. Chest 2013;143:758–66.

23. Chen Y, Guo H, Xu D, et al. Left ventricular failure produces profound lung remodeling and pulmonary hypertension in mice. Hypertension 2012;59:1170–8.

24. Guazzi M, Naeije R. Pulmonary hypertension in heart failure. J Am Coll Cardiol 2017;69:1718–34.

25. Lundgren J, Algotsson L, Kornhall B, et al. Preoperative pulmonary hypertension and its impact on survival after heart transplantation. Scand Cardiovasc J 2014;48:47–58.

26. Tedford RJ, Hassoun PM, Mathai SC, et al. Pulmonary capillary wedge pressure augments right ventricular pulsatile loading. Circulation 2012;125:289–97.

27. Vonk Noordegraaf A, Westerhof BE, Westerhof N. The relationship between the right ventricle and its load in pulmonary hypertension. J Am Coll Cardiol 2017;69:236–43.

28. Pellegrini P, Rossi A, Pasotti M, et al. Prognostic relevance of pulmonary arterial compliance in patients with chronic heart failure. Chest 2014;145:1064–70.

29. Al-Naamani N, Preston IR, Paulus JK, et al. Pulmonary arterial capacitance is an important predictor of mortality in heart failure with a preserved ejection fraction. JACC Heart Fail 2015;3:467–74.

30. Thenappan T, Prins KW, Pritzker MR, et al. The critical role of pulmonary arterial compliance in pulmonary hypertension. Ann Am Thorac Soc 2016;13:276–84.

31. Gaynor SL, Maniar HS, Bloch JB, et al. Right atrial and ventricular adaptation to chronic right ventricular pressure overload. Circulation 2005;112:I212–8.

32. Ferrara F, Gargani L, Ostenfeld E, et al. Imaging the right heart pulmonary circulation unit: Insights from advanced ultrasound techniques. Echocardiography 2017;34:1216–31.

33. Baker BJ, Wilen MM, Boyd CM, et al. Relation of right ventricular ejection fraction to exercise capacity in chronic left ventricular failure. Am J Cardiol 1984;54:596–9.

34. Salvo TG Di, Mathier M, Semigran MJ, et al. Preserved right ventricular ejection fraction predicts exercise capacity and survival in advanced heart failure. J Am Coll Cardiol 1995;25:1143–53.

35. Ghio S, Recusani F, Klersy C, et al. Prognostic usefulness of the tricuspid annular plane systolic excursion in patients with congestive heart failure secondary to idiopathic or ischemic dilated cardiomyopathy. Am J Cardiol 2000;85:837–42.

36. Ghio S, Guazzi M, Scardovi AB, et al, all investigators. Different correlates but similar prognostic implications for right ventricular dysfunction in heart failure patients with reduced or preserved ejection fraction. Eur J Heart Fail 2017;19:873–9.

37. Grünig E, Benjamin N, Krüger U, et al. General measures and supportive therapy for pulmonary arterial hypertension: updated recommendations from the Cologne Consensus Conference 2018. Int J Cardiol 2018;272:30–6.

38. Wolsk E, Bakkestrøm R, Thomsen JH, et al. The influence of age on hemodynamic parameters during rest and exercise in healthy individuals. JACC Heart Fail 2017;5:337–46.

39. Guazzi M, Vicenzi M, Arena R, et al. Pulmonary hypertension in heart failure with preserved ejection fraction. Circulation 2011;124:164–74.

40. Hoendermis ES, Liu LCY, Hummel YM, et al. Effects of sildenafil on invasive haemodynamics and exercise capacity in heart failure patients with preserved ejection fraction and pulmonary hypertension: a randomized controlled trial. Eur Heart J 2015;36:2565–73.

41. Bermejo J, Yotti R, García-Orta R, et al. Sildenafil for improving outcomes in patients with corrected valvular heart disease and persistent pulmonary hypertension: a multicenter, double-blind, randomized clinical trial. Eur Heart J 2018;39:1255–64.

42. Vachiéry J-L, Delcroix M, Al-Hiti H, et al. Macitentan in pulmonary hypertension due to left ventricular dysfunction. Eur Respir J 2018;51:1701886.

43. Marra AM, Halank M, Benjamin N, et al. Right ventricular size and function under riociguat in pulmonary arterial hypertension and chronic thromboembolic pulmonary hypertension (the RIVER study). Respir Res 2018;19:258.

44. Marra AM, Egenlauf B, Ehlken N, et al. Change of right heart size and function by long-term therapy with riociguat in patients with pulmonary arterial hypertension and chronic thromboembolic pulmonary hypertension. Int J Cardiol 2015;195:19–26.

45. Bonderman D, Ghio S, Felix SB, et al, Left Ventricular Systolic Dysfunction Associated With Pulmonary Hypertension Riociguat Trial (LEPHT) Study Group. Riociguat for patients with pulmonary hypertension caused by systolic left ventricular dysfunction: a phase IIb double-blind, randomized, placebo-controlled, dose-ranging hemodynamic study. Circulation 2013;128:502–11.

46. Mascherbauer J, Grünig E, Halank M, et al. Evaluation of the pharmacoDYNAMIC effects of riociguat in subjects with pulmonary hypertension and heart failure with preserved ejection fraction : Study protocol for a randomized controlled trial. Wien Klin Wochenschr 2016;128:882–9.

47. Fonarow GC, Adams KF, Abraham WT, et al, ADHERE Scientific Advisory Committee, Study Group, and Investigators. Risk stratification for in-hospital mortality in acutely decompensated heart failure classification and regression tree analysis. JAMA 2005;293:572.

48. Adamson PB, Abraham WT, Bourge RC, et al. Wireless pulmonary artery pressure monitoring guides management to reduce decompensation in heart failure with preserved ejection fraction. Circ Heart Fail 2014;7:935–44.

49. Grünig E, Biskupek J, D'Andrea A, et al. Reference ranges for and determinants of right ventricular area in healthy adults by two-dimensional echocardiography. Respiration 2015;89:284–93.

50. Harjola V-P, Mebazaa A, Čelutkienė J, et al. Contemporary management of acute right ventricular failure: a statement from the Heart Failure Association and the Working Group on Pulmonary Circulation and Right Ventricular Function of the European Society of Cardiology. Eur J Heart Fail 2016;18:226–41.

51. Bursi F, Barbieri A, Grigioni F, et al. Prognostic implications of functional mitral regurgitation according to the severity of the underlying chronic heart failure: a long-term outcome study. Eur J Heart Fail 2010;12:382–8.

52. Stone GW, Lindenfeld J, Abraham WT, et al, COAPT Investigators. Transcatheter mitral-valve repair in patients with heart failure. N Engl J Med 2018;379:2307–18.

53. Obadia J-F, Messika-Zeitoun D, Leurent G, et al. Percutaneous repair or medical treatment for secondary mitral regurgitation. N Engl J Med 2018;379:2297–306.

54. Nishimura RA, Bonow RO. Percutaneous repair of secondary mitral regurgitation–a tale of two trials. N Engl J Med 2018;379:2374–6.

55. Ponikowski P, Voors AA, Anker SD, et al, Authors/Task Force Members, Document Reviewers. 2016 ESC guidelines for the diagnosis and treatment of acute and chronic heart failure. Eur J Heart Fail 2016;18:891–975.

56. Olsson KM, Halank M, Egenlauf B, et al. Decompensated right heart failure, intensive care and perioperative management in patients with pulmonary hypertension. Dtsch Med Wochenschr 2016;141(S 01):S42–7.

57. Olsson KM, Halank M, Egenlauf B, et al. Decompensated right heart failure, intensive care and perioperative management in patients with pulmonary hypertension: updated recommendations from the Cologne Consensus Conference 2018. Int J Cardiol 2018;272:46–52.

58. Hoeper MM, Granton J. Intensive care unit management of patients with severe pulmonary hypertension and right heart failure. Am J Respir Crit Care Med 2011;184:1114–24.

59. Mereles D, Ehlken N, Kreuscher S, et al. Exercise and respiratory training improve exercise capacity and quality of life in patients with severe chronic pulmonary hypertension. Circulation 2006;114:1482–9.

60. Ferrara F, Gargani L, Armstrong WF, et al. The Right Heart International Network (RIGHT-NET): rationale, objectives, methodology, and clinical implications. Heart Fail Clin 2018;14:443–65.

61. Marra AMAM, Egenlauf B, Bossone E, et al. Principles of rehabilitation and reactivation: pulmonary hypertension. Respiration 2015;89:265–73.

62. Benjamin N, Marra AM, Eichstaedt C, et al. Exercise training and rehabilitation in pulmonary hypertension. Heart Fail Clin 2018;14(3):425–30.

63. Grünig E, Eichstaedt C, Barberà J-A, et al. ERS statement on exercise training and rehabilitation in patients with severe chronic pulmonary hypertension. Eur Respir J 2019;53:1800332.

64. Kitzman DW, Brubaker P, Morgan T, et al. Effect of caloric restriction or aerobic exercise training on peak oxygen consumption and quality of life in obese older patients with heart failure with preserved ejection fraction. JAMA 2016;315:36.

Cardiac Cachexia Revisited
The Role of Wasting in Heart Failure

Miroslava Valentova, MD, PhD[a,b], Stefan D. Anker, MD, PhD[c],
Stephan von Haehling, MD, PhD[a,b,*]

KEYWORDS

• Heart failure • Cachexia • Sarcopenia • Wasting • Body composition • Congestion

KEY POINTS

- Cachexia is a systemic metabolic disorder defined as involuntary nonedematous weight loss of 6% or more of total body weight within the previous 6 to 12 months.
- The prevalence of cardiac cachexia ranges between 10% to 39%.
- Cachexia is an independent predictor of mortality in heart failure.
- Cachexia is strongly related to congestive right ventricular dysfunction, activation of the renin–angiotensin–aldosterone system and sympathetic nervous system, and elevation of proinflammatory cytokines.

INTRODUCTION

Development and prognosis of chronic heart failure (HF) are related to nutritional status. Obesity has been regarded as a traditional risk factor for developing HF, mainly in the presence of the metabolic syndrome.[1,2] However, the unfavorable effect of obesity disappears once HF is established, as first demonstrated in 2001 by Horwich and colleagues[3] in patients with preexisting HF. Actually, patients with overweight or obesity before the onset of HF have been shown to have better survival once HF develops compared with patients with normal weight.[4] This reverse epidemiology has been termed the obesity paradox and has been meanwhile confirmed in large meta-analyses in patients with HF with reduced ejection fraction (HFrEF) and patients with HF with preserved ejection fraction (HFpEF).[5,6] It may even be prudent to speak of an obesity paradigm rather than of a paradox, because the relationship is extremely consistent across several analyses and chronic diseases.[7]

In 1997, before the introduction of the obesity paradox, cardiac cachexia had been identified as the first marker of nutritional status predicting outcomes in patients with HF.[8] Anker and colleagues[8] found that involuntary weight loss in outpatients with HFrEF was associated with a 3-fold higher risk of all-cause mortality compared with patients with stable weight or weight gain. In the last 2 decades, several hypotheses explaining the development of cardiac cachexia have been suggested and shifted the understanding of cachexia away from a simple nutritional problem to a complex metabolic disorder. Indeed, nutritional supplementation alone cannot cure cachexia. Based on evidence by Anker and colleagues, guidelines of

This article originally appeared in *Heart Failure Clinics*, Volume 16, Issue 1, January 2020.
Disclosure Statement: The authors have nothing to disclose.
[a] Department of Cardiology and Pneumology, University Medical Center Göttingen, Robert-Koch-Street 40, 37075 Göttingen, Germany; [b] DZHK (German Centre for Cardiovascular Research), Partner Site Göttingen, Robert-Koch-Street 40, 37075 Göttingen, Germany; [c] Division of Cardiology and Metabolism, Department of Cardiology (CVK), Berlin-Brandenburg Center for Regenerative Therapies (BCRT), German Centre for Cardiovascular Research (DZHK) Partner Site Berlin, Charité Universitätsmedizin Berlin, Augustenburger Platz 1, 13353 Berlin, Germany
* Corresponding author. Department of Cardiology and Pneumology, University Medical Center Göttingen, Robert-Koch-Street 40, 37075 Göttingen, Germany.
E-mail address: stephan.von.haehling@med.uni-goettingen.de

Cardiol Clin 40 (2022) 199–207
https://doi.org/10.1016/j.ccl.2021.12.008

the European Society of Cardiology (ESC) have started to mention cardiac cachexia in 2001 and recognized cachexia as comorbidity of HF later on in 2012.[9,10] Moreover, since 2016 the ESC does no longer recommend weight reduction in obese and overweight patients with preexisting HF.[11] Although both body mass index (BMI) and cachexia are nutritional–metabolic markers, it is important to understand the difference between them: cachexia is defined by weight loss rather than absolute weight. This allows identifying patients at risk in every BMI category, even in obese patients, and it makes it a more sensitive prognostic tool compared with BMI alone.

PREVALENCE AND PROGNOSIS OF CARDIAC CACHEXIA

Cachexia (from the Greek *kakos* for *bad*, and *hexis* for *condition*) is a systemic metabolic disorder characterized by a nonintentional weight loss owing to wasting of all body compartments, that is, fat tissue, skeletal muscle, and bone tissue.

The prevalence of cachexia among patients with HF ranges between 10% and 39%, depending on the study design, diagnostic criteria of cachexia, and stage of HF (**Table 1**). Cachexia is more frequent in patients with advanced disease and HFrEF. The prevalence of cachexia in patients with HFpEF has not been sufficiently addressed in studies so far. Based on our clinical experience, patients with HFpEF are affected by cachexia in late stages of the disease too, although less frequently, which is likely explained by the activation of different biological pathways in HFrEF and HFpEF, as shown recently in a study analyzing biomarker profiles.[12]

The prognosis for patients with cardiac cachexia is dismal with mortality reaching 50% in 18 months.[8] Cachexia is associated with markers of more advanced disease such as reduced functional capacity and higher New York Heart Association functional class. However, the relation between cachexia and mortality is independent.[8]

CHANGES OF BODY COMPOSITION IN CARDIAC CACHEXIA

The human body consists of 3 major body compartments, that is, lean, fat, and bone tissue. A different density of each of these compartments allows a precise assessment of body composition. The most common technique used for measurement of body composition in studies assessing patients with cardiac cachexia is dual energy x-ray absorptiometry. Dual energy x-ray absorptiometry quantifies the fat-free mass (which contains mainly the skeletal muscle), fat mass, and bone mineral content.[13] However, it needs to be kept in mind that congestion and the presence of edema may lead to an overestimation of the fat-free mass. During the course of HF, wasting of individual body compartments seems to follow a specific pattern that is characterized by an earlier loss of skeletal muscle than fat tissue.[14,15] The loss of skeletal muscle starts already in early stages of HF, long before a significant weight loss and cachexia become apparent. A prospective study that investigated body composition in 2815 healthy participants using dual energy x-ray absorptiometry revealed that participants who developed HF during the follow-up period experienced a greater loss of muscle mass over time compared with those without HF, whereas fat mass remained relatively preserved.[14]

In cachexia, which is a marker of advanced HF, fat rather than muscle becomes the predominantly wasted tissue. This finding is supported by several clinical studies that compared the body composition of noncachectic and cachectic patients with HF and showed that lower total body mass in cachectic patients was attributed mainly to lower fat mass.[16–18] In contrast, lean mass seemed to be less affected or even preserved in cachectic compared with noncachectic patients.[16–18] However, particularly the loss of muscle mass leads to reduced exercise capacity and strength.[19] Beyond skeletal muscle, wasting in cachexia also regards the myocardium as shown in a clinical study that compared left ventricular mass of cachectic and noncachectic patients using MRI.[20] Loss of myocardium may be one of the mechanisms explaining the intrinsic relationship between cachexia and decreased survival.

Studies investigating loss of the third body compartment, that is, bone tissue, during cardiac cachexia are scarce and have yielded controversial findings so far.[16,21]

DEFINITION OF CARDIAC CACHEXIA

A number of chronic diseases other than HF can be complicated by the development of cachexia, the most important being cancer, chronic obstructive lung disease, chronic kidney disease, and rheumatoid arthritis.[22] Several definitions of cachexia have appeared in the past 2 decades, which complicates the comparison between studies. The key diagnostic component that is shared by all definitions is the presence of a nonintentional weight loss. Beyond the weight loss, some definitions have also implemented additional minor criteria to enhance specificity. Considering cachexia in HF, the first established cut-off point

Table 1
Overview of clinical studies reporting the prevalence of cardiac cachexia

Study	Definition of Cachexia	Study Cohort	Prevalence of Cachexia (%)
Anker et al,[8] 1997	Weight loss ≥7.5% over a period of ≥6 mo	171 outpatients with LV dysfunction	16
Nagaya et al,[67] 2001	Weight loss of >7.5% over a period of ≥6 mo	74 outpatients with an LVEF <40%	39
Anker et al,[23] 2003	Weight loss of ≥6% at any time during follow-up	1929 outpatients with an LVEF of ≤35%	36
Davos et al,[68] 2003	Weight loss of >7.5% over a period of ≥6 mo	589 patients hospitalized with HF, LV dysfunction	11
Castillo-Martínez et al,[46] 2005	Weight loss of ≥6.0% in 6 mo	73 outpatients with LV dysfunction	19
Habedank et al,[69] 2013	BMI of <21 kg/m² or weight loss >6% within 1 y	249 outpatients with an LVEF of <40%	10
Christensen et al,[34] 2013	Weight loss of >5% over ≥6 mo	328 nondiabetic outpatients with LVEF of <45%	11
Melenovsky et al,[17] 2013	Weight loss of >5% within 6 mo by simultaneous presence of abnormal biochemistry[a]	408 outpatients with an LVEF of <50%	19
Szabó et al,[70] 2014	BMI of <20 kg/m² or a weight loss of ≥5% within 1 year plus presence of abnormal biochemistry[a]	111 nondiabetic outpatients with an LVEF of ≤45%	16
Sandek et al,[53] 2014	Weight loss of ≥5% within the previous 6–12 mo	65 outpatients with an LVEF of ≤40%	19
Valentova et al,[16] 2016	Weight loss of ≥5% over a period of ≥6 mo plus minor criteria[b]	165 outpatients with an LVEF of ≤40%	18
Gaggin et al,[35] 2016	Weight loss of ≥5% or final BMI <20 kg/m² within 10 mo	108 outpatients with an LVEF of ≤40%	19
Santos et al,[71] 2018	Weight loss of ≥5% in the previous 12 mo or a BMI of <20 kg/m² plus minor criteria[b]	156 patients hospitalized owing to HF	37
Emami et al,[19] 2018	Weight loss of ≥6% over a period of ≥1 y	207 outpatients with HFrEF and HFpEF	19

Abbreviations: LV, left ventricular; LVEF, left ventricular ejection fraction.
[a] C-reactive protein greater than 5 mg/L or hemoglobin less than 120 g/L or albumin less than 32 g/L.
[b] According to the consensus definition.[24]

for weight loss was introduced by Anker and colleagues[8] in 1997 and was set arbitrarily at 7.5% or greater. In 2003, Anker and colleagues[23] refined the cut-off based on a study that compared the diagnostic accuracy of weight loss at several cut-off points (5%, 6%, 7.5%, 10%, and 15%) and showed that a weight loss of 6% or greater predicted survival with the highest accuracy. Based on this piece of evidence, the ESC defines cardiac cachexia as an involuntary nonedematous weight loss of 6% or more of total body weight within the previous 6 to 12 months.[11]

Beside this HF-specific definition, many clinicians and scientists use another broadly established definition, which applies to cachectic patients independently of the underlying disease. This definition was elaborated by a panel of experts from different fields of medicine during a meeting in Washington, DC, in 2006 and was published in 2008.[24] It recommends diagnosing cachexia in the presence of 5% or greater weight loss within the previous 12 months. The cut-off point of 5% or greater was based mainly on expert opinion and evidence coming from one prospective observational study in 900 nursing home residents, which showed a reduced survival in residents who lost 5% of body weight or more during the follow-up (owing to any disease) compared with residents who gained weight.[25] Although this cut-off point is more liberal compared with the ESC recommendation, the consensus definition is in fact stricter because it also requires the presence of at least 3 additional criteria beyond weight loss. These so-called minor criteria reflect decreased muscle mass and strength as well as nutritional and inflammatory abnormalities that typically accompany cachexia (**Box 1**).

According to the consensus definition, in cases where the weight history is not available, the presence of a BMI of less than 20 kg/m^2 can be used to establish the diagnosis.[24]

Box 1
Diagnostic criteria of cachexia according to the consensus definition

Major criterion

Involuntary nonedematous weight loss of $\geq$5% within the previous 12 months

PLUS

Minor criteria ($\geq$3 of 5):

1. Fatigue
2. Limited food intake (ie, total caloric intake of <20 kcal/kg body weight/d; <70% of usual food intake) or poor appetite
3. Decreased muscle strength (in the lowest tertile)
4. Depletion of skeletal muscle mass measured by:
   a. Appendicular skeletal muscle index by dual energy x-ray absorptiometry (<5.45 kg/m^2 in females and <7.25 kg/m^2 in males)
   b. Lumbar muscle cross-sectional area by computer tomography or MRI[72]
   c. Mid-upper arm muscle circumference (<10th percentile for age and gender or <20 cm in females and <24 cm in males)

Adapted from Evans WJ, Morley JE, Argilés J, et al. Cachexia: A new definition. Clin Nutr 2008;27(6):796; with permission.

Several pitfalls need to be taken into account when assessing weight history. First of all, the weight loss has to be unintentional, which means that weight reductions achieved by diet or exercise are excluded. Second, weight loss should be corrected for edema. This point is particularly important in patients with HF who often present with fluid retention. The presence of edema can hamper the diagnosis of cachexia in 2 ways. The elimination of edema by diuretic treatment can be misinterpreted as significant weight loss and patients can be falsely diagnosed with cachexia. In contrast, progressive edema can mask the loss of tissue and delay or even disable recognizing cachexia. To avoid this bias, many studies that investigated cardiac cachexia enrolled only patients who were edema free at baseline. Of course, this approach is not applicable in clinical practice. Instead, a continuous recording of both weight as well as the presence and severity of edema may help to assess the nonedematous weight loss in the clinical setting. Third, the time period in which the unintentional weight loss occurred should be assessed. Weight loss in patients with cardiac cachexia typically develops slowly within the preceding 6 to 12 months. In cases where the weight loss develops faster, other reasons such as cancer or elimination of edema should be considered.

DIFFERENTIAL DIAGNOSIS OF INVOLUNTARY WEIGHT LOSS

All patients with cachexia have involuntary weight loss; however, not all patients with involuntary weight loss have cachexia. Therefore, cachexia needs to be distinguished from other conditions such as malnutrition, anorexia, malabsorption, and hyperthyroidism.

Malnutrition and anorexia are caused solely by decreased food intake, implying that weight loss can be completely reversed by increasing calorie intake. Similarly, weight loss owing to malabsorption can be reversed by overcoming problems of a digestion and absorption of nutrients. In contrast, cachexia cannot be resolved by optimizing nutrition.[26]

Another important differential diagnosis of cachexia is sarcopenia. Sarcopenia is characterized by a mere muscle wasting that is accompanied by decreased strength and functional capacity.[27] The prevalence of sarcopenia varies between 20% and 50%.[28–30] It has been identified in patients with HFrEF as well as in patients with HFpEF.[28–30] Patients with dilated cardiomyopathy may be particularly prone to losing skeletal muscle, because a close interaction with myopathy may be present in these patients.[30] Sarcopenia is not associated with weight loss, so if weight loss becomes apparent, then the diagnosis of cachexia should be made instead. Indeed, transition from sarcopenia to cachexia may be common in HF.[19]

CHARACTERISTICS OF CARDIAC FUNCTION IN PATIENTS WITH CACHEXIA

Cachexia seems to be strongly related to congestive right ventricular dysfunction (RVD), whereas left-sided dimensions and LV systolic and diastolic function were found to be similar to noncachectic patients with advanced HF.[16,17,31] This finding is striking because the right ventricle has been treated as a bystander chamber for decades. Although it is not possible to differentiate whether RVD is a marker or mediator of cachexia, splanchnic congestion arising from RVD offers a mechanistically plausible explanation for many mechanisms involved in cachexia including excessive activation of immune response, malabsorption, and loss of appetite.[16] The importance of RVD in cachexia is also supported by the fact that cachexia can be found in patients with isolated RVD owing to atrial septal defect or primary pulmonary hypertension.[32,33]

PATHOPHYSIOLOGY OF CARDIAC CACHEXIA

Cachexia is a complication of HF that does not exist as a solitary disorder, in contrast to other comorbidities such as diabetes, anemia, or chronic kidney disease. Therefore, it seems to be logical that the catabolic–anabolic imbalance observed in cachexia arises from the activation of a complex network of metabolic, immune, and neurohormonal factors characteristic for HF. Most of these factors are activated early in the development of HF, but result in wasting first when HF had advanced into an inexorable state of congestive HF. The decompensated state of HF in cachectic patients is demonstrated by significantly increased levels of natriuretic peptides.[17,34,35] Several lines of evidence have considerably expanded our understanding of mechanisms that regulate cell metabolism in cachexia in the past 2 decades. However, some caution is needed when extrapolating study results to patients with HF, because many clinical and the majority of the experimental studies were conducted in cancer cachexia.[36] In contrast, the intracellular pathways seem to be very similar in cardiac and cancer cachexia. The extracellular factors are more disease specific.

INTRACELLULAR PATHWAYS OF MUSCLE AND FAT WASTING IN HEART FAILURE

The signaling pathway that seems to be most involved in muscle wasting is the protein degradation mediated by expression of the transcription factor nuclear factor-κB.[37] Nuclear factor-κB upregulates the transcription of members of the proteolytic ubiquitin–proteasome pathway that is responsible for protein degradation in the myofibrils (**Fig. 1**). Recently, the role of microRNAs in muscle wasting in HF yielded an increasing interest.[38] These noncoding RNAs regulate gene expression post-transcriptionally and have been shown to critically control wasting of skeletal muscle and myocardium.[38]

The most predominant process involved in wasting of adipose tissue seems to be an increased lipolysis.[39] Analysis of messenger RNA from adipose tissue of patients with cancer revealed a 2-fold higher expression of hormone-sensitive lipase compared with controls.[39] In contrast, expression of proteins involved in lipid synthesis was similar to healthy subjects.[39] The lipolysis is stimulated by several factors, among them catecholamines, cortisol, and natriuretic peptides (see **Fig. 1**).[18,40]

EXTRACELLULAR MECHANISMS OF CARDIAC CACHEXIA

Processes that are involved in the modulation of the intracellular pathways of cardiac cachexia include neurohormonal derangements, proinflammatory immune activation, anorexia, malabsorbtion, and anabolic hormone resistance.

The compensatory activation of the renin–angiotensin–aldosterone system and the sympathetic nervous system are the hallmark of HF along with their well-known deleterious effects that evolve in case of sustained activation.[41] Excessive sympathetic activity leads to cardiac remodeling and systolic dysfunction as well as to activation of the renin–angiotensin–aldosterone system (see **Fig. 1**).[42] Angiotensin II is a potent mediator of muscle loss via stimulation of several pathways, including the proteolytic pathway, expression of proinflammatory cytokines, inhibition of anabolic insulin growing factor I, and insulin responsiveness and inhibition of feeding centers in the hypothalamus resulting in decreased appetite.[43]

Other potential mediators of wasting are proinflammatory cytokines whose levels are increased in patients with cardiac cachexia compared with their noncachectic counterparts.[18] Similar to angiotensin II, cytokines stimulate proteolysis via

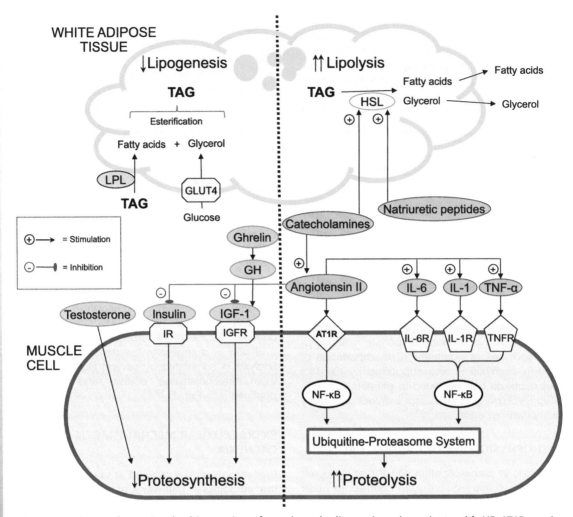

Fig. 1. Signaling pathways involved in wasting of muscle and adipose tissue in patients with HF. AT1R, angiotensin II type-1 receptor; GH, growth hormone; GLUT4, glucose transporter type 4; HSL, hormone sensitive lipase; IGF-1, insulin-like growth factor 1; IR, insulin receptor; LPL, lipoprotein lipase; NF-κB, nuclear factor κB; TAG, triglycerides; TNF-α, tumor necrosis factor -α.

ubiquitin–proteasome pathway and anorexigenic neurons in hypothalamus.[18,44,45]

Notably, the energy intake in patients with cardiac cachexia seems to be comparable with non-cachectic patients.[46] However, considering the energy deficit in cachexia, the feeding centers in hypothalamus seem to respond inadequately.[47] The underlying mechanism is probably an excessive anorexigenic stimulation through leptin and cytokines and a relative deficit of pro-orexigenic hormone ghrelin.[47,48]

Another potential mediator of decreased anabolic drive in cachexia is malabsorption of nutrients. Findings from several clinical studies suggest that cardiac cachexia is related to impaired absorption of carbohydrates and fat.[49–51] Whether malabsorption of proteins also plays a role remains unclear.[50,52] The malabsorption in HF is

well-explained by the intestinal congestion and hypoperfusion that are most pronounced in cachectic patients.[16,53] The absorptive capacity of the gut may be further impaired owing to alterations of the gut microbiome, because the gut microbiota fulfill important energy harvesting functions.[54,55] However, the role of gut microbiome in cardiac cachexia has still to be investigated.

TREATMENT OPTIONS

The treatment options for wasting in HF remain poorly defined. Optimal HF treatment is certainly one of the mainstays of therapy.[56,57] Exercise is generally advisable, because studies have shown reduced skeletal muscle degradation during periods of exercise such as bicycle training.[58] High-calorie nutritional supplements have been used to maintain or to increase body weight in patients with cardiac cachexia. Rozentryt and colleagues[59] used 600 kcal/d on top of patients' standard diet to increase body weight and to reduce inflammatory activity. Intravenous ferric carboxymaltose[60,61] and intramuscular testosterone[62–64] have been used to improve exercise capacity in patients with HF outside of cachexia, but their administration may help to improve exercise capacity in patients with wasting as well. Indeed, iron deficiency also yields to an insult of skeletal muscle.[65,66] In the absence of large-scale randomized trials, treatment recommendations need to take into account the specific problems of a given patient. Certainly, additional studies are required to help establish treatment of wasting in affected patients.

REFERENCES

1. Kenchaiah S, Evans JC, Levy D, et al. Obesity and the risk of heart failure. N Engl J Med 2002;347(5):305–13.
2. Voulgari C, Tentolouris N, Dilaveris P, et al. Increased heart failure risk in normal-weight people with metabolic syndrome compared with metabolically healthy obese individuals. J Am Coll Cardiol 2011; 58(13):1343–50.
3. Horwich TB, Fonarow GC, Hamilton MA, et al. The relationship between obesity and mortality in patients with heart failure. J Am Coll Cardiol 2001; 38(3):789–95.
4. Khalid U, Ather S, Bavishi C, et al. Pre-morbid body mass index and mortality after incident heart failure: the ARIC Study. J Am Coll Cardiol 2014;64(25): 2743–9.
5. Oreopoulos A, Padwal R, Kalantar-Zadeh K, et al. Body mass index and mortality in heart failure: a meta-analysis. Am Heart J 2008;156(1):13–22.
6. Zhang J, Begley A, Jackson R, et al. Body mass index and all-cause mortality in heart failure patients with normal and reduced ventricular ejection fraction: a dose–response meta-analysis. Clin Res Cardiol 2019;108(2):119–32.
7. Doehner W, von Haehling S, Anker SD. Protective overweight in cardiovascular disease: moving from "paradox" to "paradigm. Eur Heart J 2015;36(40): 2729–32.
8. Anker SD, Ponikowski P, Varney S, et al. Wasting as independent risk factor for mortality in chronic heart failure. Lancet 1997;349(9058):1050–3.
9. Remme WJ, Swedberg K. Guidelines for the diagnosis and treatment of chronic heart failure. Eur Heart J 2001;22(17):1527–60.
10. McMurray JJV, Adamopoulos S, Anker SD, et al. ESC Guidelines for the diagnosis and treatment of acute and chronic heart failure 2012. Eur Heart J 2012;33(14):1787–847.
11. Ponikowski P, Voors AA, Anker SD, et al. 2016 ESC Guidelines for the diagnosis and treatment of acute and chronic heart failure. Eur J Heart Fail 2016; 18(8):891–975.
12. Tromp J, Westenbrink BD, Ouwerkerk W, et al. Identifying pathophysiological mechanisms in heart failure with reduced versus preserved ejection fraction. J Am Coll Cardiol 2018;72(10):1081–90.
13. Buckinx F, Landi F, Cesari M, et al. Pitfalls in the measurement of muscle mass: a need for a reference standard. J Cachexia Sarcopenia Muscle 2018;9(2):269–78.
14. Forman DE, Santanasto AJ, Boudreau R, et al. Impact of incident heart failure on body composition over time in the health ABC study population. Circ Heart Fail 2017;10(9) [pii:e003915].
15. von Haehling S. The wasting continuum in heart failure: from sarcopenia to cachexia. Proc Nutr Soc 2015;74(4):367–77.
16. Valentova M, von Haehling S, Bauditz J, et al. Intestinal congestion and right ventricular dysfunction: a link with appetite loss, inflammation, and cachexia in chronic heart failure. Eur Heart J 2016;37(21):1684–91.
17. Melenovsky V, Kotrc M, Borlaug BA, et al. Relationships between right ventricular function, body composition, and prognosis in advanced heart failure. J Am Coll Cardiol 2013;62(18):1660–70.
18. Anker SD, Ponikowski PP, Clark AL, et al. Cytokines and neurohormones relating to body composition alterations in the wasting syndrome of chronic heart failure. Eur Heart J 1999;20(9):683–93.
19. Emami A, Saitoh M, Valentova M, et al. Comparison of sarcopenia and cachexia in men with chronic heart failure: results from the Studies Investigating Co-morbidities Aggravating Heart Failure (SICA-HF). Eur J Heart Fail 2018;20(11):1580–7.
20. Florea VG, Moon J, Pennell DJ, et al. Wasting of the left ventricle in patients with cardiac cachexia: a cardiovascular magnetic resonance study. Int J Cardiol 2004;97(1):15–20.
21. Anker SD, Clark AL, Teixeira MM, et al. Loss of bone mineral in patients with cachexia due to chronic heart failure. Am J Cardiol 1999;83(4):612–5.
22. von Haehling S, Anker MS, Anker SD. Prevalence and clinical impact of cachexia in chronic illness in Europe, USA, and Japan: facts and numbers update 2016. J Cachexia Sarcopenia Muscle 2016;7(5): 507–9.
23. Anker SD, Negassa A, Coats AJ, et al. Prognostic importance of weight loss in chronic heart failure and the effect of treatment with angiotensin-converting-enzyme inhibitors: an observational study. Lancet 2003;361(9363):1077–83.
24. Evans WJ, Morley JE, Argilés J, et al. Cachexia: a new definition. Clin Nutr 2008;27(6):793–9.
25. Sullivan DH, Johnson LE, Bopp MM, et al. Prognostic significance of monthly weight fluctuations

among older nursing home residents. J Gerontol A Biol Sci Med Sci 2004;59(6):M633–9.

26. Anker SD, Morley JE. Cachexia: a nutritional syndrome? J Cachexia Sarcopenia Muscle 2015;6(4): 269–71.

27. von Haehling S. Muscle wasting and sarcopenia in heart failure: a brief overview of the current literature. ESC Heart Fail 2018;5(6):1074–82.

28. Fülster S, Tacke M, Sandek A, et al. Muscle wasting in patients with chronic heart failure: results from the studies investigating co-morbidities aggravating heart failure (SICA-HF). Eur Heart J 2013;34(7): 512–9.

29. Bekfani T, Pellicori P, Morris DA, et al. Sarcopenia in patients with heart failure with preserved ejection fraction: impact on muscle strength, exercise capacity and quality of life. Int J Cardiol 2016;222: 41–6.

30. Hajahmadi M, Shemshadi S, Khalilipur E, et al. Muscle wasting in young patients with dilated cardiomyopathy. J Cachexia Sarcopenia Muscle 2017;8(4): 542–8.

31. Florea VG, Henein MY, Rauchhaus M, et al. The cardiac component of cardiac cachexia. Am Heart J 2002;144(1):45–50.

32. Giannakopoulos G, Roffi M, Frangos C, et al. Symptom improvement and cachexia reversal in an 84-year-old woman after percutaneous closure of atrial septal defect. J Am Geriatr Soc 2015; 63(2):416–8.

33. le Roux CW, Ghatei MA, Gibbs JSR, et al. The putative satiety hormone PYY is raised in cardiac cachexia associated with primary pulmonary hypertension. Heart 2005;91(2):241–2.

34. Christensen HM, Kistorp C, Schou M, et al. Prevalence of cachexia in chronic heart failure and characteristics of body composition and metabolic status. Endocrine 2013;43(3):626–34.

35. Gaggin HK, Belcher AM, Gandhi PU, et al. Serial echocardiographic characteristics, novel biomarkers and cachexia development in patients with stable chronic heart failure. J Cardiovasc Transl Res 2016;9(5–6):429–31.

36. Ishida J, Saitoh M, Doehner W, et al. Animal models of cachexia and sarcopenia in chronic illness: cardiac function, body composition changes and therapeutic results. Int J Cardiol 2017;238:12–8.

37. Argilés JM, Busquets S, Stemmler B, et al. Cancer cachexia: understanding the molecular basis. Nat Rev Cancer 2014;14(11):754–62.

38. Bei Y, Xiao J. MicroRNAs in muscle wasting and cachexia induced by heart failure. Nat Rev Cardiol 2017;14(9):566.

39. Thompson MP, Cooper ST, Parry BR, et al. Increased expression of the mRNA for hormone-sensitive lipase in adipose tissue of cancer patients. Biochim Biophys Acta 1993;1180(3):236–42.

40. Moro C, Galitzky J, Sengenes C, et al. Functional and pharmacological characterization of the natriuretic peptide-dependent lipolytic pathway in human fat cells. J Pharmacol Exp Ther 2004;308(3): 984–92.

41. Anker SD, Sharma R. The syndrome of cardiac cachexia. Int J Cardiol 2002;85(1):51–66.

42. Ferrara R, Mastrorilli F, Pasanisi G, et al. Neurohormonal modulation in chronic heart failure. Eur Heart J Suppl 2002;4(suppl_D):D3–11.

43. Yoshida T, Delafontaine P. Mechanisms of cachexia in chronic disease states. Am J Med Sci 2015; 350(4):250–6.

44. Jackman RW, Kandarian SC. The molecular basis of skeletal muscle atrophy. Am J Physiol Cell Physiol 2004;287(4):C834–43.

45. Braun TP, Marks DL. Pathophysiology and treatment of inflammatory anorexia in chronic disease. J Cachexia Sarcopenia Muscle 2010;1(2):135–45.

46. Castillo-Martínez L, Orea-Tejeda A, Rosales MT, et al. Anthropometric variables and physical activity as predictors of cardiac cachexia. Int J Cardiol 2005;99(2):239–45.

47. Suzuki H, Asakawa A, Amitani H, et al. Cancer cachexia—pathophysiology and management. J Gastroenterol 2013;48(5):574–94.

48. Barazzoni R, Gortan Cappellari G, Palus S, et al. Acylated ghrelin treatment normalizes skeletal muscle mitochondrial oxidative capacity and AKT phosphorylation in rat chronic heart failure. J Cachexia Sarcopenia Muscle 2017;8(6):991–8.

49. King D, Smith ML, Chapman TJ, et al. Fat malabsorption in elderly patients with cardiac cachexia. Age Ageing 1996;25(2):144–9.

50. Arutyunov GP, Kostyukevich OI, Serov RA, et al. Collagen accumulation and dysfunctional mucosal barrier of the small intestine in patients with chronic heart failure. Int J Cardiol 2008;125(2):240–5.

51. Sandek A, Bjarnason I, Volk H-D, et al. Studies on bacterial endotoxin and intestinal absorption function in patients with chronic heart failure. Int J Cardiol 2012;157(1):80–5.

52. King D, Smith ML, Lye M. Gastro-intestinal protein loss in elderly patients with cardiac cachexia. Age Ageing 1996;25(3):221–3.

53. Sandek A, Swidsinski A, Schroedl W, et al. Intestinal blood flow in patients with chronic heart failure: a link with bacterial growth, gastrointestinal symptoms, and cachexia. J Am Coll Cardiol 2014;64(11): 1092–102.

54. Turnbaugh PJ, Ley RE, Mahowald MA, et al. An obesity-associated gut microbiome with increased capacity for energy harvest. Nature 2006; 444(7122):1027–31.

55. Luedde M, Winkler T, Heinsen F-A, et al. Heart failure is associated with depletion of core intestinal microbiota. ESC Heart Fail 2017;4(3):282–90.

56. Clark AL, Coats AJS, Krum H, et al. Effect of beta-adrenergic blockade with carvedilol on cachexia in severe chronic heart failure: results from the CO-PERNICUS trial. J Cachexia Sarcopenia Muscle 2017;8(4):549–56.

57. Cohen-Solal A, Jacobson AF, Piña IL. Beta blocker dose and markers of sympathetic activation in heart failure patients: interrelationships and prognostic significance. ESC Heart Fail 2017;4(4):499–506.

58. Stephan G, Marcus S, Irina K, et al. Exercise training attenuates MuRF-1 expression in the skeletal muscle of patients with chronic heart failure independent of age. Circulation 2012;125(22):2716–27.

59. Rozentryt P, von Haehling S, Lainscak M, et al. The effects of a high-caloric protein-rich oral nutritional supplement in patients with chronic heart failure and cachexia on quality of life, body composition, and inflammation markers: a randomized, double-blind pilot study. J Cachexia Sarcopenia Muscle 2010;1(1):35–42.

60. Anker SD, Comin Colet J, Filippatos G, et al. Ferric carboxymaltose in patients with heart failure and iron deficiency. N Engl J Med 2009;361(25):2436–48.

61. Ponikowski P, van Veldhuisen DJ, Comin-Colet J, et al. Beneficial effects of long-term intravenous iron therapy with ferric carboxymaltose in patients with symptomatic heart failure and iron deficiency†. Eur Heart J 2015;36(11):657–68.

62. Caminiti G, Volterrani M, Iellamo F, et al. Effect of long-acting testosterone treatment on functional exercise capacity, skeletal muscle performance, insulin resistance, and baroreflex sensitivity in elderly patients with chronic heart failure a double-blind, placebo-controlled, randomized study. J Am Coll Cardiol 2009;54(10):919–27.

63. Iellamo F, Volterrani M, Caminiti G, et al. Testosterone therapy in women with chronic heart failure: a pilot double-blind, randomized, placebo-controlled study. J Am Coll Cardiol 2010;56(16):1310–6.

64. Stout M, Tew GA, Doll H, et al. Testosterone therapy during exercise rehabilitation in male patients with chronic heart failure who have low testosterone status: a double-blind randomized controlled feasibility study. Am Heart J 2012;164(6):893–901.

65. Dziegala M, Josiak K, Kasztura M, et al. Iron deficiency as energetic insult to skeletal muscle in chronic diseases. J Cachexia Sarcopenia Muscle 2018;9(5):802–15.

66. Tkaczyszyn M, Drozd M, Węgrzynowska-Teodorczyk K, et al. Depleted iron stores are associated with inspiratory muscle weakness independently of skeletal muscle mass in men with systolic chronic heart failure. J Cachexia Sarcopenia Muscle 2018;9(3):547–56.

67. Noritoshi N, Masaaki U, Masayasu K, et al. Elevated circulating level of ghrelin in cachexia associated with chronic heart failure. Circulation 2001;104(17):2034–8.

68. Davos CH, Doehner W, Rauchhaus M, et al. Body mass and survival in patients with chronic heart failure without cachexia: the importance of obesity. J Card Fail 2003;9(1):29–35.

69. Habedank D, Meyer FJ, Hetzer R, et al. Relation of respiratory muscle strength, cachexia and survival in severe chronic heart failure. J Cachexia Sarcopenia Muscle 2013;4(4):277–85.

70. Szabó T, Scherbakov N, Sandek A, et al. Plasma adiponectin in heart failure with and without cachexia: catabolic signal linking catabolism, symptomatic status, and prognosis. Nutr Metab Cardiovasc Dis 2014;24(1):50–6.

71. Santos NFD, Pinho CPS, Cardoso AJPF, et al. Cachexia in hospitalized patients with heart failure. Nutr Hosp 2018;35(3):669–76.

72. Beaudart C, McCloskey E, Bruyère O, et al. Sarcopenia in daily practice: assessment and management. BMC Geriatr 2016;16(1):170.

The Impact of Obesity in Heart Failure

Salvatore Carbone, PhD[a,b],*, Carl J. Lavie, MD[c], Andrew Elagizi, MD[c], Ross Arena, PhD[d,e], Hector O. Ventura, MD[f]

KEYWORDS

- Obesity • Heart failure • Obesity paradox • Body composition • Cardiorespiratory fitness

KEY POINTS

- Obesity is a strong risk factor for heart failure, particularly heart failure with preserved ejection fraction.
- The increased risk of heart failure resulting from obesity seems to be mediated by cardiorespiratory fitness. Recent evidence suggests that after adjustments for cardiorespiratory fitness obesity is no longer significantly associated with a greater risk for heart failure.
- Based on several epidemiologic studies, patients with overweight and class I-II obesity and established heart failure present a more favorable short- and mid-term prognosis compared to those who are normal weight and underweight, but only in those individuals with severely reduced cardiorespiratory fitness.
- Therapeutics such as aerobic with resistance exercise training, increased physical activity, sustained weight loss and improvements in quality of diet have the potential to improve cardiorespiratory fitness in patients with obesity and heart failure, particularly heart failure with preserved ejection fraction.

INTRODUCTION

Overweight and obesity have reached global epidemic proportions, adversely impacting health worldwide.[1] In fact, in 2016, the prevalence of obesity on the basis of body mass index (BMI) of 30 kg/m^2 or greater in the United States was 39.6% in adults, and even more disturbing is the prevalence of class III or severe obesity (BMI ≥40 kg/m^2), which has increased to 7.7%.[2]

Clearly, obesity has many adverse effects on population health and health care economics.[1]

In the United States, more than 6 million adults currently have heart failure (HF) and the prevalence is projected to increase nearly 50% between 2012 and 2030. This projected increase is related to aging of the population and the increased prevalence of the comorbidity phenotype (ie, ≥2 chronic conditions) that increases HF risk, that latter of which

This article originally appeared in *Heart Failure Clinics*, Volume 16, Issue 1, January 2020.

Funding Support: S. Carbone is supported by a Career Development Award 19CDA34660318 from the American Heart Association.

Disclosures: The authors have nothing to disclose.

[a] Department of Kinesiology & Health Sciences, College of Humanities & Sciences, Virginia Commonwealth University, 1020 W Grace St, 500 Academic Centre, Room 113c, Richmond, VA 23220, USA; [b] Department of Internal Medicine, Division of Cardiology, VCU Pauley Heart Center, Virginia Commonwealth University, 1200 E Broad St, Richmond, VA 23219, USA; [c] John Ochsner Heart and Vascular Institute, Ochsner Clinical School-The University of Queensland School of Medicine, 1514 Jefferson Highway, New Orleans, LA 70121-2483, USA; [d] Department of Physical Therapy, College of Applied Health Sciences, University of Illinois at Chicago, 1919 W Taylor Street, Chicago, IL 60612, USA; [e] TotalCardiology Research Network, Calgary, Alberta, Canada; [f] Cardiomyopathy and Heart Transplantation, Department of Cardiovascular Diseases, John Ochsner Heart and Vascular Institute, Ochsner Clinical School, University of Queensland School of Medicine, 1514 Jefferson Highway, New Orleans, LA 70121-2483, USA

* Corresponding author.

E-mail address: scarbone@vcu.edu

Cardiol Clin 40 (2022) 209–218

https://doi.org/10.1016/j.ccl.2021.12.009

includes the marked increase in obesity and its severity.[1,3,4] In recent decades, 2 distinct HF phenotypes have been described: HF with reduced left ventricular ejection fraction (LVEF; HF with reduced ejection fraction [HFrEF]) and HF with preserved LVEF (HFpEF), the latter being "heavily" influenced by obesity.[1,3,5,6]

> **Box 1**
> **Impact of obesity on hemodynamics and cardiac structure and function**
>
> *Hemodynamics*
>
> Increased blood volume
>
> Increased stroke volume
>
> Increased arterial pressure
>
> Increased LV wall stress
>
> Pulmonary artery hypertension
>
> *Cardiac structure*
>
> LV concentric remodeling
>
> LV hypertrophy
>
> Left atrial enlargement
>
> Right ventricular hypertrophy
>
> *Cardiac function*
>
> LV diastolic dysfunction
>
> LV systolic function
>
> Right ventricular failure
>
> *Neurohumoral*
>
> Insulin resistance and hyperinsulinemia
>
> Leptin insensitivity and hyperleptinemia
>
> Reduced adiponectin
>
> Sympathetic nervous system activation
>
> Renin–angiotensin–aldosterone system activation
>
> Peroxisome proliferator-activator receptor over expression
>
> *Inflammation*
>
> Increased C-reactive protein
>
> Overexpression of tumor necrosis factor
>
> *Cellular*
>
> Hypertrophy
>
> Apoptosis
>
> Fibrosis
>
> *Abbreviation:* LV, left ventricular.
> *From* Lavie CJ, Laddu D, Arena R, et al. Healthy weight and obesity prevention: JACC health promotion series. J Am Coll Cardiol. 2018;72(13):1509; with permission.

Obesity has numerous adverse effects on coronary heart disease risk factors, including increased blood pressure and the prevalence of hypertension, 2 strong risk factors for HF.[3,5,6] Additionally, obesity has many adverse effects on cardiac structure and function (**Box 1**), which clearly increases the prevalence of cardiac dysfunction and HF (**Fig. 1**), which are reviewed in detail elsewhere.[1,3,5–7]

The current review addresses (1) the impact of obesity, physical activity (PA)/physical inactivity and low cardiorespiratory fitness (CRF) on the risk of HF; and (2) the impact of these factors on prognosis once an HF diagnosis is confirmed, including in the "obesity paradox." The critical role of CRF on HF prognosis and the impact on the obesity paradox, the role of body composition in obesity and HF, including the importance of muscle mass, sarcopenia, sarcopenic obesity and cachexia, and the impact of exercise and dietary interventions in obesity and HF are also reviewed.

BODY MASS INDEX AND HEART FAILURE RISK

One of the largest studies to assess HF risk and obesity is from Kenchaiah and colleagues[4] from the Framingham Heart Study, demonstrating in a cohort of 5881 participants that HF increased by 7% in women and 5% in man for every 1 kg/m[2] increase in BMI. In a subgroup of the same study, Ho and colleagues[8] showed that BMI was a stronger predictor of HFpEF than HFrEF. Similarly, in an analysis using 3 large longitudinal cohort studies, Pandey and colleagues[9] demonstrated a graded association between high BMI and risk of HFpEF; compared with normal BMI subjects, overweight and obese class I (BMI 30.0–34.9 kg/m[2]) subjects had 38% and 56% higher risk, respectively (**Fig. 2**).

PHYSICAL INACTIVITY, LOW CARDIORESPIRATORY FITNESS, AND HEART FAILURE RISK

Physical inactivity and low CRF both increase the risk of HF.[3] Several studies show consistent dose-dependent associations between PA, CRF, and HF risk and suggest that this relationship is also stronger for HFpEF than HFrEF.[3,9–11] Also, improvements in PA and CRF over time are associated with lower risk of incident HF. In fact, a 1 metabolic equivalent (METs) improvement in CRF during follow-up lowered HF risk by 17%.[12]

OBESITY PARADOX AND HEART FAILURE

Despite the adverse effects that obesity has on cardiovascular structure and function and on

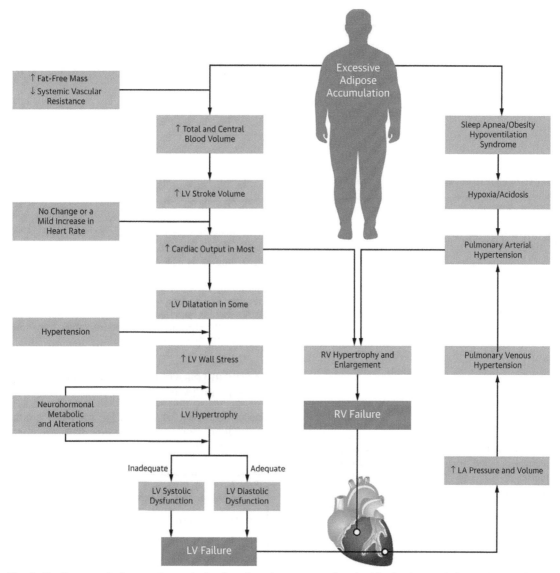

Fig. 1. Cardiac morphology and ventricular function changes associated with obesity. LA, left atrial; LV, left ventricular; RV, right ventricular. (*From* Lavie CJ, Laddu D, Arena R, et al. Healthy weight and obesity prevention: JACC health promotion series. J Am Coll Cardiol. 2018;72(13):1510; with permission.)

strong HF risk factors, such as hypertension and coronary heart disease, which all increase the risk of HF,[1,3,5,6] numerous studies in both HFpEF but, especially, HFrEF have demonstrated a strong obesity paradox, where patients with HF who are overweight or obese have a much better clinical prognosis than underweight (ie, BMI <18.5 kg/m²) as well as normal (ie, BMI 18.5–24.9 kg/m²) weight patients with HF.[1,3,5,6,13] Horwich and colleagues[14] first described this finding almost 20 years ago, and this association has now been confirmed in many studies and meta-analyses.[5,6,15] Sharma and colleagues[15] reported a meta-analysis of 6 studies in nearly 23,000 patients with HF that assessed

cardiovascular disease mortality, all-cause mortality, and rehospitalization during a 2.9-year mean follow-up (**Fig. 3**), and prognosis was worse with a low BMI, whereas the least risk was observed in overweight patients. Some studies have suggested that this paradox may be stronger in women, whereas others have suggested that it is gender independent.[16,17] Other studies have suggested that this may be explained by confounding factors.[18] One study of close to 1500 patients with HF even showed that BMI measured 6 or more months (average 4.3 years) before HF incidence still showed that pre-HF overweight and obese individuals had 28% and 30% lower mortality than did patients

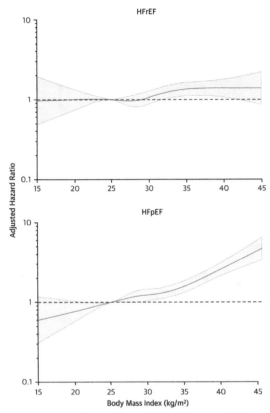

Fig. 2. BMI and HF risk. Association between BMI and risk of HFrEF (*top*) and HFpEF (*bottom*). (*From* Pandey A, LaMonte M, Klein L, et al. Relationship between physical activity, body mass index, and risk of heart failure. J Am Coll Cardiol. 2017;69(9):1138; with permission.)

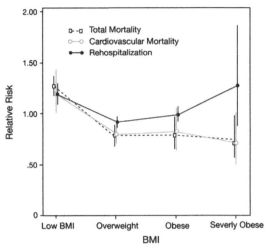

Fig. 3. Impact of BMI on cardiovascular mortality, all-cause mortality, and hospitalizations in HF. (*From* Sharma A, Lavie CJ, Borer JS, et al. Meta-analysis of the relation of body mass index to all-cause and cardiovascular mortality and hospitalization in patients with chronic heart failure. Am J Cardiol. 2015;115(10):1430; with permission.)

CARDIORESPIRATORY FITNESS AND THE OBESITY PARADOX

The assessment of CRF in HF provides crucial information for an accurate cardiovascular risk status stratification, even in the setting of

with HF with normal BMI, respectively, suggesting that being overweight or obese even before HF is associated with better survival after HF is diagnosed.[19]

Most of the studies assessing the obesity paradox have only used BMI,[3,5,6,15] but some studies using percent fat mass (FM)[20] and waist circumference[21,22] have also demonstrated an obesity paradox. Moreover, the evidence for the obesity paradox seems stronger in HFrEF than HFpEF, although many studies show an obesity paradox also in HFpEF.[23] One recent study shows an obesity paradox for both BMI and waist circumference in univariate analysis, but showed the opposite for waist circumference or central obesity (direct relationship with increasing mortality) in a multivariate analysis.[24]

The constellation of findings, however, suggests a better prognosis among patients with HF who are overweight or at least mildly obese compared with lean HF subjects. Potential mechanisms for this paradox are listed in **Box 2**.[5,25]

Box 2
Potential reasons for the obesity paradox in HF

1. Unintentional weight loss
2. Greater metabolic reserves
3. Less cachexia
4. Protective cytokines
5. Earlier presentation[a]
6. Attenuated response to the renin–angiotensin–aldosterone system
7. Higher blood pressure leading to more cardiac medications
8. Different cause of HF
9. Increased muscle mass and muscular strength
10. Implications related to cardiorespiratory fitness

[a] Caused by lower natriuretic peptide levels, restrictive lung disease, venous insufficiency and other comorbidities.
From Lavie CJ, Alpert MA, Arena R, et al. Impact of obesity and the obesity paradox on prevalence and prognosis in heart failure. JACC Heart Fail. 2013;1(2):98; with permission.

obesity.[26] The gold-standard CRF assessment is through cardiopulmonary exercise testing (CPX); peak oxygen consumption (Vo_2) is a primary CRF measure obtained from CPX.[26] Other assessments of CRF have also been implemented to assess exercise capacity, such as estimated METs of task (MET; 1 MET = 3.5 $mLO_2 \cdot kg^{-1} \cdot min^{-1}$).[26] CRF modulates the effects of obesity in both the prevention of HF and its prognosis in patients with established HF. In a recent analysis of 20,254 male veterans, obesity was associated with a significant 22% relative risk increase to develop HF.[27] However, after adjustment for CRF (ie, peak METs), the positive influence of obesity was no longer significant, suggesting that the increased risk of HF in individuals with obesity may be mediated by the reduced CRF observed in individuals with obesity.[27] Furthermore, increased CRF was associated with a progressive lower risk for HF, independent of BMI.[27] These results provide evidence that therapeutics targeting of CRF in patients with obesity have the potential to decrease the risk of HF.

In individuals with obesity but without HF as well as those with a confirmed HF diagnosis, the assessment of CRF allows for improved cardiovascular risk stratification, refining the identification of those individuals in which an obesity paradox may be apparent. In a multicenter CPX database study of 2066 patients with HFrEF and a BMI of 18.5 kg/m^2 or greater, those with a markedly reduced CRF, defined as a peak Vo_2 of less than 14 $mL \cdot kg^{-1} \cdot min^{-1}$ and concomitant overweight (BMI $\geq$25 kg/m^2 and <30 kg/m^2) or obesity (BMI $\geq$30 kg/m^2), demonstrated a significantly improved 5-year prognosis compared with those within normal range of body weight (BMI $\geq$18.5 kg/m^2 and <25 kg/m^2).[28] In those with a higher CRF (ie, peak Vo_2 $\geq$14 $mL \cdot kg^{-1} \cdot min^{-1}$), the obesity paradox was not apparent, because the different BMI categories presented with a similar prognosis.[28] Similarly, in a recent analysis of 774 patients with HFrEF and HFpEF followed for up to 12 years, those with preserved CRF, defined as having an estimated METs of 4 or more, presented with a similar prognosis independent of BMI. In contrast, in those with a lower CRF (<4 METs), an obesity paradox was reported.[29] Taken together, these results suggest that the obesity paradox is highly relevant in those individuals with reduced CRF, proposing the addition of measured or estimated CRF for a more accurate risk stratification in patients with HF.

The reason why obesity is protective in the setting of reduced CRF remains the object of intense scrutiny. Because obesity by definition is characterized by an excess body mass, particularly FM, the use of peak Vo_2 adjusted by total body weight may underestimate the CRF in patients with obesity.[30] Such a limitation may explain why in the lower CRF levels, those with obesity present with a more favorable prognosis, because their absolute Vo_2 would in fact be greater than their leaner counterparts, although still lower than healthy individuals.[30,31] To overcome the limitation, a peak Vo_2 adjusted by fat-free mass, also known as lean peak Vo_2, has been proposed for a more accurate risk stratification in individuals with obesity. In fact, in 225 patients with HFrEF,[32] a lean peak Vo_2 of more than 19 $mL \cdot kg$ fat-free mass $^{-1} \cdot min^{-1}$ was a stronger prognosticator than the most commonly used peak Vo_2 $\geq$14 $mL \cdot kg^{-1} \cdot min^{-1}$.[33]

THE ROLE OF BODY COMPOSITION IN OBESITY AND HEART FAILURE

The exclusive use of BMI for nutritional status stratification relies on the assumption that the distribution of FM and fat-free mass remains constant throughout our lives and that individuals with the same BMI present with similar body composition compartment distribution. Although this may be proven correct in most healthy individuals, where BMI represents a good surrogate for total body adiposity,[34] in those at high risk or with established cardiovascular disease, relying exclusively on BMI may result in nutritional and overall cardiovascular disease risk status misclassification. Changes in body composition resulting in diverse body composition phenotypes can affect the risk to develop cardiovascular disease, including HF, in a different manner. Excess FM, particularly visceral FM, typically reported in obese individuals seems to be responsible, at least in part, for the increased HF risk, particularly HFpEF.[9] Adipose tissue produces several proinflammatory cytokines, such as IL-1 and IL-18, which have direct cardiodepressant properties, therefore increasing the risk of cardiac dysfunction and ultimately HF.[35] Similarly, adipose tissue can produce hormones named adipokines, such as leptin, adiponectin, and resistin.[36] Although these hormones have been highly involved in the regulation of body weight and glucose metabolism, their role in HF remains largely unclear.

Leptin regulates food intake by inducing satiety at the central level.[37] However, individuals with obesity develop a leptin resistance state, resulting in a decrease in the satiety signal leading to increased food intake, contributing to a further increase of FM.[37] For this reason, increased levels of leptin typically reflect increased FM, which may explain why leptin is associated with an increased risk for HF.[38] Once HF is diagnosed, however, the role of leptin may be more complex. Increased leptin is, in fact, associated with reduced peak V_{O_2} in HFpEF,[39] which is not surprising considering its association with adiposity. However, in HFrEF leptin has been associated with an increased minute ventilation/carbon dioxide production slope,[40] a measure obtained from CPX and a strong marker of increased risk in HF. The minute ventilation/carbon dioxide production slope is negatively associated with FM, but positively associated with leptin, suggesting alternative mechanisms independent of increased adiposity through which leptin may affect ventilatory efficiency.[40] Of note, leptin can induce the synthesis of aldosterone,[41] which may contribute to the increased volume expansion and exercise intolerance reported in individuals with obesity.[42]

Similar to leptin, resistin is associated with the development of HF.[43] Its role in the setting of established HF remains, however, largely unknown. Preclinical models suggest that resistin is expressed in the heart and its overexpression may induce cardiac hypertrophy and impaired contractility.[44] Nevertheless, both leptin and resistin have been associated with increased N-terminal prohormone of brain natriuretic peptide in patients with cardiomyopathy,[45] suggesting a detrimental effect of these adipokines in the progression of HF.

Adiponectin presents a complex relationship with the development and progression of HF. Although increased adiponectin does not seem to predict the risk for HF,[43] in patients with established HF increased adiponectin levels portend a poor prognosis.[46,47] Similar to leptin and resistin, adiponectin has also been associated with increased N-terminal prohormone of brain natriuretic peptide.[48] Of note, adiponectin can also be produced by the heart itself,[49] and its synthesis is promoted by N-terminal prohormone of brain natriuretic peptide.[50]

At a tissue level, FM and lean mass are also strong determinants of CRF. FM is strongly and inversely associated with CRF in HF, especially in HFpEF,[39] in which intra-abdominal adiposity and intermuscular fat are strong predictors of CRF.[51] Although in the past such effects were thought to be mediated by the same proinflammatory effects of FM responsible for the initial increased risk for HF, the same associations may not be relevant once an HF diagnosis is established. In fact, in a cross-sectional analysis of patients with obesity or severe obesity and concomitant HFpEF, BMI and more accurate measures of adiposity such as FM index were strongly and inversely associated with CRF (ie, peak V_{O_2}), but not with cardiac function parameters assessed by Doppler echocardiography measured at rest and peak exercise.[39] In contrast, cardiac diastolic function remains a strong predictor for CRF in patients with HFpEF.[52] Such evidence suggests that obesity and cardiac diastolic dysfunction may often be described in the setting of HF, but that they may not necessarily be affected by each other, proposing the 2 conditions as comorbidities that often coexist and independently contribute to exercise intolerance.[53]

Contrary to FM, deceased lean mass, and particularly appendicular lean mass (ie, lean mass of the extremities), which is considered the best surrogate for skeletal muscle mass,[54] is associated with worse CRF and muscle strength in both HFrEF and HFpEF.[55,56] Such condition characterized by reduced lean mass, when associated with reduced lean mass functionality, is defined as sarcopenia. When lean mass abnormalities are paired with an excess FM (ie, obesity), this body composition phenotype is defined as sarcopenic obesity, which portends an even worse prognosis and exercise capacity compared with sarcopenia alone.[57,58]

Skeletal muscle mass amount, mitochondrial activity, oxidative fibers, and enzyme expression contribute to the overall diffusion capacity of the skeletal muscle, which in turn, largely contributes to the O_2 pathway.[59] In addition to decreased cardiac output, which results in a decreased peak V_{O_2}, patients with HF can present with abnormalities in skeletal muscle diffusion capacity,[59] proposing that lean mass-targeted therapeutics may result in improved CRF, not necessarily by improving cardiac function but rather body composition compartments,[60] particularly in patients with HFpEF and concomitant obesity. Nevertheless, improvements in cardiac function, with and without improvements in body composition compartments are also desirable in HF, in which favorable changes in cardiac function can also result in improved CRF.[61]

EXERCISE AND DIETARY INTERVENTIONS IN OBESITY AND HEART FAILURE

The role of nonpharmacologic interventions for the treatment of patients with obesity and HF has received much attention in the last few years, particularly in patients with HFpEF for which pharmacologic strategies have largely failed. Exercise training improves exercise capacity in a large spectrum of individuals with different forms of HF and BMI. The mechanisms through which exercise training improves CRF in patients with HF may differ in patients with HFrEF from those with HFpEF. In patients with HFrEF, exercise training improves peak V_{O_2} by improvements in cardiac function. Specifically, in HFrEF, exercise training improves cardiac output by improving systolic function defined as LVEF and cardiac remodeling, reducing LV end-diastolic volume and LV end-systolic volume.[62,63] Exercise training, however, can also improve several noncardiac peripheral factors,[58] further contributing to the improvements in exercise capacity and CRF.[63] Importantly, exercise training-induced changes in both cardiac and noncardiac factors are independent of changes in body weight,[64] further supporting the targeting CRF should remain a priority for the treatment of individuals with obesity and concomitant HFrEF.

In addition to investigating the effects of exercise training on CRF, in patients with HFrEF with an LVEF of 35% or less, the role of this lifestyle intervention on clinical outcomes has also been investigated in Heart Failure: A Controlled Trial Investigating Outcomes of Exercise Training (HF-ACTION).[65] HF-ACTION demonstrated that aerobic exercise associated with home-based exercise training can improve CRF and clinical outcomes, specifically the composite outcome of all-cause mortality and all-cause hospitalizations after prespecified adjustments for key prognostic factors.[65] HF-ACTION, however, demonstrated that adherence to exercise training remains a major challenge, because only 30% of patients met the weekly goal for exercise training, causing a much smaller improvement in peak V_{O_2} (approximately 4%)[65] compared with the predicted 10% to 15% improvement.[66] In fact, in those individuals achieving the prespecified goals of weekly exercise training, improvements in CRF were significantly greater and led to a greater reduction in adverse clinical outcomes,[67] suggesting that improvements in adherence to exercise training could result in significantly greater benefits. Importantly, HF-ACTION has also confirmed the safety of exercise training in HFrEF, which to that point had not been explored in a large multicenter randomized controlled trial.

In patients with HFpEF, the effects of exercise training have only been investigated on CRF and quality of life, but not clinical outcomes. The improvements in CRF have been consistent in different phenotypes, including in those who are overweight, obese, and severely obese,[68,69] which, taken together, can be found in up to 80% of individuals with HFpEF. Contrary to what has been described in HFrEF, exercise training elicits improvements in CRF through mechanisms that are for the most part associated with improvements in noncardiac factors, such as an increase in systemic arterial–venous oxygen difference, leg blood flow, and O_2 delivery.[70] Of note, many of the studies investigating the effects of exercise training on CRF did not perform an assessment of cardiac function at peak exercise. In fact, in patients with HFpEF, the assessment of resting cardiac diastolic function may not be sufficient to detect diastolic dysfunction or even potential changes after an intervention, often requiring the need for its assessment during or at peak exercise.[61]

The role of dietary interventions in patients with HF with concomitant obesity has been less investigated. Although unintentional weight loss is associated with a worse prognosis,[71] intentional weight loss may exert beneficial effects. In HFrEF, small pilot studies suggest that weight loss induced by caloric restriction may improve cardiac systolic and diastolic function and reduce LV mass and left atrial dimension.[72,73] However, randomized controlled trials are lacking to confirm these initial promising findings.

In 100 individuals with HFpEF and obesity randomized to a 20-week caloric restriction dietary intervention and/or aerobic exercise training, intentional weight loss induced by a dietary energy deficit of about 400 kcal/d resulted in improved CRF (1.3 mL·kg^{-1}·min^{-1} increase in peak V_{O_2}), which was further improved when associated with aerobic exercise training 3 times per week for an average of 49 minutes per session (2.5 mL·kg^{-1}·min^{-1} increase in peak V_{O_2}).[69] Importantly, the improvements in CRF were associated with changes in body composition and markers of systemic inflammation, but not cardiac function measured with Doppler echocardiography and cardiac magnetic resonance, except for minor although statistically significant improvements in LV mass in the caloric restriction group but not in the exercise group, further supporting the concept that in patients with HFpEF and concomitant obesity, improvements in CRF may be achieved independent of cardiac function improvements.

The effects of long-term weight loss strategies on clinical outcomes remain, however, unknown. Weight loss induced by caloric restriction alone can also result in a significant reduction in lean mass,[74] which in the long-term could potentially be detrimental, especially in older adults who are at greater risk for sarcopenia or sarcopenic obesity.[75] A weight loss dietary intervention study associated with aerobic and resistance exercise training to minimize lean mass loss in HFpEF is currently ongoing (NCT02636439). In addition to weight loss strategies, improvements in quality of diet have also shown promising results. In a cross-sectional analysis of 23 patients with obesity and HFpEF, the consumption of unsaturated fatty acids, typically found in food like extra virgin olive oil, canola oil, nuts, and avocados, has been associated with a favorable CRF response.[76] Importantly, in a pilot study of 9 patients with obesity and HFpEF, supplementation strategy aimed at increasing unsaturated fatty acids was feasible and, in fact, associated with potential improvements in CRF.[77] A randomized controlled trial aimed at increasing the consumption of dietary unsaturated fatty acids to improve CRF in patients with obesity and HFpEF is currently ongoing (NCT: 03966755).

SUMMARY

Obesity remains a major risk factor for HF, particularly for HFpEF. However, the increased risk seems to be mediated by reduced PA and CRF, proposing therapies aimed at increasing both PA and CRF for the prevention of HF in individuals with obesity as viable options. In those with established HF, obesity has been associated with improved prognosis in several epidemiologic studies (ie, obesity paradox), which may be partially explained by the increased lean mass typically reported in nonsarcopenic obese individuals, which is associated with a higher CRF. Even in the setting of HF, increased CRF has been associated with improved prognosis, supporting the concept that interventions that improve CRF, such as dietary interventions (ie, caloric restriction, improvement in diet quality) and exercise training, may improve clinical outcomes. Randomized controlled trials are warranted, particularly in HFpEF, in which pharmacologic strategies have failed in the last several decades.

REFERENCES

1. Lavie CJ, Laddu D, Arena R, et al. Healthy weight and obesity prevention: JACC health promotion series. J Am Coll Cardiol 2018;72(13):1506–31.
2. Hales CM, Fryar CD, Carroll MD, et al. Trends in obesity and severe obesity prevalence in US youth and adults by sex and age, 2007-2008 to 2015-2016. JAMA 2018;319(16):1723–5.
3. Pandey A, Patel KV, Vaduganathan M, et al. Physical activity, fitness, and obesity in heart failure with preserved ejection fraction. JACC Heart Fail 2018; 6(12):975–82.
4. Kenchaiah S, Evans JC, Levy D, et al. Obesity and the risk of heart failure. N Engl J Med 2002;347(5): 305–13.
5. Lavie CJ, Sharma A, Alpert MA, et al. Update on obesity and obesity paradox in heart failure. Prog Cardiovasc Dis 2016;58(4):393–400.
6. Horwich TB, Fonarow GC, Clark AL. Obesity and the obesity paradox in heart failure. Prog Cardiovasc Dis 2018;61(2):151–6.
7. Alpert MA, Karthikeyan K, Abdullah O, et al. Obesity and cardiac remodeling in adults: mechanisms and clinical implications. Prog Cardiovasc Dis 2018; 61(2):114–23.
8. Ho JE, Lyass A, Lee DS, et al. Predictors of new-onset heart failure: differences in preserved versus reduced ejection fraction. Circ Heart Fail 2013; 6(2):279–86.
9. Pandey A, LaMonte M, Klein L, et al. Relationship between physical activity, body mass index, and risk of heart failure. J Am Coll Cardiol 2017;69(9): 1129–42.
10. Pandey A, Garg S, Khunger M, et al. Dose-response relationship between physical activity and risk of heart failure: a meta-analysis. Circulation 2015; 132(19):1786–94.
11. Berry JD, Pandey A, Gao A, et al. Physical fitness and risk for heart failure and coronary artery disease. Circ Heart Fail 2013;6(4):627–34.
12. Pandey A, Patel M, Gao A, et al. Changes in mid-life fitness predicts heart failure risk at a later age independent of interval development of cardiac and noncardiac risk factors: the Cooper Center Longitudinal Study. Am Heart J 2015;169(2): 290–7.e1.
13. Carbone S, Lavie CJ, Arena R. Obesity and heart failure: focus on the obesity paradox. Mayo Clin Proc 2017;92(2):266–79.
14. Horwich TB, Fonarow GC, Hamilton MA, et al. The relationship between obesity and mortality in patients with heart failure. J Am Coll Cardiol 2001; 38(3):789–95.
15. Sharma A, Lavie CJ, Borer JS, et al. Meta-analysis of the relation of body mass index to all-cause and cardiovascular mortality and hospitalization in patients with chronic heart failure. Am J Cardiol 2015; 115(10):1428–34.
16. Lavie CJ, Ventura HO. The obesity paradox in heart failure: is it all about fitness, fat, or sex? JACC Heart Fail 2015;3(11):927–30.
17. Vest AR, Wu Y, Hachamovitch R, et al. The heart failure overweight/obesity survival paradox: the missing sex link. JACC Heart Fail 2015;3(11):917–26.
18. Shah R, Gayat E, Januzzi JL Jr, et al. Body mass index and mortality in acutely decompensated heart failure across the world: a global obesity paradox. J Am Coll Cardiol 2014;63(8):778–85.
19. Khalid U, Ather S, Bavishi C, et al. Pre-morbid body mass index and mortality after incident heart failure: the ARIC Study. J Am Coll Cardiol 2014;64(25): 2743–9.
20. Lavie CJ, Osman AF, Milani RV, et al. Body composition and prognosis in chronic systolic heart failure: the obesity paradox. Am J Cardiol 2003;91(7): 891–4.
21. Clark AL, Fonarow GC, Horwich TB. Waist circumference, body mass index, and survival in systolic heart failure: the obesity paradox revisited. J Card Fail 2011;17(5):374–80.

22. Clark AL, Chyu J, Horwich TB. The obesity paradox in men versus women with systolic heart failure. Am J Cardiol 2012;110(1):77–82.

23. Lavie CJ, Milani RV, Ventura HO. Adipose composition and heart failure prognosis: paradox or not? J Am Coll Cardiol 2017;70(22):2750–1.

24. Tsujimoto T, Kajio H. Abdominal obesity is associated with an increased risk of all-cause mortality in patients with HFpEF. J Am Coll Cardiol 2017; 70(22):2739–49.

25. Lavie CJ, Alpert MA, Arena R, et al. Impact of obesity and the obesity paradox on prevalence and prognosis in heart failure. JACC Heart Fail 2013;1(2):93–102.

26. Ross R, Blair SN, Arena R, et al. Importance of assessing cardiorespiratory fitness in clinical practice: a case for fitness as a clinical vital sign: a scientific statement from the American Heart Association. Circulation 2016;134(24):e653–99.

27. Kokkinos P, Faselis C, Franklin B, et al. Cardiorespiratory fitness, body mass index and heart failure incidence. Eur J Heart Fail 2019;21(4):436–44.

28. Lavie CJ, Cahalin LP, Chase P, et al. Impact of cardiorespiratory fitness on the obesity paradox in patients with heart failure. Mayo Clin Proc 2013; 88(3):251–8.

29. McAuley PA, Keteyian SJ, Brawner CA, et al. Exercise capacity and the obesity paradox in heart failure: the FIT (Henry Ford Exercise Testing) Project. Mayo Clin Proc 2018;93(6):701–8.

30. Krachler B, Savonen K, Komulainen P, et al. VO2max/kg is expected to be lower in obese individuals! Int J Cardiol 2015;189:234.

31. Hothi SS, Tan DK, Partridge G, et al. Is low VO2max/kg in obese heart failure patients indicative of cardiac dysfunction? Int J Cardiol 2015;184:755–62.

32. Osman AF, Mehra MR, Lavie CJ, et al. The incremental prognostic importance of body fat adjusted peak oxygen consumption in chronic heart failure. J Am Coll Cardiol 2000;36(7):2126–31.

33. Mancini DM, Eisen H, Kussmaul W, et al. Value of peak exercise oxygen consumption for optimal timing of cardiac transplantation in ambulatory patients with heart failure. Circulation 1991;83(3): 778–86.

34. Gallagher D, Visser M, Sepúlveda D, et al. How useful is body mass index for comparison of body fatness across age, sex, and ethnic groups? Am J Epidemiol 1996;143(3):228–39.

35. Carbone S. Obesity and diastolic heart failure: is inflammation the link? Translational Medicine 2013; 03(03):e124.

36. Tchernof A, Despres JP. Pathophysiology of human visceral obesity: an update. Physiol Rev 2013; 93(1):359–404.

37. Sainz N, Barrenetxe J, Moreno-Aliaga MJ, et al. Leptin resistance and diet-induced obesity: central and peripheral actions of leptin. Metabolism 2015;64(1): 35–46.

38. Lieb W, Sullivan LM, Harris TB, et al. Plasma leptin levels and incidence of heart failure, cardiovascular disease, and total mortality in elderly individuals. Diabetes Care 2009;32(4):612–6.

39. Carbone S, Canada JM, Buckley LF, et al. Obesity contributes to exercise intolerance in heart failure with preserved ejection fraction. J Am Coll Cardiol 2016;68(22):2487–8.

40. Wolk R, Johnson BD, Somers VK. Leptin and the ventilatory response to exercise in heart failure. J Am Coll Cardiol 2003;42(9):1644–9.

41. Huby AC, Otvos L Jr, Belin de Chantemele EJ. Leptin induces hypertension and endothelial dysfunction via aldosterone-dependent mechanisms in obese female mice. Hypertension 2016;67(5): 1020–8.

42. Packer M. The conundrum of patients with obesity, exercise intolerance, elevated ventricular filling pressures and a measured ejection fraction in the normal range. Eur J Heart Fail 2019;21(2):156–62.

43. Frankel DS, Vasan RS, D'Agostino RB Sr, et al. Resistin, adiponectin, and risk of heart failure the Framingham offspring study. J Am Coll Cardiol 2009; 53(9):754–62.

44. Kim M, Oh JK, Sakata S, et al. Role of resistin in cardiac contractility and hypertrophy. J Mol Cell Cardiol 2008;45(2):270–80.

45. Bobbert P, Jenke A, Bobbert T, et al. High leptin and resistin expression in chronic heart failure: adverse outcome in patients with dilated and inflammatory cardiomyopathy. Eur J Heart Fail 2012;14(11): 1265–75.

46. Tamura T, Furukawa Y, Taniguchi R, et al. Serum adiponectin level as an independent predictor of mortality in patients with congestive heart failure. Circ J 2007;71(5):623–30.

47. Kistorp C, Faber J, Galatius S, et al. Plasma adiponectin, body mass index, and mortality in patients with chronic heart failure. Circulation 2005;112(12): 1756–62.

48. George J, Patal S, Wexler D, et al. Circulating adiponectin concentrations in patients with congestive heart failure. Heart 2006;92(10):1420–4.

49. Takano H, Obata JE, Kodama Y, et al. Adiponectin is released from the heart in patients with heart failure. Int J Cardiol 2009;132(2):221–6.

50. Tsukamoto O, Fujita M, Kato M, et al. Natriuretic peptides enhance the production of adiponectin in human adipocytes and in patients with chronic heart failure. J Am Coll Cardiol 2009;53(22):2070–7.

51. Haykowsky MJ, Nicklas BJ, Brubaker PH, et al. Regional adipose distribution and its relationship to exercise intolerance in older obese patients who have heart failure with preserved ejection fraction. JACC Heart Fail 2018;6(8):640–9.

52. Trankle C, Canada JM, Buckley L, et al. Impaired myocardial relaxation with exercise determines peak aerobic exercise capacity in heart failure with preserved ejection fraction. ESC Heart Fail 2017; 4(3):351–5.

53. Carbone S, Pandey A, Lavie CJ. Editorial commentary: obesity and heart failure with preserved ejection fraction: a single disease or two co-existing conditions? Trends Cardiovasc Med 2018;28(5): 328–9.

54. Prado CM, Heymsfield SB. Lean tissue imaging: a new era for nutritional assessment and intervention. JPEN J Parenter Enteral Nutr 2014;38(8):940–53.

55. Emami A, Saitoh M, Valentova M, et al. Comparison of sarcopenia and cachexia in men with chronic heart failure: results from the Studies Investigating Co-morbidities Aggravating Heart Failure (SICA-HF). Eur J Heart Fail 2018;20(11):1580–7.

56. Fulster S, Tacke M, Sandek A, et al. Muscle wasting in patients with chronic heart failure: results from the studies investigating co-morbidities aggravating heart failure (SICA-HF). Eur Heart J 2013;34(7): 512–9.

57. Ventura HO, Carbone S, Lavie CJ. Muscling up to improve heart failure prognosis. Eur J Heart Fail 2018;20(11):1588–90.

58. Carbone S, Billingsley HE, Rodriguez-Miguelez P, et al. Lean mass abnormalities in heart failure: the role of sarcopenia, sarcopenic obesity and cachexia. Curr Probl Cardiol 2019. https://doi.org/10.1016/j.cpcardiol.2019.03.006. [Epub ahead of print].

59. Houstis NE, Eisman AS, Pappagianopoulos PP, et al. Exercise intolerance in heart failure with preserved ejection fraction: diagnosing and ranking its causes using personalized O_2 pathway analysis. Circulation 2018;137(2):148–61.

60. Lavie CJ, Ozemek C, Carbone S, et al. Sedentary behavior, exercise and cardiovascular health. Circ Res 2019;124(5):799–815.

61. Kosmala W, Rojek A, Przewlocka-Kosmala M, et al. Effect of aldosterone antagonism on exercise tolerance in heart failure with preserved ejection fraction. J Am Coll Cardiol 2016;68(17):1823–34.

62. Haykowsky MJ, Liang Y, Pechter D, et al. A meta-analysis of the effect of exercise training on left ventricular remodeling in heart failure patients: the benefit depends on the type of training performed. J Am Coll Cardiol 2007;49(24):2329–36.

63. Sullivan MJ, Higginbotham MB, Cobb FR. Exercise training in patients with severe left ventricular dysfunction. Hemodynamic and metabolic effects. Circulation 1988;78(3):506–15.

64. Horwich TB, Broderick S, Chen L, et al. Relation among body mass index, exercise training, and outcomes in chronic systolic heart failure. Am J Cardiol 2011;108(12):1754–9.

65. O'Connor CM, Whellan DJ, Lee KL, et al. Efficacy and safety of exercise training in patients with chronic heart failure: HF-ACTION randomized controlled trial. JAMA 2009;301(14):1439–50.

66. Ismail H, McFarlane JR, Nojoumian AH, et al. Clinical outcomes and cardiovascular responses to different exercise training intensities in patients with heart failure: a systematic review and meta-analysis. JACC Heart Fail 2013;1(6):514–22.

67. Keteyian SJ, Leifer ES, Houston-Miller N, et al. Relation between volume of exercise and clinical outcomes in patients with heart failure. J Am Coll Cardiol 2012;60(19):1899–905.

68. Pandey A, Parashar A, Kumbhani D, et al. Exercise training in patients with heart failure and preserved ejection fraction: meta-analysis of randomized control trials. Circ Heart Fail 2015;8(1):33–40.

69. Kitzman DW, Brubaker P, Morgan T, et al. Effect of caloric restriction or aerobic exercise training on peak oxygen consumption and quality of life in obese older patients with heart failure with preserved ejection fraction: a randomized clinical trial. JAMA 2016;315(1):36–46.

70. Haykowsky MJ, Brubaker PH, John JM, et al. Determinants of exercise intolerance in elderly heart failure patients with preserved ejection fraction. J Am Coll Cardiol 2011;58(3):265–74.

71. Zamora E, Diez-Lopez C, Lupon J, et al. Weight loss in obese patients with heart failure. J Am Heart Assoc 2016;5(3):e002468.

72. Alpert MA, Lambert CR, Panayiotou H, et al. Relation of duration of morbid obesity to left ventricular mass, systolic function, and diastolic filling, and effect of weight loss. Am J Cardiol 1995;76(16):1194–7.

73. Alpert MA, Terry BE, Mulekar M, et al. Cardiac morphology and left ventricular function in normotensive morbidly obese patients with and without congestive heart failure, and effect of weight loss. Am J Cardiol 1997;80(6):736–40.

74. Houston DK, Miller ME, Kitzman DW, et al. Long-Term effects of randomization to a weight loss intervention in older adults: a pilot study. J Nutr Gerontol Geriatr 2019;38(1):83–99.

75. Miller SL, Wolfe RR. The danger of weight loss in the elderly. J Nutr Health Aging 2008;12(7):487–91.

76. Carbone S, Canada JM, Buckley LF, et al. Dietary fat, sugar consumption, and cardiorespiratory fitness in patients with heart failure with preserved ejection fraction. JACC Basic Transl Sci 2017;2(5): 513–25.

77. Carbone S, Billingsley HE, Canada JM, et al. Unsaturated Fatty Acids to Improve Cardiorespiratory Fitness in Patients With Obesity and HFpEF: The UFA-Preserved Pilot Study. JACC Basic Transl Sci. 2019 Aug 26;4(4):563–5. https://doi.org/10.1016/j.jacbts.2019.04.001.

The Cardiorenal Syndrome in Heart Failure

Maria Rosa Costanzo, MD, FESC

KEYWORDS

- Cardiorenal syndrome • Heart failure • Diuretics • Ultrafiltration • Acute kidney injury
- Worsening renal function • Creatinine • Fluid overload

KEY POINTS

- The heart and the kidney are highly interdependent in health and disease.
- In acute heart failure, transient elevations of serum creatinine represent a physiologic response to fluid removal and should not trigger discontinuation of symptom-improving and/or life-saving decongestive therapies.
- Accurate quantitative measurement of fluid volume is vital to individualizing therapy for patients with congestive heart failure.
- The inherent diuretic unresponsiveness of patients with fluid-overloaded heart failure should stimulate investigation of alternative decongestive therapies.
- Investigation of new fluid-management technologies should focus on safety, ease of use, candidates' selection, and cost.

INTRODUCTION

This discussion is focused on the interactions during acute and chronic heart failure (HF) between heart and kidney, which are highly interdependent in health and disease. In normal individuals the kidney depends on the blood flow and perfusion pressure provided by the heart, whose performance is contingent on the kidney's regulation of the body's content of salt and water.[1] In HF, fluid overload produces mutually harmful and self-perpetuating interactions between the heart and the kidney, which lead to deterioration of both organs and increased morbidity and mortality. The term "cardiorenal syndrome" has evolved to encompass all maladaptive relationships between heart and kidney occurring with diverse and sometimes overlapping diseases.[1] Although countless articles have attempted to capture the diagnosis, pathophysiology, prognosis, and treatment of the cardiorenal syndrome, knowledge gaps persist in all these areas.

EPIDEMIOLOGIC AND PROGNOSTIC CONSIDERATIONS

Approximately 50% of patients with chronic HF with both reduced and preserved left ventricular ejection fraction (LVEF) have an estimated glomerular filtration rate (eGFR) of less than 60 L/min/1.73 m², consistent with underlying chronic kidney disease.[2] Multivariate analyses from the SOLVD (Study of Left Ventricular Dysfunction) trials first demonstrated that moderate renal insufficiency (defined as eGFR <60 mL/min/1.73 m² by the Cockroft-Gault equation) was associated with increased risk for all-cause mortality, pump-failure death, and the combined end point of death or hospitalization for HF.[3] Among 372 patients enrolled in the Second Prospective Randomized Study of Ibopamine on Mortality and Efficacy, eGFR, and not LVEF, had the greatest prognostic value: subjects in the lowest eGFR quartile (<44 mL/min) had almost 3-times the mortality

This article originally appeared in *Heart Failure Clinics*, Volume 16, Issue 1, January 2020.
Disclosures: Dr M.R. Costanzo receives consulting honoraria from CHF-Solutions, Fresenius, Abbott, Medtronic, Boston Scientific, and Axon Technologies. Dr M.R. Costanzo's Institution, the Advocate Heart Institute, receives research grant funding from Abbott, Boehringer Ingelheim, V-Wave Medical, and Merck.
Heart Failure Research, Advocate Heart Institute, Edward Hospital Center for Advanced Heart Failure, 801 South Washington Street, Naperville, IL, USA
E-mail address: mariarosa.costanzo@advocatehealth.com

cardiology.theclinics.com

risk (relative risk, 2.85; $P<.001$) of those in the highest quartile (>76 mL/min).[4] These findings have been repeatedly confirmed.[2]

Unlike chronic HF, the significance of renal function changes in acute HF remain controversial because of the assumption that "increased serum creatinine (sCr)/cystatin C," "worsening renal function" (WRF), and "acute kidney injury" (AKI) are different names of the same pathologic entity.[5] In fact, transient sCr increases may represent a benign, and potentially reversible hemodynamically driven reduction in GFR, reflective of effective decongestion, which portends improved outcomes.[6] In aggressively diuresed patients, increases in either sCr or markers of tubular damage were poorly correlated with each other and with diuretic effect, and may have worsened patients' outcomes by triggering premature discontinuation of decongestive therapies.[7] Assessment of renal status by sCr is not straightforward, because defective excretion of sCr can result from extrarenal hypovolemia, impaired blood perfusion, intrinsic kidney etiology, or postrenal disease.[8] It is implausible, therefore, that creatinine, an end product of muscle catabolism freely filtered by the glomerulus and secreted by the tubule, can discriminate between causes of renal dysfunction. Although measurement of sCr is cheap, widely available, and standardized, its disadvantages include the many inducers of elevated sCr, and the numerous conditions affecting its non-GFR determinants (renal reserve, muscle metabolism, protein intake, volume of distribution, medications, and extrarenal degradation).[8] Equations estimating GFR using sCr have variable bias across populations and are imprecise despite standardization of sCr assays and inclusion of age, sex, race, and body size as surrogates for creatinine generation.[8] These equations assume that sCr is a steady-state marker of creatinine production and disposal, conditions that do not apply to AKI or HF. An alternative to creatinine, cystatin C, is a protein produced in all nucleated cells and distributed in extracellular fluid. It is freely filtered and mostly reabsorbed and catabolized by the proximal tubule. Although not affected by modifiers of sCr, smoking, inflammation, adiposity, thyroid diseases, malignancy, and glucocorticoids influence cystatin C levels, diminishing their value as a measure of renal excretory performance.[8] Estimation of GFR using creatinine, cystatin C, or both have not been validated in acutely ill patients.[9] It is disappointing, therefore, that the severity of AKI is classified by changes in sCr or cystatin C.[8,10] A patient may have tubular damage without significant changes in sCr because of renal reserve. Conversely, the correlation of an increase in sCr levels with better outcomes during HF treatment suggests that elevation of this analyte identifies physiologic, volume-sensitive responses to diuretics, rather than AKI.[6]

Advances in kidney transcriptomics and urinary proteomics suggest that kidney genes and their encoded proteins can be specific for certain stimuli and cellular targets. Serum creatinine is not in this category because it can be similarly elevated in different experimental and clinical situations. Different genetic signatures are activated by renal ischemia versus volume depletion in both animal models and patients with a broad range of illnesses.[11,12] The intrinsic characteristics of sCr (delayed, insensitive, not specific to tubular damage) contrast with the genetic responses of the kidney (rapid, sensitive, cell- and stimulus-specific).[11,13,14] Therefore, an obvious question is why biomarkers of tubular injury are not widely used in patients with decompensated HF to distinguish true AKI from changes in renal clearance resulting from diuresis-driven hemoconcentration. In predictive modeling, the performance of AKI biomarkers is undermined by both use of sCr as the "gold standard" comparator and disregard for disease prevalence in the target population.[14] Assuming that, at a certain cutoff value, sCr is 90% sensitive and 90% specific and disease prevalence is 20%, a new biomarker with 100% sensitivity and 100% specificity may seem to have only 69% sensitivity and 97% specificity compared with the "imperfect gold standard."[14] Therefore, changes in acute HF therapy based only on sCr increases may trigger adjustment or discontinuation of symptom-improving and/or life-saving antineurohormonal drugs and prevent effective decongestion.[5,15] Mounting evidence shows that unresolved congestion trumps renal function as a predictor of poor HF outcomes.[5–7,15]

MECHANISMS OF FLUID ACCUMULATION IN HEART FAILURE AND THE CARDIORENAL SYNDROME

In chronic HF, renal retention of sodium and water causes intravascular and interstitial fluid-volume expansion and redistribution. Renal sodium excretion decreases early in response to an absolute or relative decrease in cardiac output (CO), which reduces arterial filling and, consequently, effective circulating blood volume (BV).[16,17] The resulting alteration of baroreceptor activity produces neurohormonal activation, which enhances renal sodium and water reabsorption. Although sympathetic-driven vasoconstriction initially maintains organ perfusion, concomitant gradual fluid accumulation in the interstitium produces a compensatory and sustained expansion of plasma volume (PV). Because with lower CO less than 30% to 40% of total BV resides in the arterial circulation, volume must expand to preserve tissue perfusion.[16] When this compensatory mechanism becomes maladaptive, volume overload and organ congestion ensue (**Fig. 1**). Hypervolemia leads to increased cardiac filling pressures and later to clinical congestion, which often becomes apparent after retention of several liters of fluid. Because diuretics incompletely eliminate fluid excess, a vicious circle occurs whereby a partial response to treatment triggers gradual reaccumulation and redistribution of fluid, leading to recurrent HF decompensation.[5,15,18–21] In untreated patients with symptomatic systolic dysfunction, indicator dilution techniques showed that interstitial and intravascular volumes expand proportionately (33%–35% above normal).[16] Normally, fluid retention expands PV because of low interstitial compliance. When this increases in HF, the interstitium can accommodate a greater amount of fluid volume, which persists after clinical congestion

appears resolved.[20,22,23] Reduced effective circulating BV and systemic blood pressure lower capillary hydrostatic pressure, facilitating fluid shifts from the interstitial to the intravascular compartment. Conversely, abnormal capillary endothelial permeability, coupled with reduced plasma oncotic pressure from albumin loss, promotes fluid shifts from the intravascular to the interstitial compartment.[19,20] Diuretic response becomes inadequate when the ratio of interstitial volume to PV exceeds by severalfold the normal 3:1 to 4:1 ratio (**Fig. 2**). Persistent hypervolemia can progress to acute HF decompensation when sympathetic-mediated vasoconstriction causes transfer of up to 1 L of fluid from the splanchnic venous reservoir into the central circulation.[18,23–27] Importantly, red blood cell volume can also contribute to volume overload. In HF, polycythemia is often masked by a low hemoglobin or hematocrit level owing to dilution in an expanded PV. In chronic HF, polycythemia is a physiologic response to low CO, tissue hypoxia, impaired oxygen exchange, and acidosis. With polycythemia, diuretics may enhance thrombotic risk and myocardial work

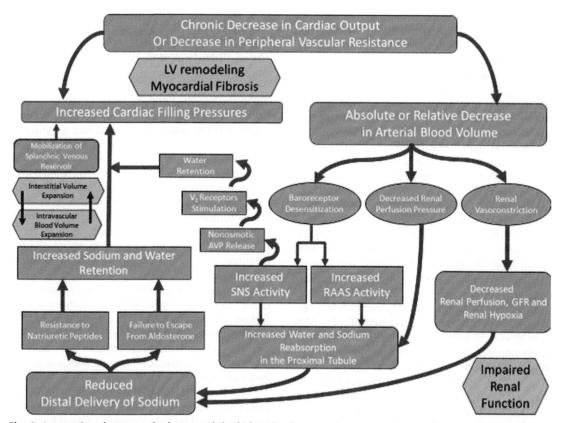

Fig. 1. Interactions between the heart and the kidney leading to volume expansion and congestion in acute and chronic heart failure. AVP, arginine vasopressin; GFR, glomerular filtration rate; LV, left ventricle; RAAS, renin-angiotensin-aldosterone system; SNS, sympathetic nervous system; V₂ Receptors, vasopressin receptors type 2.

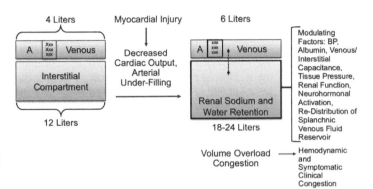

Fig. 2. Mechanisms of interstitial and intravascular volume expansion in chronic heart failure. BP, blood pressure; CO, cardiac output. (*From* Miller WL. Fluid volume overload and congestion in heart failure. time to reconsider pathophysiology and how volume is assessed. Circ Heart Fail. 2016;9:e002922; with permission.)

because of increased blood viscosity.[28–30] These facts underscore that accurate quantitative measurement of both red blood cell volume and PV are vital to the individualization of therapy for patients with congestive HF.

Methods for assessing fluid volume are described later in this article.

PATHOPHYSIOLOGIC EVENTS IN THE KIDNEY IN THE SETTING OF HEART FAILURE

The kidney filtration function is the sum of single nephrons' GFR. This depends on the area and permeability characteristics of the glomerular membrane and Starling forces in the glomerular capillary, and Bowman's space favoring and opposing filtration. Normal single-nephron GFR and filtration fraction (FF) are 40 to 70 mL/min and 20% to 25%, respectively. When renal blood flow (RBF) is high, the glomerular capillary colloid osmotic pressure (πGC) increases slowly from the proximal to the distal end of the glomerular capillary and a filtration pressure gradient persists over the length of the capillaries. When RBF decreases, the PV exposed to the filtration pressure gradient per area unit of the capillary wall is smaller. The faster increase of πGC along the glomerular capillary results in an increased πGC at the level of the efferent arteriole and, hence, an increase in FF. This will attenuate the absolute drop in a single nephron's GFR, independent of changes in glomerular capillary hydrostatic pressure. However, when the maximum FF of ~60% is achieved, a further decrease in RBF causes single-nephron GFR to drop linearly so that the filtration pressure gradient cannot be maintained over the length of the glomerular capillary (wasted capillary). These mechanisms are amplified by the neurohormonal activation occurring in HF.[31]

In the proximal tubules, different transporters mediate active movement of sodium across their luminal side. However, because the proximal tubular epithelium is leaky, back flux occurs and net sodium reabsorption depends on passive Starling forces between peritubular capillaries and interstitium. These processes can occur independent of, but are exaggerated by, neurohumoral activity. In HF, because of increased FF, peritubular capillary colloid osmotic pressure is higher, which stimulates sodium and water reabsorption. Moreover, owing to fluid overload and encapsulation of the kidney, interstitial fluid hydrostatic pressure and peritubular capillary hydrostatic pressure both increase, whereas interstitial fluid colloid osmotic pressure decreases because of removal of interstitial proteins by increased lymph flow (Q_L). This further facilitates net sodium and water reabsorption.[31]

Normally, the macula densa senses increased chloride delivery because active chloride transport triggers metabolism of adenosine triphosphate (ATP) to adenosine, which has a paracrine vasoconstrictive effect on the afferent arteriole. This tubule-glomerular feedback protects the nephron from hyperfiltration. In HF, diminished chloride delivery to the macula densa caused by increased proximal reabsorption stimulates nitric oxide synthetase I and cyclo-oxygenase-2, and release of nitric oxide and prostaglandin E_2. The latter 2 act on the granulosa cells of the afferent arteriole, causing renin release and vasodilation resulting from relaxation of smooth muscle cells. Renin activates angiotensin II, which initiates a vicious cycle of neurohumoral activation and further sodium and water retention. Notably, loop diuretics inhibit the $Na^+/K^+/2Cl^-$ cotransporter, further reducing intracellular chloride levels in the macula densa and thus escalating renin secretion.[31]

The distal convoluted tubules and collecting ducts reabsorb only ≤10% of the total amount of sodium filtered by the glomerulus. Distal fractional sodium reabsorption rates vary according to tubular flow rate, and aldosterone and arginine vasopressin levels.[32–34] In normal subjects, high doses of aldosterone initially increase renal sodium retention so that the volume of extracellular fluid is increased by 1.5 to 2 L. However, renal sodium retention then ceases, sodium balance is reestablished, and no edema occurs. This escape from mineralocorticoid-mediated sodium retention depends, at least in part, on an increase in delivery of sodium to aldosterone's site of action in the collecting ducts. Owing to increased proximal sodium reabsorption, such escape fails to occur in HF patients, who continue to retain sodium in response to aldosterone. Hence, substantial natriuresis can be expected in HF with mineralocorticoid antagonists.[35]

CONTRIBUTIONS OF THE ABDOMINAL CIRCULATION TO THE CARDIORENAL SYNDROME IN HEART FAILURE

The capacitance veins of the splanchnic vasculature ensure a stable cardiac preload despite changes in volume status. If arteriolar perfusion decreases, sympathetic stimulation from centrally perceived hypovolemia causes α-mediated vasoconstriction of splanchnic capacitance veins and β_2-mediated vasodilation of the hepatic veins, causing autotransfusion to the central circulation to maintain effective intravascular volume.[27,36] In the splanchnic microcirculation, net filtration prevails over the length of the capillaries. Fluid overload increases capillary hydrostatic pressure, further augmenting net filtration pressure. Increased abdominal Q_L drains fluid, solutes, and proteins, decreasing interstitial fluid oncotic pressure and opposing filtration. Once Q_L is maximal and interstitial compliance increases, protein-rich edema compresses lymphatics, further impairing Q_L and promoting fluid accumulation.[36–38]

In the liver, adenosine, continuously produced from ATP by hepatocytes, accumulates in the perisinusoidal space and is drained by lymphatics. When portal blood flow is reduced by α-receptor–mediated vasoconstriction, Q_L decreases and intrahepatic adenosine concentrations increases. The resulting stimulation of hepatic afferent nerves, which are synapsed with renal efferent nerves, promotes further sodium retention.[36]

The spleen also contributes to the regulation of intravascular volume. Because splenic sinusoids are permeable to plasma proteins, their colloid osmotic pressure is the same as that of the lymphatic matrix, so that fluid transport between the 2 spaces is determined by differences in hydrostatic pressure. Transient splanchnic venous system congestion results in increased hydrostatic pressure in the splenic sinusoids. Therefore, more fluid is drained to the lymphatic matrix and buffered in the splenic lymphatic reservoirs. However, with increased cardiac filling pressures and atrial natriuretic peptide production, splenic arterial vasodilation and venous vasoconstriction facilitate fluid shifts into the perivascular splenic third space. This leads to perceived central hypovolemia and further neurohumoral activation.[36] Moreover, overload of the lymphatic system results in interstitial edema.

The countercurrent system of the intestinal microcirculation allows extensive exchange between arterioles and venules. Therefore, oxygen short-circuits from arterioles to venules, creating a gradient with the lowest oxygen partial pressure at the villus tip. In HF, the low-flow state in the splanchnic microcirculation caused by hypoperfusion, increased venous stasis, and sympathetically mediated arteriolar vasoconstriction increases oxygen exchange between arterioles and venules, augmenting the gradient between the villus base and tip. The resulting ischemia causes loss of the intestinal barrier function of the epithelial cells, which permits lipopolysaccharide and endotoxin, produced by gram-negative bacteria in the gut lumen, to enter the systemic circulation and further increase generalized inflammation and hemodynamic abnormalities.[39]

METHODS FOR THE ASSESSMENT OF FLUID VOLUME IN THE CARDIORENAL SYNDROME OCCURRING IN HEART FAILURE
Blood Volume Measurement and the Indicator Dilution Principle

Indicator dilution techniques measure an unknown volume when a known volume of a known concentration of a tracer is added to an unknown volume of fluid.[40] After complete mixing, the concentration of the tracer is measured in a sample taken from the unknown volume. The size of the unknown volume is inversely proportional to the concentration of the tracer in the sample because the latter becomes progressively more diluted as the size of the unknown volume increases. This can be calculated as $C_1V_1 = C_2V_2$, where C_1 is the concentration of tracer injected, V_1 is the volume of tracer injected, C_2 is the concentration of the tracer in a sample from the unknown volume, and V_2 is the unknown volume. Nuclear medicine techniques can accurately measure a radioisotope tracer concentration in fluid samples using the indicator dilution technique, which allows assessment of PV with ^{131}iodine-tagged human serum albumin. A propensity-score control matching analysis by demographics, comorbidity, and time of treatment was performed in 245 consecutive HF admissions undergoing BV analysis and controls derived from the Center for Medicare and Medicaid data and matched 10:1 for demographics, comorbidity, and year of treatment. Decongestion strategy targeted total BV to 6%–8% above patient-specific norm.[41] Compared with controls, subjects receiving BV analysis-guided therapy experienced lower 30-day readmissions (12.2% vs 27.7%, $P<.001$), 30-day mortality (2.0% vs 11.1%, $P<.001$), and 1-year mortality (4.9% vs 35.5%, $P<.001$) rates.[41] Independent validation that increased adoption of BV analysis provides incremental benefit with a favorable cost-benefit profile is required.

Bioelectrical Impedance Analysis Methods

The human body is akin to a conducting cylinder.[42] Both intracellular fluid and extracellular fluid are ionic solutions and are therefore good electricity conductors (low impedance to passage of an alternating current). The protein-lipid-protein layers of cell membranes function as capacitors. Bone and adipose tissue act as resistors (high impedance to the passage of an alternating current). Therefore, living soft tissues form a complex network of resistive and capacitive conductors arranged in parallel and in series. When an alternating current is applied to them, bioelectrical impedance depends on tissue composition and the current's frequency. Driving electrodes deliver the alternating current while sensing electrodes measure the voltage according to Ohm's law:

$$V = (R + X_c)I$$

where V is the voltage, I is the current, and $R + X_c$ is the complex impedance consisting of resistance (R) and reactance (X_c), which accounts for the movement of electrons determined by the characteristics of the tissue where they reside.[42] In humans, driving and sensing electrodes can be placed sufficiently far apart to measure whole-body impedance, or closer to each other to measure impedance of a body segments. Alternating current can be applied at single (50 kHz), dual (50 and 200 kHz), or multiple frequencies (5–1000 kHz).

A device manufactured by RSMM (Tel Aviv, Israel) that measures net lung impedance was used in a single-blind 2-center trial (NCT01315223) wherein 256 HF patients with LVEF ≤35%, New York Heart Association (NYHA) class II to IV, and a recent HF hospitalization were randomized to controls (clinical assessment alone) or to a lung impedance-guided therapy group.[43] Net lung impedance typically

decreased 3 weeks before hospitalization. Over 48 months, compared with controls, the monitored group had fewer hospitalizations (rate per patient-year follow-up: 1.03 vs 1.68, hazard ratio [HR] 0.66, 95% confidence interval [CI] 0.59–0.74, $P<.001$) and deaths (HR 0.52, 95% confidence interval 0.35–0.78, $P = .002$).[43] The study's limitations include possible influence of treatment assignment on hospitalization, no independent adjudication of events, and a high event rate (0.94/patient-year) in a population with 50% of subjects being NYHA class II.[44]

Bioreactance

Bioreactance measures phase shifts of the electrical currents traversing the thorax and may provide a more accurate estimation of hemodynamics thanks to its higher signal-to-noise ratio. Preliminary investigations suggest that bioreactance methods can discriminate between cardiac and noncardiac dyspnea, assess the efficacy of ultrafiltration (UF) during hemodialysis, and predict fluid responsiveness in spontaneously breathing patients.[42]

Pulmonary Artery Pressure Sensors

Elevated cardiac filling pressures increase the risk for hospitalizations and mortality.[45,46] Regardless of LVEF, filling pressures gradually increase more than 2 weeks before HF-related hospitalizations.[47,48] In the CHAMPION trial (CardioMEMS Heart Sensor Allows Monitoring of Pressure to Improve Outcomes in Class III Heart Failure), HF treatment guided by pulmonary artery (PA) pressures measured by the CardioMEMS sensor was associated with a reduction in HF hospitalization rates of 28% and 37% at 6 and 15 months, respectively, compared with clinical management.[49,50] The CHAMPION-HF trial algorithm recommended use of sequential doses of diuretics and vasodilators to lower and maintain the PA diastolic pressure below 20 mm Hg and provided guidance for de-escalation of diuretics if the filling pressures were low, to prevent hypovolemia and renal dysfunction.[51] More than twice as many medication changes (both increases and decreases) occurred in the active monitoring group compared with the blind therapy group. Although the average diuretic doses from baseline to 6 months were higher in the active monitoring group, the eGFR was similar in the 2 arms, indicating that the decrease in HF hospitalizations because of PA pressure–guided therapy did not occur at the expense of WRF.[50,51] A recent CHAMPION-HF analysis showed that hemodynamically guided HF management also reduces mortality in patients with reduced LVEF receiving guideline-directed medical therapy, highlighting the important synergy of hemodynamic and neurohormonal targets of HF therapy.[52] The PA pressure–guided therapy had similar benefits in subjects with preserved and reduced LVEF.[53] The favorable outcomes of CHAMPION-HF have been replicated in clinical practice.[54,55] The Hemodynamic-GUIDEd Management of Heart Failure (GUIDE-HF) trial (NCT03387813) is testing the effects of PA pressure–guided therapy in broader HF populations.

Data from Cardiac Implanted Electronic Devices

Approximately 40% of HF patients with reduced LVEF receive a cardiac implantable electronic device (CIED). Some CIEDs can estimate thoracic fluid content when a small alternating current passes between the case and the lead. The greater is the amount of fluid in the path of the electrical impulse, the lower the measured impedance.[56] Studies using this feature have yielded conflicting results.[57] More recent analyses have assessed whether combinations of CIEDs data are superior to measurement of a single variable in risk-stratifying HF patients. To develop the HeartLogic alert algorithm, available in the COGNIS (Boston Scientific, St Paul, MN) CIED, data from multiple device sensors were used in combination with clinical baseline and HF events data. Initial analyses identified heart sounds (S1 and S3), thoracic impedance, respiration, heart rate, and activity as predictive of an HF event.[58] Changes in these features from each patient's baseline were aggregated and weighted based on an individual's daily risk for worsening HF. The HeartLogic index is updated daily, and an alert is issued when the nominal threshold of 16 is crossed.[58] In the Multisensor Chronic Evaluation in Ambulatory Heart Failure Patients (MultiSENSE) study, this alert index forecasted HF events with a 70% sensitivity and a median of 34-day warning.[58] The ongoing Multiple Cardiac Sensors for the Management of Heart Failure (MANAGE-HF) study compares remote monitoring with versus without HeartLogic alerts to drive HF care (NCT03237858). However, the data obtainable from CIEDs have limitations: (1) estimation only of fluid in the thorax; (2) imprecise quantitation of excess volume and its changes with fluid removal; (3) applicability only to patients with CIED indications, which excludes patients preserved LVEF, constituting greater than 50% of the HF population.[59]

Ultrasound Methods

Lung ultrasonography

Lung ultrasonography (LUS) can assess extravascular lung water (ELW), determined by lung permeability and cardiac filling pressures, with the analysis of B-line artifacts.[60] These are discrete vertical hyperechoic reverberation artifacts that arise from the pleural line, extend to the bottom of the ultrasound screen, and move with lung sliding.[60] Comparison with data from computed tomography and invasive hemodynamics confirms a direct relationship between B lines and ELW. LUS can be performed with any type of echography device at any transducer frequency, is reproducible, and is easy to learn.[60] In one metaanalysis, 3 or more B lines in 2 or more bilateral lung zones were diagnostic for pulmonary edema (sensitivity, 94%; specificity, 92%).[60] A B-line score cutoff of $\geq$15 is significantly correlated with clinical congestion scores, E/E′ ratio, natriuretic peptide levels, increased LV filling pressure, larger LV volumes, LV mass index, left atrial volume index, tricuspid regurgitation velocity, and estimated systolic PA pressure.[60] In 6 studies including 438 acutely decompensated HF patients, B lines decreased as early as 3 hours after therapy initiation and were cleared within 4 days.[61] A decrease of 2.7 B lines occurs with every 500 mL of fluid removed by UF.[62] In HF patients, the number of B lines is correlated with natriuretic peptide levels.[63,64] However, because B lines lack specificity, because those caused by edema versus interstitial fibrosis are similar, they must be considered in the context of clinical, hemodynamic, and echocardiographic assessments.

Inferior vena cava ultrasonography

The diameter of the inferior vena cava (IVC) changes with respiration, reflecting the elasticity of this capacitance vessel. In spontaneously breathing subjects, intrathoracic pressure decreases during inspiration, thereby increasing venous return and causing collapse of the IVC. During expiration, venous return decreases, leading to increased IVC diameter.[65] In acutely decompensated HF, when volume overload dilates the IVC to the limits of its elasticity, respirations produce only minimal changes in IVC diameter.[65] A respiratory variation of IVC diameter of $\leq$15% was highly sensitive and specific for the diagnosis of acutely decompensated HF.[66] Ultrasonography of the IVC is a rapid, simple, and noninvasive method for bedside monitoring of intravascular volume during UF and adjustment of fluid-removal rate. Accuracy of IVC measurements is influenced by the patient's position and ability to follow instructions as well as intraobserver and interobserver variability.

Biomarkers

The use of natriuretic peptides to assess and guide the treatment of fluid overload is not recommended, given the multiple causes of increased levels of these biomarkers.[67,68] Removal of fluid to achieve prespecified natriuretic peptide levels is untested in acute HF. The limitations of sCr as a biomarker of AKI during fluid removal have been previously discussed.

The staggering number of HF rehospitalizations underscores the inability to accurately estimate fluid excess and determine when euvolemia has been achieved. The most accurate method to measure extracellular fluid is BV analysis. Unfortunately, this approach is not widely used because of the perceived complexity and lack of studies correlating BV analysis with other measures of fluid-volume assessment (hematocrit, biomarkers, hemodynamics, and bioelectrical impedance). All bioelectrical impedance or bioreactance methods lack rigorous comparison with invasive hemodynamics; therefore, their accuracy in quantifying fluid excess and changes with treatment remains unknown. Therapy guided by implanted PA pressure sensors is associated with reductions in rehospitalizations regardless of LVEF, with a pointer toward decreased mortality in NYHA class III HF patients. Although risk scores from CIED data may forecast HF events with enough warning to avert hospitalizations, they cannot provide quantitation of fluid volume and be used in patients without CIED indications. Ultrasound methods have not been meaningfully compared with other methods of fluid-volume determination. Owing to the multitude of factors contributing to their elevation, biomarkers such as natriuretic peptides cannot precisely quantitate fluid excess or guide HF therapy. The use of elevation in sCr, WRF, and AKI as interchangeable terms causes premature discontinuation of decongestive therapies and the resulting poorer outcomes in hospitalized HF patients.

The initial step is to confirm the ability of BV analysis to quantitate fluid excess and diagnose the achievement of euvolemia after treatment; BV analysis should then be compared with methods that can performed easily, serially, and inexpensively: hemodynamically guided therapy can be used for early detection of fluid overload and prevention of HF hospitalizations; CIED data may forecast the risk of HF events early enough to trigger interventions to prevent HF decompensation; and noninvasive wearable devices detecting variables similar to those obtainable from CIEDs may soon become available for all HF patients, regardless of LVEF. As for CIED-derived risk indices, those from wearable devices must provide targets sufficiently specific to trigger appropriate therapies.

REFRACTORINESS TO DIURETICS IN HEART FAILURE

Still the cornerstone of decongestive therapy, diuretics' effectiveness decreases with progression of HF.[69,70] Impaired absorption, decreased RBF, azotemia, and proteinuria result in reduced diuretic concentrations in the tubular lumen[70] (Fig. 3). Definitions of diuretic resistance include: persistent congestion despite escalating diuretic doses equivalent to ≥80 mg/d furosemide;

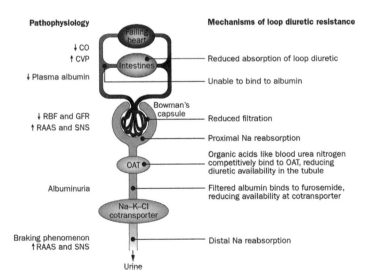

Fig. 3. Mechanisms of diuretic unresponsiveness in patients with heart failure. CO, cardiac output; CVP, central venous pressure; GFR, glomerular filtration rate; OAT, organic anion transporter; RAAS, renin-angiotensin-aldosterone system; RBF, renal blood flow; SNS, sympathetic nervous system. (*From* ter Maaten JM, Valente MA, Damman K, et al. Diuretic response in acute heart failure—pathophysiology, evaluation, and therapy. Nat Rev Cardiol 2015;12:184–92; with permission.)

amount of sodium excretion as a percentage of filtered load less than 0.2%; and failure to excrete ≥90 mmol of sodium within 72 h of a 160-mg twice-daily furosemide dose. Metrics of diuretic response include: weight loss per 40 mg of furosemide or equivalent; net fluid loss per milligram of loop diuretic; and urinary sodium-to-urinary furosemide ratio.[70] Hallmarks of diuretic resistance are insufficient symptom relief, higher risk of in-hospital HF worsening, increased mortality after discharge, and a 3-fold increase in rehospitalization rates.[70,71] Among more than 50,000 patients enrolled in the ADHERE (Acute Decompensated Heart Failure National Registry) study, only 33% lost ≤2.27 kg (5 lb), and 16% gained weight during hospitalization.[72] With conventional diuretic therapies, nearly 50% of hospitalized HF patients are discharged with residual fluid excess.[72] Regardless of diuretic strategy, 42% of acutely decompensated HF subjects in the DOSE (Diuretic Optimization Strategies Evaluation) trial reached the composite end point of death, rehospitalization, or emergency department visit at 60 days.[73] Vasopressin and adenosine-A1 receptor antagonists, exogenous natriuretic peptides, and low-dose dopamine, studied as complement or replacement for diuretics, decrease short-term fluid overload but fail to improve long-term outcomes.[74–76] Therefore, there is an unmet clinical need for more effective fluid-removal methods for HF patients (**Table 1**).

EXTRACORPOREAL ULTRAFILTRATION

Ultrafiltration consists of the production of plasma water from whole blood across a semipermeable membrane (hemofilter) in response to a transmembrane pressure gradient. Newer, simplified UF devices afford the advantages of small size, portability, low blood-flow rates, extracorporeal

BV less than 50 mL, and a wide range of UF rates (0–500 mL/h) without requiring cannulation of a central vein and stay in intensive care units.[5]

As ultrafiltrate is isotonic to plasma, approximately 134 to 138 mmol of sodium is removed with each liter of ultrafiltrate.[77] Knowledge that refill of the intravascular space from the interstitium decreases as fluid is removed led to the hypothesis that UF initiation before reduction of capillary refill by previously administered diuretics might decongest HF patients more effectively than intravenous loop diuretics. Hence, in the UNLOAD (Ultrafiltration vs Intravenous Diuretics Decompensated Heart Failure) trial, randomization occurred within 24 h of hospitalization, and after a maximum of 2 intravenous doses of loop diuretic.[78] Compared with standard care, the UF group had greater weight loss and similar improvement in dyspnea score at 48 h. The percentage of patients with increases in serum creatinine ≥0.3 mg/dL was similar between groups.[78] The 90-day HF events were fewer in the UF than in the diuretic group. Total body sodium and excess fluid removal by UF may be more effective than withdrawal of hypotonic fluid by diuretic agents or free water by arginine vasopressin V_2 receptor antagonists.[73–76] Prehospitalization diuretics use itself may impair natriuretic response to intravenous administration.[70] UNLOAD lacked treatment targets, BV assessments, cost analysis, and independent adjudication of events.

The CARRESS-HF (Cardiorenal Rescue Study in Acute Decompensated Heart Failure) trial compared a fixed UF rate of 200 mL/h with stepped pharmacologic therapy (adjustable doses of intravenous loop diuretics, thiazide diuretics, vasodilators, and inotropes) in acutely decompensated HF patients with prerandomization increase in sCr.[79] CARRESS-HF's primary end point was the bivariate change in serum creatinine and

Table 1	
Differential characteristics of loop diuretics and isolated ultrafiltration	
Loop Diuretics	**Isolated Ultrafiltration**
Direct neurohormonal activation	No direct neurohormonal activation
Elimination of hypotonic urine	Removal of isotonic plasma water
Unpredictable elimination of sodium and water	Precise control of rate and amount of fluid removal
Development of diuretic resistance with prolonged administration	Restoration of diuretic responsiveness
Risk of hypokalemia and hypomagnesemia	No effect on plasma concentration of potassium and magnesium
Peripheral venous access	Peripheral or central venous catheter
No need for anticoagulation	Need for anticoagulation
No extracorporeal circuit	Need for extracorporeal circuit

body weight from baseline to 96 h.[79] According to CARRESS-HF's design, this assumes that weight loss is a measurement of effective fluid removal and that an increase in sCr represents AKI. In CARRESS-HF, both groups lost an equivalent amount of weight, but greater increases in sCr occurred with UF.[79] Although more patients in the UF group experienced serious adverse events, the high crossover rate in CARRESS-HF intention-to-treat analysis impairs their adjudication to one or the other therapy.[79] A per-protocol analysis including only patients who had ultrafiltrate collected if randomized to UF, or no ultrafiltrate collected if randomized to the pharmacologic arm, revealed that UF was associated with higher net fluid loss ($P = .001$) and weight reduction ($P = .02$).[80,81]

In the CUORE (Continuous Ultrafiltration for Congestive Heart Failure) trial, UF-treated patients had a lower incidence of HF rehospitalizations through 1 year than those receiving standard care, despite similar weight loss at discharge. In CUORE, diuretics were continued during UF in the belief that this approach enhances natriuresis.[82] In previous studies, diuretics were stopped during UF to give patients a "diuretic holiday," during which loop diuretic–induced neurohormonal activation is absent.[78,83,84]

The hypothesis of the AVOID-HF (Aquapheresis vs Intravenous Diuretics and Hospitalization for Heart Failure) trial was that patients hospitalized for HF and treated with adjustable UF would have a longer time to first HF event within 90 days than those receiving adjustable intravenous loop diuretics.[85] The trial was terminated unilaterally by the sponsor (Baxter Healthcare, Deerfield, IL) after enrollment of 224 patients (27.5% of the planned sample). Detailed algorithms guided investigators on how to adjust both therapies according to patients' vital signs, renal function, and urine output.[85] The adjustable UF group had a trend to longer time to first HF event than patients in the diuretics group (62 vs 34 days; $P = .106$). At 30 days UF patients had significantly fewer independently adjudicated HF and cardiovascular events.[86] Adjustments of UF rates to individual patients' hemodynamics and renal function may explain the lack of differences in sCr between groups, despite greater net fluid loss with UF.[86] Restoration of diuretic responsiveness may be a key mechanism by which UF delays the recurrence of HF events.[86] Serious therapy-related adverse events occurred at higher rates in the UF group than in the diuretics group (14.6% vs 5.4%; $P = .026$).[86] Although in AVOID-HF, UF-related adverse events were fewer than in CARRESS-HF, the excess of UF-related

complications is a serious concern.[79,86] More studies are needed to identify strategies that minimize access-related and other potentially preventable complications.[78,86]

The key features of the trials discussed here are summarized in **Table 2**.

The conflicting results from UF studies suggest that patient selection and fluid-removal targets are incompletely understood.[79,86] Practice guidelines recommend that inadequate response to an initial dose of intravenous loop diuretic be treated with an increased dose.[87,88] If this is ineffective, invasive hemodynamic assessment is suggested. Persistent fluid excess can then be treated with the addition of thiazide diuretics, aldosterone antagonists, or continuous intravenous infusion of a loop diuretic. Only if all these measures fail can UF be considered.[87,88] A similar degree of diuretic resistance characterized CARRESS-HF's subjects, whose poor outcomes may be partially related to the lack of therapy adjustment according to individual patients' characteristics.[79] In AVOID-HF, fine-tuning of UF rates in response to vital signs, renal function, or urine output resulted in greater net fluid loss and was associated with fewer 30-day HF events without a greater increase in sCr levels compared with the diuretics group.[86] Additional investigation of UF as both first-line and rescue therapy is needed, provided that UF rates are individualized.[78,86] Use of UF is not recommended in de novo HF patients who are likely to respond to intravenous diuretics. The lingering question concerns which patients who develop HF decompensation despite daily oral diuretics should be considered for UF instead of intravenous diuretic agents. One important general recommendation is that the chosen initial UF rate should be either maintained or reduced because capillary refill decreases with fluid removal.[5] In general, UF rates of greater than 250 mL/h are not recommended.[85,86] Patients with predominantly right-sided HF or HF with preserved LVEF are exquisitely susceptible to intravascular volume depletion and may only tolerate low UF rates (50–100 mL/h).[89] Clinical experience teaches us that extracorporeal fluid removal is better tolerated when conducted with low UF rates over prolonged periods of time.[5]

A frequently used approach is to compare patients' current weight with that preceding signs and symptoms of congestion and to use this "dry weight" as the fluid removal. No consensus exists on whether removal of only 60% to 80% of excess fluid by UF and continuation of loop diuretics during therapy results in less hemodynamic instability and greater urinary sodium excretion.[82,86]

Table 2
Overview of selected ultrafiltration clinical trials

Study Name, Publication Year	Patient Population	UF Arm	Comparison Arm	Primary Efficacy End Point	Primary End Point Result	Reported Clinical Outcomes	Mortality	Adverse Events
UNLOAD, 2007[78]	N = 200 Hospitalized with HF, ≥2 signs of fluid overload	Aquadex System 100[a] Mean fluid-removal rate 241 mL/h for 12.3 ± 12 h	Standard care: intravenous diuretics. For each 24-h period at least twice the prehospitalization daily oral dose	Weight loss and dyspnea assessment at 48 h after randomization	Weight loss: 5.0 ± 3.1 (UF) vs 3.1 ± 3.5 kg (standard care), P = .001 Dyspnea score: 5.4 ± 1.1 (UF) vs 5.2 ± 1.2 (standard care), P = .588	90 d: HF rehospitalization: 18% (UF) vs 32% (standard care), P = .022; HR 0.56, 95% CI 0.28–0.51, P = .04 Unscheduled clinic/ emergency visits: 21% (UF) vs 44% (standard care), P = .009	90 d: 9(9.6%) UF vs 11 (11.6) standard care	No significant between group differences, except bleeding (1 UF vs 7 standard care, P = .032). UF group: 1 catheter infection, 5 filter clotting events, 1 patient transitioned to hemodialysis due to insufficient response to UF
CARRESS-HF, 2012[79]	N = 188 Hospitalized with HF, ≥2 signs of congestion, and recent ≥0.3 mg/dL sCr increase	Aquadex System 100[a] at a fixed rate of 200 mL/h Median duration 40 h	SPT with intravenous diuretics dosed to maintain urine output 3–5 L/d	Bivariate response of change in sCr and change in weight 96 h after randomization	Mean sCr change: +0.23 ± 0.70 mg/dL (UF) vs −0.04 ± 0.53 mg/dL (SPT) Mean weight loss: 5.7 ± 3.9 (UF) vs 5.5 ± 5.1 kg (SPT), P = .58	Crossover: STP: 6 patients STP: (6%) also received UF (2 before 96 h) UF: 8 patients (9%) received diuretics instead of UF: 28 patients (30%) also received diuretics before 96 h 7 d: No difference in death, worsening or persistent HF, hemodialysis, SAE, or crossover (23% UF vs 18% SPT, P = .45) 60 d HF hospitalization 26% (UF) vs 26% (SPT) P = .97	60 d: 17% UF vs 13% SPT, P = .47	60-d SAE: 72% UF vs 57% SPT, P = .03, attributed to renal failure, bleeding, or catheter complications

(continued on next page)

Table 2
(continued)

Study Name, Publication Year	Patient Population	UF Arm	Comparison Arm	Primary Efficacy End Point	Primary End Point Result	Reported Clinical Outcomes	Mortality	Adverse Events
CUORE, 2014[82]	N = 56 NYHA III or IV, LVEF ≤40%, ≥4 kg weight gain from peripheral fluid overload, over 2 mo	Dedyca device[b] Mean treatment duration 19 ± 90 h, volume removed 4254 ± 4842 mL	Intravenous diuretics according to guideline recommendations (standard care)	HF rehospitalization at 1 y	3 (11%) UF vs 14 (48%) standard care; HR 0.14, 95% CI 0.04–0.48, P = .002	Length of index hospitalization: 7.4 ± 4.6 (UF) vs 9.1 ± 1.9 d (standard care), P = .23 Combined death or HF rehospitalization HR for UF vs standard care 0.35, 95% CI 0.15–0.69, P = .0035	1-y: 7 (26%) UF vs 11 (38%) standard care, P = .33	Premature clotting of filter in 6 patients
AVOID-HF, 2016[86]	N = 224 Hospitalized with HF; ≥2 criteria for fluid overload; receiving daily oral loop diuretics	AUF with Aquadex FlexFlow System[c]; adjustment per protocol guidelines based on vital signs and renal function Mean fluid-removal rate 138 ± 47 mL/h for 80 ± 53 h	ALD with adjustment per protocol guidelines based on vital signs and renal function Mean furosemide-equivalent dose 271.26 ± 263.06 mg for 100 ± 78 h	Time to first HF event (HF rehospitalization or unscheduled outpatient or emergency treatment with intravenous loop diuretics or UF) within 90 d of hospital discharge	25% AUF vs 35% ALD (P = .11); HR 0.66%, 95% CI 0.4–1.1	Length of index hospitalization: median 6 (AUF) vs 5 (ALD) days, P = .106 30-d HF rehospitalizations/d at risk: 11/2876 (AUF) vs 24/2882 (ALD), P = .06 30-d CV rehospitalizations/d at risk: 17/2882 (AUF) vs 33/2891 (ALD), P = .037 For both HF and CV events: fewer patients re-hospitalized; fewer number of days re-hospitalized/d at risk	90 d 15% AUF vs 13% ALD, P = .83	At least 1 SAE: 66% (AUF) vs 60% (ALD), P = .4 SAEs of special interest: 23% (AUF) vs 14% (ALD), P = .122 Related SAEs: 14.6% (UF) vs 5.4% (ALD), P = .026

Abbreviations: ALD, adjustable loop diuretic agent; AUF, adjustable ultrafiltration; CI, confidence interval; HF, heart failure; HR, hazard ratio; LVEF, left ventricular ejection fraction; NYHA, New York Heart Association; SAE, serious adverse event; sCr, serum creatinine; SPT, stepped pharmacologic therapy; UF, ultrafiltration.
[a] CHF solutions, Minneapolis, MN, USA.
[b] Dellco, Mirandola, Italy.
[c] Baxter International, Deerfield, IL, USA.

NOVEL STRATEGIES TO OVERCOME DIURETIC RESISTANCE

Novel methods to decongest diuretic-resistant HF patients with fluid overload and the cardiorenal syndrome are outlined in **Fig. 4**.

Controlled Diuresis

The Reprieve Cardiovascular (Reprieve Cardiovascular, Milford, MA) therapy is designed to maintain venous return in a controlled manner to prevent intravascular hypovolemia and consequent neurohormonal activation. The device replaces a physician-set portion of urine volume generated by the patient in response to diuretics. The partial, controlled replacement of volume may allow intravascular volume to be maintained at an optimal level. Pilot studies with this technology are ongoing in Poland.[90]

Peritoneal Ultrafiltration Methods

Direct peritoneal sodium removal
Traditional peritoneal dialysis solutions have sodium concentrations nearly isotonic to plasma, so that sodium removal is almost entirely driven by solute drag with UF rather than diffusion down a concentration gradient. A novel approach consists in the use of a salt-free peritoneal solution and the eventual combination with a fully implanted, automatic, programmable pump that can be charged transcutaneously, adjusted wirelessly, and equipped with a catheter that can deliver the salt-rich fluid generated by the concentration gradient directly to the bladder. Preclinical studies show that direct peritoneal sodium removal can withdraw large amounts of fluid and sodium with relatively small intraperitoneal volumes.[91]

Hydrostatic pressure gradient ultrafiltration device
This novel approach consists of the implantation of a permeable absorption chamber in the peritoneum. A pump induces a negative hydrostatic pressure in the absorption chamber, triggering UF of fluid through the peritoneal membranes into the chamber. A microcatheter draining fluid from the absorption chamber is routed to a percutaneous port. Ongoing work will enable drainage of the accumulated extracellular fluid into the urinary system.[92]

"Decongestive Pumps"

The Aortix device (Procyrion, Houston, TX) is a catheter-deployed pump that is placed in the descending aorta and decouples the heart and the kidneys, with the aim of resting the heart while improving RBF. First-in-man use in patients undergoing high-risk percutaneous coronary intervention showed improvement in hemodynamics and urine output.[93]

The transcatheter renal venous decongestion system (Magenta Medical, Kadima, Israel) consists in the placement of a small continuous flow pump in each renal vein to directly reduce renal venous pressure. This should result in improved responsiveness to diuretics and, therefore, greater diuresis and natriuresis.

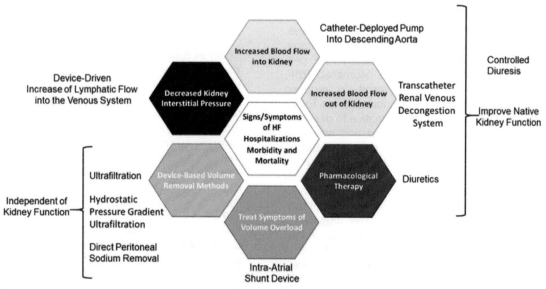

Fig. 4. Novel strategies to overcome diuretic resistance. HF, heart failure.

Preclinical data support this therapeutic concept. A European multicenter clinical trial is ongoing.[94]

The novel methods outlined herein underscore the evolution in fluid management of congestive HF patients. The focus is shifting from the unpredictable removal of hypotonic fluid by diuretics to decongestive methods that avoid intravascular volume depletion and consequent renal hypoperfusion.

The novel fluid-management methods have variable degrees of invasiveness, ranging from the requirement of a peripheral venous access and a urinary catheter to that for intravascular and intraperitoneal implant procedures. Overall novel fluid-management therapies are at an early stage of development, with some still in preclinical trials and others having been studied in first-in-man trials with a small number of subjects. Further investigation of novel fluid-management methods should focus on assessment of safety, ease of use, candidate selection, reproducibility of effects across HF populations, and costs.

SUMMARY

In HF, fluid overload is the main culprit of mutually harmful and self-perpetuating interactions between the heart and the kidney, which cause disease progression and poor outcomes. In acute HF, transient elevations of sCr represent a physiologic response to fluid removal and should not trigger discontinuation of symptom-improving and/or life-saving decongestive therapies. Accurate quantitative measurement of fluid volume is vital to individualizing therapy for congestive HF patients. BV analysis and PA pressure monitoring appear to be the most reliable methods to assess fluid volume and guide decongestive therapies. Still the cornerstone of decongestive therapy, diuretics' effectiveness decreases with HF progression. Impaired absorption, decreased RBF, azotemia, and proteinuria result in reduced diuretic concentrations in the tubular lumen. Extracorporeal ultrafiltration, an alternative to diuretics, removes fluid isotonic to plasma and has been shown to reduce HF events in some studies. Fluid-removal rates by UF should be adjusted according to patients' hemodynamic and renal profiles. Research on new fluid-management technologies should focus on safety, ease of use, candidate selection, and cost. The urgency of these investigations is underscored by the alarming prognostic and economic implications of recurrent HF hospitalizations, which remain unacceptably high with conventional pharmacologic therapies.

REFERENCES

1. Ronco C, Haapio M, House AA, et al. Cardiorenal syndrome. J Am Coll Cardiol 2008;52:1527–39.
2. Damman K, Valente MA, Voors AA, et al. Renal impairment, worsening renal function, and outcome in patients with heart failure: an updated meta-analysis. Eur Heart J 2014;35:455–69.
3. Dries DL, Exner DV, Domanski MJ, et al. The prognostic implications of renal insufficiency in asymptomatic and symptomatic patients with left ventricular systolic dysfunction. J Am Coll Cardiol 2000;35:681–9.
4. Hillege HL, Girbes AR, de Kam PJ, et al. Renal function, neurohormonal activation, and survival in patients with chronic heart failure. Circulation 2000; 102:203–10.
5. Costanzo MR, Ronco C, Abraham WT, et al. Extracorporeal ultrafiltration for fluid overload in heart failure: current status and prospects for further research. J Am Coll Cardiol 2017;69:2428–45.
6. Brisco MA, Zile MR, Hanberg JS, et al. Relevance of changes in serum creatinine during a heart failure trial of decongestive strategies: insights from the DOSE trial. J Card Fail 2016;22:753–60.
7. Ahmad T, Jackson K, Rao VS, et al. Worsening renal function in acute heart failure patients undergoing aggressive diuresis is not associated with tubular injury. Circulation 2018;137:2016–28.
8. Levey AS, Inker LA. Assessment of glomerular filtration rate in health and disease: a state of the art review. Clin Pharmacol Ther 2017;102:405–19.
9. Bragadottir G, Redfors B, Ricksten SE. Assessing glomerular filtration rate (GFR) in critically ill patients with acute kidney injury–true GFR versus urinary creatinine clearance and estimating equations. Crit Care 2013;17:R108.
10. Kidney Disease: Improving Global Outcomes (KDIGO) Acute Kidney Injury Work Group. KDIGO clinical practice guideline for acute kidney injury. Kidney Int Suppl 2012;2:1–138.
11. Xu K, Rosenstiel P, Paragas N, et al. Unique transcriptional programs identify subtypes of AKI. J Am Soc Nephrol 2017;28:1729–40.
12. Nickolas TL, Schmidt-Ott KM, Canetta P, et al. Diagnostic and prognostic stratification in the emergency department using urinary bio markers of nephron damage: a multicenter prospective cohort study. J Am Coll Cardiol 2012;59:246–55.
13. Barasch J, Zager R, Bonventre JV. Acute kidney injury: a problem of definition. Lancet 2017;389:779–81.
14. Waikar SS, Betensky RA, Emerson SC, et al. Imperfect gold standards for kidney injury biomarker evaluation. J Am Soc Nephrol 2012;23:13–21.
15. Costanzo MR. Verdict in: congestion guilty! JACC Heart Fail 2015;3:762–4.

16. Miller WL. Fluid volume overload and congestion in heart failure. time to reconsider pathophysiology and how volume is assessed. Circ Heart Fail 2016; 9:e002922.

17. Schrier RW. Body fluid volume regulation in health and disease: a unifying hypothesis. Ann Intern Med 1990;113:155–9.

18. Rothe CF. Reflex control of veins and vascular capacitance. Physiol Rev 1983;63:1281–342.

19. Miller WL, Mullan BP. Understanding the heterogeneity in volume overload and fluid distribution in decompensated heart failure is key to optimal volume management: role for blood volume quantitation. JACC Heart Fail 2014;2:298–305.

20. Seymour WB, Pritchard WH, Longley LP, et al. Cardiac output, blood and interstitial fluid volumes, total circulating serum protein, and kidney function during cardiac failure and after improvement. J Clin Invest 1942;21:229–40.

21. Setoguchi S, Stevenson LW, Schneeweiss S. Repeated hospitalizations predict mortality in the community population with heart failure. Am Heart J 2007;154:260–6.

22. Androne SA, Hryniewicz K, Hudaihed A, et al. Relation of unrecognized hypervolemia in chronic heart failure to clinical status, hemodynamics, and patient outcomes. Am J Cardiol 2004;93: 1254–9.

23. Cotter G, Metra M, Milo-Cotter O, et al. Fluid overload in acute heart failure—re-distribution and other mechanisms beyond fluid accumulation. Eur J Heart Fail 2008;10:165–9.

24. Metra M, Dei Cas L, Bristow MR. The pathophysiology of acute heart failure—it is a lot about fluid accumulation. Am Heart J 2008;155:1–5.

25. Gheorghiade M, Filippatos G, De Luca L, et al. Congestion in acute heart failure syndromes: an essential target of evaluation and treatment. Am J Med 2006;119(12 suppl 1):S3–10.

26. Tyberg JV. How changes in venous capacitance modulate cardiac output. Pflugers Arch 2002;445: 10–7.

27. Fallick C, Sobotka PA, Dunlap ME. Sympathetically mediated changes in capacitance: redistribution of the venous reservoir as a cause of decompensation. Circ Heart Fail 2011;4:669–75.

28. Sharma R, Francis DP, Pitt B, et al. Haemoglobin predicts survival in patients with chronic heart failure: a substudy of the ELITE II trial. Eur Heart J 2004;25:1021–8.

29. Gagnon DR, Zhang TJ, Brand FN, et al. Hematocrit and the risk of cardiovascular disease—the Framingham study: a 34-year follow-up. Am Heart J 1994;127:674–82.

30. Androne AS, Katz SD, Lund L, et al. Hemodilution is common in patients with advanced heart failure. Circulation 2003;107:226–9.

31. Verbrugge FH, Dupont M, Steels P, et al. The kidney in congestive heart failure: "are natriuresis, sodium, and diuretics really the good, the bad and the ugly?". Eur J Heart Fail 2014;16:133–42.

32. Lote CJ, Snape BM. Collecting duct flow rate as a determinant of equilibration between urine and renal papilla in the rat in the presence of a maximal antidiuretic hormone concentration. J Physiol 1977;270: 533–44.

33. Allen GG, Barratt LJ. Effect of aldosterone on the transepithelial potential difference of the rat distal tubule. Kidney Int 1981;19:678–86.

34. Woodhall PB, Tisher CC. Response of the distal tubule and cortical collecting duct to vasopressin in the rat. J Clin Invest 1973;52:3095–108.

35. Schreier RW, Abraham WT. Hormones and hemodynamics in heart failure. N Engl J Med 1999;341: 577–85.

36. Verbrugge FH, Dupont M, Steels P, et al. Abdominal contributions to cardiorenal dysfunction in congestive heart failure. J Am Coll Cardiol 2013;62:485–95.

37. Aukland K, Reed RK. Interstitial-lymphatic mechanisms in the control of extracellular fluid volume. Physiol Rev 1993;73:1–78.

38. Guyton AC. Interstitial fluid pressure. II. Pressure-volume curves of interstitial space. Circ Res 1965; 16:452–60.

39. Sandek A, Rauchhaus M, Anker SD, et al. The emerging role of the gut in chronic heart failure. Curr Opin Clin Nutr Metab Care 2008;11:632–9.

40. Manzone TA, Dam HQ, Soltis D, et al. Blood volume analysis: a new technique and new clinical interest reinvigorate a classic study. J Nucl Med Technol 2007;35:55–63.

41. Strobeck JE, Feldshuh J, Miller WL. Heart failure outcomes with volume-guided management. JACC Heart Fail 2018;6:940–8.

42. Bera TK. Bioelectrical impedance methods for noninvasive health monitoring: a review. J Med Eng 2014. https://doi.org/10.1155/2014/381251.

43. Shotan A, Blondheim DS, Kazatsker M, et al. Noninvasive lung IMPEDANCE-guided preemptive treatment in chronic heart failure patients: a randomized controlled trial (IMPEDANCE-HF trial). J Card Fail 2016;22:713–22.

44. Burkhoff D. Bioimpedance: has its time finally come. J Card Fail 2016;22:723–4.

45. Drazner MH, Rame JE, Stevenson LW, et al. Prognostic importance of elevated jugular venous pressure and a third heart sound in patients with heart failure. N Engl J Med 2001;345:574–81.

46. Zile MR, Bennett TD, St. John Sutton M, et al. Transition from chronic compensated to acute decompensated heart failure: pathophysiological insights obtained from continuous monitoring of intracardiac pressures. Circulation 2008;118: 1433–41.

47. Abraham WT, Stough WG, Piña IL, et al. Trials of implantable monitoring devices in heart failure: which design is optimal? Nat Rev Cardiol 2014;11: 576–85.

48. Stevenson LW, Zile M, Bennett TD, et al. Chronic ambulatory intracardiac pressures and future heart failure events. Circ Heart Fail 2010;3:580–7.

49. Adamson PB, Abraham WT, Aaron M, et al. CHAMPION trial rationale and design: the longterm safety and clinical efficacy of a wireless pulmonary artery pressure monitoring system. J Card Fail 2011;17:3–10.

50. Abraham WT, Adamson PB, Bourge RC, et al. Wireless pulmonary artery haemodynamic monitoring in chronic heart failure: a randomized controlled trial. Lancet 2011;377:658–66.

51. Costanzo MR, Stevenson LW, Adamson PB, et al. Interventions linked to decreased heart failure hospitalizations during ambulatory pulmonary artery pressure monitoring. JACC Heart Fail 2016;4: 333–44.

52. Givertz MM, Stevenson LW, Costanzo MR, et al, on behalf of the CHAMPION Trial Investigators. Pulmonary artery pressure-guided management of patients with heart failure and reduced ejection fraction. J Am Coll Cardiol 2017;70:1875–86.

53. Adamson PB, Abraham WT, Bourge RC, et al. Wireless pulmonary artery pressure monitoring guides management to reduce decompensation in heart failure with preserved ejection fraction. Circ Heart Fail 2014;7:935–44.

54. Heywood JT, Jermyn R, Shavelle D, et al. Impact of practice-based management of pulmonary artery pressures in 2000 patients implanted with the CardioMEMS sensor. Circulation 2017;135: 1509–17.

55. Desai AS, Bhimaraj A, Bharmi R, et al. Ambulatory hemodynamic monitoring reduces heart failure hospitalizations in "real-world" clinical practice. J Am Coll Cardiol 2017;69:2357–65.

56. Yu CM, Wang L, Chau E, et al. Intrathoracic impedance monitoring in patients with heart failure: correlation with fluid status and feasibility of early warning preceding hospitalization. Circulation 2005;112: 841–8.

57. van Veldhuisen DJ, Braunschweig F, Conraads V, et al, for the DOT-HF Investigators. Intrathoracic impedance monitoring, audible patient alerts, and outcome in patients with heart failure. Circulation 2011;124:1719–26.

58. Boehmer JP, Hariharan R, Devecchi FG, et al. A multisensor algorithm predicts heart failure events in patients with implanted devices: results from the MultiSENSE Study. JACC Heart Fail 2017;5:216–25.

59. Costanzo MR. The luck of having a cardiac implantable electronic device. Circ Heart Fail 2018. https:// doi.org/10.1161/CIRCHEARTFAILURE.118.004894.

60. Price S, Platz E, Cullen L, et al. for the Acute Heart Failure Study Group of the European Society of Cardiology Acute Cardiovascular Care Association Echocardiography and lung ultrasonography for the assessment and management of acute heart failure. Nat Rev Cardiol 2017;14:422–40.

61. Platz E, Hempel D, Pivetta E, et al. Echocardiographic and lung ultrasound characteristics in ambulatory patients with dyspnea or prior heart failure. Echocardiography 2014;31:133–9.

62. Trezzi M, Torzillo D, Ceriani E, et al. Lung ultrasonography for the assessment of rapid extravascular water variation: evidence from hemodialysis patients. Intern Emerg Med 2013;8:409–15.

63. Volpicelli G, Caramello V, Cardinale L, et al. Bedside ultrasound of the lung for the monitoring of acute decompensated heart failure. Am J Emerg Med 2008; 26:585–91.

64. Gargani L, Frassi F, Soldati G, et al. Ultrasound lung comets for the differential diagnosis of acute cardiogenic dyspnoea: a comparison with natriuretic peptides. Eur J Heart Fail 2008;10:70–7.

65. Guiotto G, Masarone M, Paladino F, et al. Inferior vena cava collapsibility to guide fluid removal in slow continuous ultrafiltration: a pilot study. Intensive Care Med 2010;36:692–6.

66. Blehar DJ, Dickman E, Gaspari R. Identification of congestive heart failure via respiratory variation of inferior vena cava diameter. Am J Emerg Med 2009;27:71–5.

67. Bayes-Genis A, Lupón J, Jaffe AS. Can natriuretic peptides be used to guide therapy? EJIFCC 2016; 27:208–16.

68. Felker GM, Ahmad T, Anstronm KJ, et al. Rationale and design of the GUIDE-IT study; guiding evidence based therapy using biomarker intensified treatment in heart failure. JACC Heart Fail 2014; 2:457–65.

69. Singh D, Shrestha K, Testani JM, et al. Insufficient natriuretic response to continuous intravenous furosemide is associated with poor long-term outcomes in acute decompensated heart failure. J Card Fail 2014;20:392–9.

70. ter Maaten JM, Valente MA, Damman K, et al. Diuretic response in acute heart failure—pathophysiology, evaluation, and therapy. Nat Rev Cardiol 2015;12:184–92.

71. Voors AA, Davison BA, Teerlink JR, et al, for the RELAX-AHF investigators. Diuretic response in patients with acute decompensated heart failure: characteristics and clinical outcome—an analysis from RELAX-AHF. Eur J Heart Fail 2014;16:1230–40.

72. Gheorghiade M, Filippatos G. Reassessing treatment of acute heart failure syndromes: the ADHERE registry. Eur Heart J Suppl 2005;7:B13–9.

73. Felker GM, Lee KL, Bull DA, et al, for the NHLBI Heart Failure Clinical Research Network. Diuretic

strategies in patients with acute decompensated heart failure. N Engl J Med 2011;364:797–805.

74. Konstam MA, Gheorghiade M, Burnett JC Jr, et al, for the Efficacy of Vasopressin Antagonism in Heart Failure Outcome Study With Tolvaptan (EVEREST) investigators. Effects of oral tolvaptan in patients hospitalized for worsening heart failure: the EVEREST outcome trial. JAMA 2007;297:1319–31.

75. Massie BM, O'Connor CM, Metra M, et al, for the PROTECT investigators and committees. Rolofylline, an adenosine A1-receptor antagonist, in acute heart failure. N Engl J Med 2010;363:1419–28.

76. O'Connor CM, Starling RC, Hernandez AF, et al. Effect of nesiritide in patients with acute decompensated heart failure. N Engl J Med 2011;365(365):32–43.

77. Ronco C, Ricci Z, Bellomo R, et al. Extracorporeal ultrafiltration for the treatment of overhydration and congestive heart failure. Cardiology 2001;96:155–68.

78. Costanzo MR, Guglin ME, Saltzberg MT, et al, for the UNLOAD trial investigators. Ultrafiltration versus intravenous diuretics for patients hospitalized for acute decompensated heart failure. J Am Coll Cardiol 2007;49:675–83.

79. Grodin JL, Carter S, Bart BA, et al. Direct comparison of ultrafiltration to pharmacological decongestion in heart failure: a per-protocol analysis of CARRESS-HF. Eur J Heart Fail 2018;20:1148–56.

80. Bart BA, Goldsmith SR, Lee KL, et al, for the Heart Failure Clinical Research Network. Ultrafiltration in decompensated heart failure with cardiorenal syndrome. N Engl J Med 2012;367:2296–304.

81. Costanzo MR, Kazory A. Better late than never: the true results of CARRESS-HF. Eur J Heart Fail 2018;20:1157–9.

82. Marenzi G, Muratori M, Cosentino ER, et al. Continuous ultrafiltration for congestive heart failure: the CUORE trial. J Card Fail 2014;20:9–17.

83. Lorenz JN, Weihprecht H, Schnermann J, et al. Renin release from isolated juxtaglomerular apparatus depends on macula densa chloride transport. Am J Physiol 1991;260:F486–93.

84. Schlatter E, Salomonsson M, Persson AE, et al. Macula densa cells sense luminal NaCl concentration via furosemide sensitive $Na^+2Cl^-K^+$ cotransport. Pflugers Arch 1989;414:286–90.

85. Costanzo MR, Negoianu D, Fonarow GC, et al. Rationale and design of the Aquapheresis Versus Intravenous Diuretics and Hospitalization for Heart Failure (AVOID-HF) trial. Am Heart J 2015;170l:471–82.

86. Costanzo MR, Negoianu D, Jaski BE, et al. Aquapheresis versus intravenous diuretics and hospitalizations for heart failure. JACC Heart Fail 2016;4:95–105.

87. Ponikowski P, Voors AA, Anker SD, et al. 2016 ESC guidelines for the diagnosis and treatment of acute and chronic heart failure: the task force for the diagnosis and treatment of acute and chronic heart failure of the European Society of Cardiology (ESC). Developed with the special contribution of the Heart Failure Association (HFA) of the ESC. Eur Heart J 2016;37:2129–200.

88. Yancy CW, Jessup M, Bozkurt B, et al. 2013 ACCF/AHA guideline for the management of heart failure: a report of the American College of Cardiology Foundation/American Heart Association task force on practice guidelines. J Am Coll Cardiol 2013;62:e147–239.

89. Schrier RW, Bansal S. Pulmonary hypertension, right ventricular failure, and kidney: different from left ventricular failure? Clin J Am Soc Nephrol 2008;3:1232–7.

90. Available at: https://reprievecardio.com/. Accessed February 28, 2019.

91. Mahoney D, Rao V, Asher J, et al. Development of a direct peritoneal sodium removal technique with salt-free solution. J Card Fail 2018;24:S34.

92. Feld Y, Hanani H, Costanzo MR. Hydrostatic pressure gradient ultrafiltration device: a novel approach for extracellular fluid removal. J Heart Lung Transplant 2018;37:794–6.

93. Vora AN, Schuyler Jones W, DeVore AD, et al. First-in-human experience with Aortix intraaortic pump. Catheter Cardiovasc Interv 2019;93:428–33.

94. Available at: http://www.magentamed.com/. Accessed February 28, 2019.

Hypertension and Heart Failure
Prevention, Targets, and Treatment

Katherine E. Di Palo, PharmD*, Nicholas J. Barone, BS

KEYWORDS

- Hypertension • Heart failure • Risk reduction • Pharmacotherapy

KEY POINTS

- Given the overt risk of cardiovascular disease development when blood pressure is left uncontrolled, it is imperative to view hypertension as pre–heart failure.
- The complex nature of cardiac remodeling attributed to hypertension can result in diastolic and systolic dysfunction.
- Although all antihypertensive pharmacologic agents inherently decrease blood pressure, there are noted differences between drug classes regarding ability to reduce risk of heart failure onset or progression.

INTRODUCTION

Heart failure continues to represent a major public health burden with prevalence expecting to increase by 46% from 2012 to 2030, resulting in more than 8 million US adults with heart failure.[1] Hypertension is possibly the most powerful, modifiable risk factor for the development of heart failure. In the Framingham Heart Study, hypertension predated disease in 91% of all patients with newly diagnosed heart failure during 20 years of follow-up.[2] Although diastolic dysfunction and heart failure with preserved ejection fraction (HFpEF) are the most common cardiac complications, hypertension also increases risk for myocardial infarction and subsequent heart failure with reduced ejection fraction (HFrEF). Hypertension treatment has been proven to prevent and decrease many clinical presentations related to heart failure, such as increased left ventricular hypertrophy (LVH) and left ventricular mass. This article focuses on mechanistic links, therapeutic goals, and treatment of patients with comorbid hypertension and heart failure.

EPIDEMIOLOGY

Using the new blood pressure threshold of 130 to 139/80 to 89 mm Hg from the 2017 American College of Cardiology (ACC)/American Heart Association (AHA) Hypertension Guidelines it is estimated from 2011 to 2014 National Health and Nutritional Examination Survey (NHANES) data that almost half of US adults 20 years of age or older have hypertension.[1,3] Severe increases in blood pressure directly correlate with higher risks of developing heart failure: the lifetime risk of heart failure doubles in patients with blood pressure greater than or equal to 160/100 mm Hg compared with those with blood pressure less than 140/90 mm Hg.[4] This risk translates to approximately 1 out of every 3 or 4 adults developing heart failure when blood pressure is greater than 160 mm Hg.[5] Similarly, patients with mild hypertension have a 2-fold to 3-fold increased risk of developing LVH compared with normotensive patients, whereas patients with the greatest severity of hypertension have a 10-fold risk.[6] Registry data, epidemiologic studies, and clinical trials signal that hypertension is the

This article originally appeared in *Heart Failure Clinics*, Volume 16, Issue 1, January 2020.
Disclosure: The authors have nothing to disclose.
Office of the Medical Director, Montefiore Medical Center, 111 East 210th Street, Bronx, NY 10467, USA
* Corresponding author.
E-mail address: kdipalo@montefiore.org

Cardiol Clin 40 (2022) 237–244
https://doi.org/10.1016/j.ccl.2021.12.011

most important cause of HFpEF, with a prevalence of 60%–89%.[7]

Differences in hypertension and heart failure incidence based on race, age, and sex are also noted. In the United States, black patients have the highest rate of hypertension, which is more causative of heart failure, in particular HFpEF, than coronary artery disease in this patient population.[8] Black and Hispanic patients also have poorer rates of blood pressure control resulting in longer risk factor exposure.[9] The occurrence of both hypertension and LVH increase significantly with age.[10] LVH is noted in nearly 33% of the male population and 50% of the female population more than 70 years of age.[11] Data from the Framingham Heart Study showed that the hazard for developing heart failure in hypertensive men was about 2-fold compared with 3-fold in hypertensive women, and the population attributable risk for heart failure imparted by hypertension was estimated to be 39% in men and 59% in women.[2] Older women with a long-standing hypertensive history are more likely to present with HFpEF.[12] Although 5-year mortality after initial diagnosis of heart failure is 50%, the combined presence of hypertension and heart failure is associated with even worse outcomes.[1] After the onset of hypertensive heart failure, 5-year mortality is 76% and 69% for men and women respectively.[13]

FROM HYPERTENSION TO HEART FAILURE

The progression from hypertension to heart failure is complex and multifaceted. Briefly, the four degrees of hypertensive heart disease as described by Messerli and colleagues[14] are (1) isolated diastolic dysfunction, (2) diastolic dysfunction with LVH, (3) HFpEF, and (4) HFrEF. Chronic hypertension is the most common cause of asymptomatic diastolic dysfunction, which encompasses abnormalities in diastolic filling, distensibility, or relaxation of the left ventricle (LV).[15] Pressure and volume overload cause different types of LV remodeling and pathophysiologic developments.[14] Cardiac remodeling as a response to principal pressure overload consists of increased cardiac mass at the expense of chamber volume caused by the parallel addition of sarcomeres resulting in concentric LVH. In contrast, cardiac remodeling as a response to principal volume overload consists of increased cardiac mass and chamber volume caused by serial addition of sarcomeres resulting in eccentric LV hypertrophy. These dichotomous remodeling patterns seem to be equally common in patients with hypertension.[16]

The link between hypertension and heart failure is also rooted in changes in the renin-angiotensin-aldosterone system (RAAS), which is overactivated by LV systolic wall stress and further contributes to cardiac hypertrophy. In addition, the sympathetic nervous system plays an idiopathic role in LVH, overt vasoconstriction, and retention of electrolytes such as sodium.[17] Once LVH develops, the risk of developing HFpEF and HFrEF increases dramatically.[18] HFpEF is the more common progression of long-standing hypertension given that diastolic dysfunction is the initial stage of hypertensive heart disease. However, a subset of patients develop systolic dysfunction, which may be the result of a so-called second hit as proposed by Borlaug and Redfield,[19] with an ischemic event often instigating the progression from HFpEF to HFrEF. The presence of hypertension has both a causal and continuous impact on myocardial infarction because risk increases with age and severity.[6] The proposed relationship between hypertension, cardiac remodeling, and heart failure is summarized in **Fig. 1**.

BLOOD PRESSURE TARGETS

Given the overt risk of cardiovascular disease development when blood pressure is left uncontrolled, it is imperative to view hypertension as pre–heart failure. The Staging Classification of Heart Failure (A, B, C, D) introduced by ACC/AHA in 2003 specifically draws attention to the preventive nature of heart failure and the importance of risk factor management.[5,20] For patients with stage A, those at high risk but without structural heart disease or symptoms, chronic pharmacotherapy to reduce both systolic and diastolic hypertension is crucial and has been shown to reduce the risk of incident heart failure by approximately 50%.[21,22] More specifically, a meta-analysis by Verdecchia and colleagues[23] reported that, for each 5-mm Hg reduction in systolic blood pressure (SBP), the risk for heart failure decreases by 24%. Similar results were seen in a meta-analysis by Ettehad and colleagues,[24] with every 10-mm Hg reduction SBP significantly reducing the risk of heart failure by 28%.

The results of SPRINT (Systolic Blood Pressure Intervention Trial) revealed a significant reduction in major cardiovascular events, including a 38% lower relative risk of heart failure, by achieving a blood pressure target of less than 120/80 mm Hg among certain patients with high cardiovascular risk.[25] Other findings included greater reduction in LVH as well as resolution of LVH. Stemming from these landmark results, blood pressure goals shifted from conservative

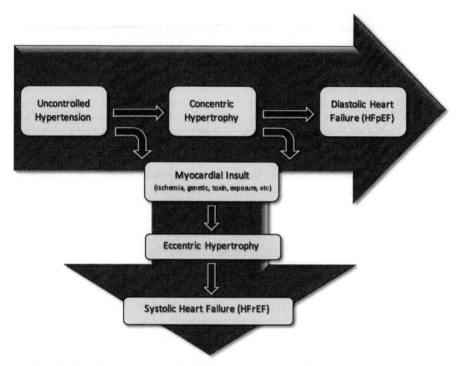

Fig. 1. Proposed mechanism for the progression of hypertensive heart disease to HFpEF or HFrEF. (*Modified from Borlaug BA, Redfield MM. Diastolic and systolic heart failure are distinct phenotypes within the heart failure spectrum. Circulation 2011;123(18).*)

(eg, 140/90 mm Hg) toward more aggressive control. The 2017 Focused Update of the 2013 Heart Failure Guidelines included a new section on treating hypertension to reduce the incidence of heart failure as well as treating hypertension in stage C HFrEF and HFpEF. A target of less than 130/80 mm Hg is recommended for all 3 groups and the threshold for therapy initiation is blood pressure greater than or equal to 130/80 mm Hg.[3,26] This target and threshold is also recommended in the 2017 High Blood Pressure Clinical Practice Guideline for patients with other comorbidities such as diabetes mellitus, chronic kidney disease, peripheral artery disease, and stable ischemic heart disease.[3]

Note that randomized clinical trials (RCTs) targeting intensive blood pressure control have not been studied in the heart failure population and SPRINT excluded patients with an ejection fraction less than 35% or a history of symptomatic heart failure within 6 months. The J-shaped relationship between SBP and mortality in hypertensive and high-risk patients, including those with heart failure, has been debated for decades.[27–29] Observational analyses have provided conflicting results. An evaluation of BEST (Beta-Blocker Evaluation of Survival Trial) found an increased risk of heart failure hospitalization, but not all-cause mortality,

in patients with HFrEF with an SBP less than 120 mm Hg.[30] A recent examination of the OPTIMIZE-HF (Organized Program to Initiate Lifesaving Treatment in Hospitalized Patients with Heart Failure) registry compared 30-day, 1-year, and overall all-cause mortality in hospitalized patients with HFpEF discharged with an SBP of less than 120 mm Hg versus 120 mm Hg or greater.[31] Lower SBP on discharge was associated with significantly higher risk of all mortality end points in addition to higher risk of heart failure readmission at 30 days. However, the exact cause of this phenomenon is unknown and may be affected by frailty, comorbidities, older age, and more advanced disease severity.[32]

PHARMACOTHERAPY

Although all antihypertensive pharmacologic agents inherently decrease blood pressure, there are noted differences between drug classes regarding ability to reduce risk of heart failure onset or progression. More importantly, there are drug classes that may predispose or exacerbate heart failure and should be avoided when possible. Primary prevention by effectively treating hypertension is the most effective method to divert physiologic remodeling and heart failure.

A meta-analysis of antihypertensive treatment ranked thiazidelike diuretics, angiotensin-converting enzyme (ACE) inhibitors, and angiotensin II receptor blockers (ARBs) to be most effective in preventing new-onset heart failure.[21] Calcium channel blockers (CCBs) and β-blockers were significantly inferior to diuretics and tended to be inferior to ACE inhibitors and ARBs. Secondary outcomes of ALLHAT (Antihypertensive and Lipid-Lowering Treatment to Prevent Heart Attack Trial) examined the role of chlorthalidone, lisinopril, and amlodipine in preventing heart failure.[33] During year 1 of treatment, there was a higher rate of incident heart failure with amlodipine and lisinopril versus chlorthalidone. After 1 year of treatment, risk continued to remain decreased in patients receiving chlorthalidone compared with amlodipine, but longer use of lisinopril was shown to have equivalent risk to chlorthalidone. Results showing the effectiveness of chlorthalidone in reducing LVH was also seen in TOMHS (Treatment of Mild Hypertension Study), which again compared the diuretic with amlodipine and lisinopril as well as doxazosin and acebutolol.[34] Given the prolonged-half life and proven trial data signaling the reduction of heart failure in additional to other cardiovascular diseases, such as stroke, chlorthalidone is the preferential thiazide diuretic, especially because no outcome data are available for hydrochlorothiazide.[3] In patients with stage B heart failure with structural heart disease or LV dysfunction but without heart failure symptoms, β-blockers can reverse remodeling and improve LV function.[35] ACE inhibitors and ARBs can prevent symptomatic heart failure in this setting as well.[36,37] Although sacubitril/valsartan is currently only US Food and Drug Administration approved for the treatment of HFrEF, promising results indicating its effectiveness at blood pressure reduction in patients without heart failure have emerged. Compared with valsartan alone, sacubitril/valsartan showed a greater reduction in systolic and diastolic blood pressure.[38]

RCTs comparing one BP-reducing agent with another for the management of hypertension in patients with comorbid symptomatic heart failure do not exist. Triple therapy to reduce morbidity and mortality in stage C HFrEF includes (1) ACE inhibitors, ARBs or angiotensin II receptor neprilysin inhibitor; (2) select β-blockers; and (3) aldosterone antagonists.[26] Therefore, these agents are guideline recommended as first-line therapy for treatment of comorbid hypertension. For patients who self-identify as black with New York Heart Association (NYHA) class II to III symptoms, hydralazine

and isosorbide dinitrate are recommended in addition to the triple-therapy backbone.[39] Therapeutic effect is dose dependent so titration is imperative to maximize blood pressure–reducing ability as well as to achieve positive heart failure outcomes. Target doses for heart failure compared with dose ranges used for hypertension for select agents are listed in **Table 1**. In successful heart failure treatment trials with these agents, it has been observed that SBP usually decreases to a normal range of 110 to 130 mm Hg.[40]

Hypotension, which may or may not be symptomatic, is often a rate-limiting step in guideline-directed medical therapy (GDMT) uptitration and subsequently most patients with advanced HFrEF do not manifest hypertension.[41] However, if additional agents are needed to treat refractory hypertension, careful consideration is warranted to avoid certain agents known to worsen heart failure. Because of its noncardioselective vasodilating properties, carvedilol is more effective in reducing blood pressure compared with the other evidence-based β-blockers metoprolol succinate and bisoprolol.[41] It is therefore reasonable to select or switch to carvedilol as part of GDMT before initiating adjunct therapy with another drug class. If not already indicated, hydralazine can be initiated but other vasodilators, such as minoxidil, should be avoided because there is evidence it affects renin-related salt and fluid retention.[42] Although dihydropyridine CCBs such as amlodipine and felodipine do not improve heart failure, they are efficacious in decreasing blood pressure and seem to be safe to use for patients with HFrEF.[43] However, pedal edema is a common dose-related side effect that is more common in women. Nondihydropyridine CCBs, such as diltiazem and verapamil, should be avoided because of negative inotropic effects. In ALLHAT, patients receiving the alpha-1 antagonist doxazosin had a 2-fold higher risk for heart failure, causing this arm of the trial to stop prematurely. Therefore, this drug class should be avoided in patients with or at risk for heart failure.[44] In addition, moxonidine was associated with increased mortality in patients with heart failure, which may preclude the use of other centrally acting agents such as clonidine.[45]

Despite decades of historical RCTs showing improved outcomes in HFrEF, currently there are no therapeutic options proved to reduce morbidity and mortality in HFpEF. Loop diuretics are a cornerstone for symptom management; however, drugs within this class are usually less effective than thiazidelike diuretics in decreasing blood pressure. ARB and

Table 1
Hypertension dose range and heart failure guideline–directed medical therapy target dose

Drug Class	Hypertension Dose Range	Heart Failure Target Dose
ACE Inhibitors		
Enalapril	5–40 mg daily or twice daily	10–20 mg twice daily
Lisinopril	10–40 mg daily	20–40 mg daily
Ramipril	2.5–20 mg daily or twice daily	10 mg daily
Captopril	12.5–150 mg twice daily or 3 times a day	50 mg 3 times a day
Perindopril	4–16 mg daily	8–16 mg daily
Fosinopril	10–40 mg daily	40 mg daily
ARBs		
Valsartan	80–320 mg daily	160 mg twice daily
Candesartan	8–32 mg daily	32 mg daily
Losartan	50–100 mg daily or twice daily	50–150 mg daily
Aldosterone Antagonists		
Spironolactone	25–100 mg twice daily	25 mg daily or twice daily
Eplerenone	50–100 mg daily or twice daily	50 mg daily
β-Blockers		
Metoprolol succinate	50–200 mg daily	200 mg daily
Bisoprolol	2.5–10 mg daily	10 mg daily
Carvedilol	12.5–50 mg twice daily	50 mg twice daily

Data from Whelton PK, Carey RM, Aronow WS, et al. 2017 ACC/AHA/AAPA/ABC/ACPM/AGS/APhA/ASH/ASPC/NMA/PCNA guideline for the prevention, detection, evaluation, and management of high blood pressure in adults: executive summary. a report of the American College of Cardiology/American Heart Association Task Force on Clinical Practice Guidelines. Hypertension. 2018;71(6):1269–1324; and Yancy CW, Jessup M, Bozkurt B, et al. 2013 ACCF/AHA guideline for the management of heart failure: a report of the American College of Cardiology Foundation/American Heart Association Task Force on Practice Guidelines. J Am Coll Cardiol. 2013;62(16):e147–e239.

aldosterone antagonist use is suggested to decrease heart failure hospitalizations and can effectively decrease blood pressure through RAAS inhibition.[26] Aldosterone antagonist target doses for hypertension are higher than for heart failure and may increase risk for hyperkalemia, which occurs in a dose-dependent fashion.[46] Refractory hypertension is more common in HFpEF than HFrEF but there is a substantial lack of evidence available to provide recommendations to support or contest therapies such as thiazidelike diuretics, β-blockers, CCBs, or alpha-1 antagonists. Nitrates should be avoided because they may worsen functional status and do not improve quality of life.[39]

Achieving adequate blood pressure control in patients with comorbid HFrEF and HFpEF is vital. However, important considerations of stringent pharmacotherapy to achieve lower blood pressure targets in the setting of maximum-dose GDMT include syncope, orthostatic hypotension, acute kidney injury, and electrolyte disturbances. These adverse drug events may be especially pronounced in older adults, so tapering should be gradual and additional monitoring may be required. In contrast, low blood pressure levels should not hinder titration of GDMT provided patients are able to tolerate dose increases. When possible, combination therapy should be used to decrease pill burden and polypharmacy, especially in patients with HFpEF. Select fixed-dose combination tablets are detailed in **Box 1**.

LIFESTYLE MODIFICATIONS

Therapeutic lifestyle changes, including sodium cognizance, smoking cessation, and cardiovascular exercise, should be addressed when treating hypertension to prevent heart failure or in patients with established systolic or diastolic dysfunction.[47] Management of other risk factors, such as obesity and sleep apnea, may also help prevent cardiac remodeling. Sodium glucose cotransporter 2 inhibitors represent a paradigm shift in the treatment of diabetes because increasing evidence reveals their ability to reduce cardiovascular risk, including heart failure. This drug class also has important physiologic effects on blood pressure

---

Box 1
Select fixed-dose combination tablets

ACE inhibitor/calcium channel blocker

    Perindopril/amlodipine

ACE inhibitor/thiazide diuretic

    Lisinopril/hydrochlorothiazide

    Enalapril/hydrochlorothiazide

    Captopril/hydrochlorothiazide

    Fosinopril/hydrochlorothiazide

ARB/calcium channel blocker

    Valsartan/amlodipine

ARB/thiazide diuretic

    Losartan/hydrochlorothiazide

    Valsartan/hydrochlorothiazide

    Candesartan/hydrochlorothiazide

Aldosterone antagonist/thiazide diuretic

    Spironolactone/hydrochlorothiazide

β-Blocker/thiazide diuretic

    Bisoprolol/hydrochlorothiazide

    Metoprolol succinate/hydrochlorothiazide

Calcium channel blocker/thiazide diuretic/ARB

    Amlodipine/hydrochlorothiazide/valsartan

Data from Whelton PK, Carey RM, Aronow WS, et al. 2017 ACC/AHA/AAPA/ABC/ACPM/AGS/APhA/ASH/ASPC/NMA/PCNA guideline for the prevention, detection, evaluation, and management of high blood pressure in adults: executive summary. a report of the American College of Cardiology/American Heart Association Task Force on Clinical Practice Guidelines. Hypertension. 2018;71(6):1269–1324.

reduction even in patients concomitantly taking antihypertensives.[48]

SUMMARY

The high prevalence of hypertension establishes it as the single greatest risk factor for heart failure from a population health standpoint. Despite this, many patients remain undiagnosed, undertreated, or untreated and fail to achieve control targets. To prevent the seemingly inevitable transition from chronic hypertension to heart failure, blood pressure should be managed in accordance with current clinical practice guidelines and evidence-based therapies should be used when available. Additional RCTs, particularly in patients with HFpEF, are needed to provide strategies for the management of comorbid hypertension and heart failure.

REFERENCES

1. Benjamin EJ, Muntner P, Bittencourt MS. Heart disease and stroke statistics-2019 update: a report from the American Heart Association. Circulation 2019;139(10):e56–528.
2. Levy D, Larson MG, Vasan RS, et al. The progression from hypertension to congestive heart failure. JAMA 1996;275(20):1557–62.
3. Whelton PK, Carey RM, Aronow WS, et al. 2017 ACC/AHA/AAPA/ABC/ACPM/AGS/APhA/ASH/ASPC/NMA/PCNA guideline for the prevention, detection, evaluation, and management of high blood pressure in adults: executive summary. a report of the American College of Cardiology/American Heart Association Task Force on Clinical Practice Guidelines. Hypertension 2018;71(6):1269–324.
4. Lloyd-Jones DM, Larson MG, Leip EP, et al. Lifetime risk for developing congestive heart failure: the Framingham Heart Study. Circulation 2002;106(24):3068–72.
5. Pfeffer MA. Heart failure and hypertension: importance of prevention. Med Clin North Am 2017;101(1):19–28.
6. Vasan RS, Levy D. The role of hypertension in the pathogenesis of heart failure: a clinical mechanistic overview. Arch Intern Med 1996;156(16):1789–96.
7. Bhuiyan T, Maurer MS. Heart failure with preserved ejection fraction: persistent diagnosis, therapeutic enigma. Curr Cardiovasc Risk Rep 2011;5(5):440–9.
8. Carnethon Mercedes R, Pu J, Howard G, et al. Cardiovascular health in African Americans: a scientific statement from the American Heart Association. Circulation 2017;136(21):e393–423.
9. Vivo RP, Krim SR, Cevik C, et al. Heart failure in Hispanics. J Am Coll Cardiol 2009;53(14):1167–75.
10. Lloyd-Jones DM, Evans JC, Levy D. Hypertension in adults across the age spectrum: current outcomes and control in the community. JAMA 2005;294(4):466–72.
11. Levy D, Anderson KM, Savage DD, et al. Echocardiographically detected left ventricular hypertrophy: prevalence and risk factors: the Framingham Heart Study. Ann Intern Med 1988;108(1):7–13.
12. Eisenberg E, Di Palo KE, Piña IL. Sex differences in heart failure. Clin Cardiol 2018;41(2):211–6.
13. Bui AL, Horwich TB, Fonarow GC. Epidemiology and risk profile of heart failure. Nat Rev Cardiol 2010;8:30.
14. Messerli FH, Rimoldi SF, Bangalore S. The transition from hypertension to heart failure: contemporary update. JACC Heart Fail 2017;5(8):543–51.
15. Sorrentino MJ. The evolution from hypertension to heart failure. Heart Fail Clin 2019;15(4):447–53.
16. Ganau A, Devereux RB, Roman MJ, et al. Patterns of left ventricular hypertrophy and geometric

remodeling in essential hypertension. J Am Coll Cardiol 1992;19(7):1550–8.

17. Wright JW, Mizutani S, Harding JW. Pathways involved in the transition from hypertension to hypertrophy to heart failure. Treatment strategies. Heart Fail Rev 2008;13(3):367–75.

18. de Simone G, Gottdiener JS, Chinali M, et al. Left ventricular mass predicts heart failure not related to previous myocardial infarction: the Cardiovascular Health Study. Eur Heart J 2008;29(6):741–7.

19. Borlaug BA, Redfield MM. Diastolic and systolic heart failure are distinct phenotypes within the heart failure spectrum. Circulation 2011;123(18):2006–14.

20. Jessup M, Brozena S. Heart failure. New Engl J Med 2003;348(20):2007–18.

21. Sciarretta S, Palano F, Tocci G, et al. Antihypertensive treatment and development of heart failure in hypertension: a Bayesian network meta-analysis of studies in patients with hypertension and high cardiovascular risk. Arch Intern Med 2011;171(5): 384–94.

22. Staessen JA, Wang J-G, Thijs L. Cardiovascular prevention and blood pressure reduction: a quantitative overview updated until 1 March 2003. J Hypertens 2003;21(6):1055–76.

23. Verdecchia P, Angeli F, Cavallini C, et al. Blood pressure reduction and renin–angiotensin system inhibition for prevention of congestive heart failure: a meta-analysis. Eur Heart J 2009;30(6):679–88.

24. Ettehad D, Emdin CA, Kiran A, et al. Blood pressure lowering for prevention of cardiovascular disease and death: a systematic review and meta-analysis. Lancet 2016;387(10022):957–67.

25. SPRINT Research Group, Wright JT Jr, Williamson JD, Whelton PK, et al. A randomized trial of intensive versus standard blood-pressure control. N Engl J Med 2015;373(22):2103–16.

26. Yancy CW, Jessup M, Bozkurt B, et al. 2017 ACC/AHA/HFSA focused update of the 2013 ACCF/AHA guideline for the management of heart failure: a report of the American College of Cardiology/American Heart Association Task Force on clinical practice guidelines and the Heart Failure Society of America. Circulation 2017;136(6):e137–61.

27. Voko Z, Bots ML, Hofman A, et al. J-shaped relation between blood pressure and stroke in treated hypertensives. Hypertension 1999;34(6):1181–5.

28. Farnett L, Mulrow CD, Linn WD, et al. The J-curve phenomenon and the treatment of hypertension: is there a point beyond which pressure reduction is dangerous? JAMA 1991;265(4):489–95.

29. Banach M, Aronow WS. Blood pressure j-curve: current concepts. Curr Hypertens Rep 2012;14(6): 556–66.

30. Desai RV, Banach M, Ahmed MI, et al. Impact of baseline systolic blood pressure on long-term outcomes in patients with advanced chronic systolic heart failure (insights from the BEST trial). Am J Cardiol 2010;106(2):221–7.

31. Tsimploulis A, Lam PH, Arundel C, et al. Systolic blood pressure and outcomes in patients with heart failure with preserved ejection fraction. JAMA Cardiol 2018;3(4):288–97.

32. Pinho-Gomes AC, Rahimi K. Management of blood pressure in heart failure. Heart 2019;105(8): 589–95.

33. Davis BR, Piller LB, Cutler JA, et al. Role of diuretics in the prevention of heart failure: the antihypertensive and lipid-lowering treatment to prevent heart attack trial. Circulation 2006;113(18):2201–10.

34. Liebson PR, Grandits GA, Dianzumba S, et al. Comparison of five antihypertensive monotherapies and placebo for change in left ventricular mass in patients receiving nutritional-hygienic therapy in the Treatment of Mild Hypertension Study (TOMHS). Circulation 1995;91(3):698–706.

35. Colucci WS, Kolias TJ, Adams KF, et al. Metoprolol reverses left ventricular remodeling in patients with asymptomatic systolic dysfunction: the REversal of VEntricular Remodeling with Toprol-XL (REVERT) trial. Circulation 2007;116(1):49–56.

36. Verdecchia P, Sleight P, Mancia G, et al. Effects of telmisartan, ramipril, and their combination on left ventricular hypertrophy in individuals at high vascular risk in the ongoing telmisartan alone and in combination with ramipril global end point trial and the telmisartan randomized assessment Study in ACE intolerant subjects with cardiovascular disease. Circulation 2009;120(14):1380–9.

37. Investigators* S. Effect of enalapril on mortality and the development of heart failure in asymptomatic patients with reduced left ventricular ejection fractions. N Engl J Med 1992;327(10):685–91.

38. Bavishi C, Messerli FH, Kadosh B, et al. Role of neprilysin inhibitor combinations in hypertension: insights from hypertension and heart failure trials. Eur Heart J 2015;36(30):1967–73.

39. Yancy CW, Jessup M, Bozkurt B, et al. 2013 ACCF/AHA guideline for the management of heart failure: a report of the American College of Cardiology Foundation/American Heart Association Task Force on practice guidelines. J Am Coll Cardiol 2013;62(16): e147–239.

40. Rosendorff C, Black HR, Cannon CP, et al. Treatment of hypertension in the prevention and management of ischemic heart disease: a scientific statement from the American Heart Association Council for High Blood Pressure Research and the Councils on Clinical Cardiology and Epidemiology and Prevention. Circulation 2007;115(21):2761–88.

41. Bozkurt B, Aguilar D, Deswal A, et al. Contributory risk and management of comorbidities of hypertension, obesity, diabetes mellitus, hyperlipidemia, and metabolic syndrome in chronic heart failure: a

scientific statement from the American Heart Association. Circulation 2016;134(23):e535–78.

42. Franciosa JA, Jordan RA, Wilen MM, et al. Minoxidil in patients with chronic left heart failure: contrasting hemodynamic and clinical effects in a controlled trial. Circulation 1984;70(1):63–8.

43. Packer M, Carson P, Elkayam U, et al. Effect of amlodipine on the survival of patients with severe chronic heart failure due to a nonischemic cardiomyopathy: results of the PRAISE-2 study (prospective randomized amlodipine survival evaluation 2). JACC Heart Fail 2013;1(4):308–14.

44. ALLHAT Officers and Coordinators for the ALLHAT Collaborative Research Group. The Antihypertensive and Lipid-Lowering Treatment to Prevent Heart Attack Trial. Major outcomes in moderately hypercholesterolemic, hypertensive patients randomized to pravastatin vs usual care: the antihypertensive and lipid-lowering treatment to prevent heart attack trial (ALLHAT-LLT). JAMA 2002;288:2981–97.

45. Cohn JN, Pfeffer MA, Rouleau J, et al. Adverse mortality effect of central sympathetic inhibition with sustained-release moxonidine in patients with heart failure (MOXCON). Eur J Heart Fail 2003;5(5):659–67.

46. Vardeny O, Claggett B, Anand I, et al. Incidence, predictors, and outcomes related to hypo-and hyperkalemia in patients with severe heart failure treated with a mineralocorticoid receptor antagonist. Circ Heart Fail 2014;7(4):573–9.

47. Georgiopoulou VV, Kalogeropoulos AP, Butler J. Heart failure in hypertension: prevention and treatment. Drugs 2012;72(10):1373–98.

48. Oliva RV, Bakris GL. Blood pressure effects of sodium–glucose co-transport 2 (SGLT2) inhibitors. J Am Soc Hypertens 2014;8(5):330–9.

Atrial Fibrillation in Heart Failure
Focus on Antithrombotic Management

Mohammed Obeidat, BMBS, MRCP (UK)[a], Malcolm Burgess, MD[a],
Gregory Y.H. Lip, MD[b,c],*

KEYWORDS

- Atrial fibrillation • Heart failure • Anticoagulation • NOAC • Direct oral anticoagulant

KEY POINTS

- Heart failure (HF) and atrial fibrillation (AF) are increasingly common in the aging population, placing a major burden on health care systems.
- Morbidity and mortality is increased when the 2 conditions are seen together. Stroke risks are significant with AF and all subtypes of HF.
- Non–vitamin K antagonist oral anticoagulants (NOACs) are effective and safe in AF and HF. Dedicated studies are still needed that demonstrate safety and efficacy comparing HF subtypes and in patients with hypertrophic cardiomyopathy.

INTRODUCTION

Heart failure (HF) and atrial fibrillation (AF) are both global pandemics.[1] Both conditions lead to significant mortality and morbidity, and represent a major burden on health care systems. HF is estimated to affect 26 million people worldwide, with a growth in incidence and prevalence year on year. AF accounts for more than one-third of cardiac rhythm disturbances and is the most common arrhythmia seen in clinical practice. Indeed, 1% to 2% of general population has AF, and adults have a 1 in 4 lifetime risk of developing the condition.[2–4]

AF presentations to hospital are expected to increase by 2.5-fold by 2050. The most significant clinical burden of AF relates to the increased risk of thromboembolic disease, particularly stroke and mortality.[5] Not only does AF increase stroke risk, but it also is associated with more severe strokes with greater disability, longer hospital stays, and increased mortality than non–AF-associated strokes.[4–6]

HF and AF are complex clinical syndromes when separate entities, and the two coexisting raises potential challenges in management. HF and AF have had a well-recognized relationship for almost a century.[7] Indeed, HF is a common coexisting condition with AF, with 32% prevalence in the AF population. Although the exact mechanism of this correlation is not entirely understood, both conditions have similar risk factor profiles: age, hypertension, obesity, diabetes, ischemia, and structural and valvular heart disease. What is known is that the complex pathophysiologic changes in AF and HF create an environment in which both conditions promote the development the other.[8–10]

This article originally appeared in *Heart Failure Clinics*, Volume 16, Issue 1, January 2020.
Disclosure Statement: G.Y.H. Lip is a consultant for Bayer/Janssen, BMS/Pfizer, Medtronic, Boehringer Ingelheim, Novartis, Verseon and Daiichi-Sankyo. He is also a speaker for Bayer, BMS/Pfizer, Medtronic, Boehringer Ingelheim, and Daiichi-Sankyo. No fees are directly received personally. The other authors have nothing to disclose.
a Department of Cardiology, Aintree Hospital, Liverpool, UK; b Liverpool Centre for Cardiovascular Science, University of Liverpool and Liverpool Heart and Chest Hospital, Liverpool, UK; c Aalborg Thrombosis Research Unit, Department of Clinical Medicine, Aalborg University, Aalborg, Denmark
* Corresponding author. Liverpool Centre for Cardiovascular Science, William Henry Duncan Building, 6 West Derby Street, Liverpool L7 8TX, UK.
E-mail address: gregory.lip@liverpool.ac.uk

0733-8651/22/© 2021 Elsevier Inc. All rights reserved.

cardiology.theclinics.com

A diagnosis of both AF and HF carries worse prognosis than either one condition alone, with HF (whether with reduced or preserved ejection fraction) in the context of AF being associated with a greater risk of all-cause mortality at 1 year, and composite end point of stroke, thromboembolic disease, transient ischemic attack (TIA), and death.[11] However, there is clear evidence of increased risk of thromboembolic disease in AF with HF.

Many risk factors exist for stroke, and the more common and validated ones have been used to formulate risk-stratification scores,[12] such as the CHA$_2$DS$_2$VASc score, which is now used in major guidelines nationally and internationally.[13-16] The use of thromboprophylaxis also has to balance the risk reduction of thromboembolic disease against the potential increased risk of bleeding.[17]

This article examines the challenges in assessing stroke risk when both these conditions coexist, examines different subtypes of HF, and explores the approach to thromboprophylaxis in these patients.

SEARCH STRATEGY

A comprehensive search of published studies was performed using electronic bibliographic databases (PubMed, Medline, EMBASE, DARE, and Cochrane database), scanning reference lists from included papers, and manually searching abstracts from national and international cardiovascular meetings. Search terms included: atrial fibrillation; heart failure; HF with preserved ejection fraction (EF) (≥50%) (HFpEF), HF with midrange EF (40%–49%) (HFmrEF), and HF with reduced EF (<40%) HFrEF; cardiac failure; antithrombotic treatment; vitamin K antagonist; dabigatran; rivaroxaban; apixaban; and edoxaban. Bibliographies of all selected papers and reviews were reviewed for other relevant papers. Finally, the supplements of major journals were searched manually to identify relevant abstracts that had not been published as peer-reviewed articles.

ATRIAL FIBRILLATION AND HEART FAILURE: PATHOPHYSIOLOGY
Relationship Between Atrial Fibrillation and Heart Failure

HF is a complex syndrome with 3 clinical subtypes being proposed: HF with preserved EF (≥50%) (HFpEF), HF with midrange EF (40%–49%) (HFmrEF), and HF with reduced EF (<40%) HFrEF.[18] With all these subtypes patients are at increased risk of AF. Moreover, this increased risk is still presented when adjusted for confounders of coinciding risk factors (ie, age, body mass index, and hypertension.)[19]

As already described, AF and HF have a reciprocal relationship (**Table 1**). The disorganized atrial depolarization in AF leads to a reduction in atrial contractility and left ventricular filling, therefore leading to a reduced cardiac output by approximately 20%.[19,20] AF with uncontrolled and rapid ventricular rates leads to worsening left ventricular EF even in patients with previously normal EF. Animal models have suggested that there are potentially several mechanisms for this, including energy depletion, cellular and extracellular matrix remodeling, myocardial ischemia, and abnormal calcium-channel activity.[21,22]

Conversely, HF may lead to an increase in left atrial pressures and, eventually, left atrial volumes.[22-29] This leads to mechanical stretching on the left atrium, leading to cellular and molecular changes that increase the automaticity and heterogeneity of atrial depolarization and repolarization. This is a well-established trigger for the development of AF.[20,23,24,26-29] Moreover, AF prevalence has been proved to increase as New York Heart Association (NYHA) class worsens.[20-29]

There are also neurohormonal mechanisms that play a part in the relationship between AF and HF. Patients with HF are in a maladaptive neurohormonal state.[29-35] The renin-angiotensin-aldosterone system, noxious hormones, and cytokines are activated in HF.[36,37] This plays a role in fibrosis of the extracellular membrane, leading to the formation of heterogeneity in atrial repolarization. The left atrium (in a normal state) plays an important part in sympathoinhibition via mechanoreceptors at the pulmonary venous-atrial junctions.[31-34] When stimulated by increased blood volume, this inhibits renal sympathetic nerve activation and leads to increased diuresis. In HF this receptor reflex is impaired, and there is development of sympathoexcitatory reflex.

In an increased sympathetic state and the presence of left atrial dysfunction, the development of AF is a common complication.[30-35] Another further mechanism that relates HF to AF is defective atrial natriuretic peptide (ANP) synthesis, which is secreted in response to stretching of the left atrium. ANP has a role in reducing hypertension, volume overload, and inhibiting the proliferation of cardiac fibroblast and, therefore, fibrosis. The defective ANP synthesis in HF increases the tendency for AF.[36,37]

Thromboembolism in Atrial Fibrillation and Heart Failure

Both AF and HF have been independently shown to demonstrate Virchow's triad: hypercoagulability (activation of platelet and clotting factors),

Table 1
Pathophysiology of atrial fibrillation and heart failure

Authors,[Ref.] Year	Study Type	N	Population	Findings
Jafri et al,[40] 1993	Prospective	147	Control, HF (70), and Coronary artery disease (41)	Patients with HF, increased plasma levels of D-dimer Etiology of HF did not affect this. Patients with severe HF were more likely to have activation of platelets and the coagulation system
Lip,[42] 1995	Cross-sectional population sample controlled study and longitudinal study of patients undergoing anticoagulation	87	Chronic AF	Increased median plasma fibrinogen and von Willebrand factor levels were found in AF. Plasma D-dimer levels were also increased, suggesting increased intravascular thrombogenesis in such patients
Cioffi et al,[30] 2010	Observational	360	Patients with HF (94), controls (100), hypertension (181), hypertrophic cardiomyopathy (40), aortic stenosis (85)	Patients with HF had significant increases in left atrial volumes
Zile et al,[28] 2011	Prospective observational	745	Patients with HFpEF	Left ventricular hypertrophy or concentric remodeling, left atrium enlargement, and diastolic dysfunction were present in most patients with HFpEF
Ng et al,[35] 2011	Animal research study	77	Dogs	In HF autonomic and electrophysiologic remodeling occurs, involving the posterior left atrium and pulmonary veins. Parasympathetic and/or sympathetic signaling may be possible therapeutic targets for AF in CHF
Shah et al,[29] 2014	Observational	935	Patients with HFpEF	53% demonstrated left atrial enlargement
Melenovsky et al,[27] 2015	Prospective	238	Patients with HF (198) and control patients (40)	Left atrium remodeling in HFpEF and HFrEF differs, with more dilation and systolic dysfunction in HFrEF and with increased stiffness, pulsatility, and predilection for AF in HFpEF

(continued on next page)

Table 1 (continued)				
Authors,[Ref.] Year	Study Type	N	Population	Findings
Masuda et al,[32] 2015	Prospective	40	Patients with AF	AF ablation restores sympathetic nervous system status via attenuation of excessive adrenergic tone in HF patients. Elevated sympathetic nervous tone 3 mo post ablation was a reliable predictor of AF recurrence

endothelial dysfunction (dilatation and fibrosis of atria), and abnormal blood flow (abnormal atrial contraction/or lack thereof).[38–43] AF is strongly associated with stroke and systemic embolism, and is influenced by associated risk factors. The loss of atrial contraction results in comparative stasis, and this effect is exaggerated with increased ventricular rate because it leads to reduced filling of the atria.[38–43]

AF has a 5-fold increase in stroke across all age groups.[44] Congestive heart failure (CHF) has been shown to be an independent risk factor for stroke in AF, and the presence of the 2 conditions has been shown to incrementally increase stroke severity and all-cause mortality (**Tables 2 and 3**).[45–50] Although stroke in HF is commonly associated with AF, HF, even in the absence of AF, also has a risk of thromboembolism and has been shown to increase platelet activation, with increased levels of procoagulant factors such as D-dimer and P-selectin.[38–43]

Many scoring systems have been developed to predict stroke risk in AF. The best evidence comes from a systematic review and evidence appraisal by the Patient-Centered Outcomes Research Institute (PCORI), which compared the $CHADS_2$, CHA_2DS_2-VASc, Framingham, and ABC scores. It concluded that $CHADS_2$, CHA_2DS_2-VASc, and ABC-stroke scores have the best prediction for stroke events, as follows: $CHADS_2$ (continuous: c-statistic of 0.69, 95% confidence interval [CI] 0.66–0.73; categorical: c-statistic of 0.66, 95% CI 0.63–0.69); CHA_2DS_2-VASc (continuous c-statistic of 0.66, 95% CI 0.63–0.69; categorical c-statistic of 0.64, 95% CI 0.58–0.70); and ABC score (c-statistic of 0.67, 95% CI 0.63–0.71).[12]

All pharmacologic treatments for stroke prevention are associated with a bleeding risk.[42] Several bleeding risk assessment scores have been devised, and the best evidence comparing the available scores comes from a PCORI systematic review and evidence appraisal, which showed the HAS-BLED score to have the best predictive value.[12] The HAS-BLED score draws attention to modifiable bleeding risks, and flags up the high-risk patients for early and more frequent review visits (eg, 4 weeks rather than 4 months).[51,52] Unfortunately, many of the risk factors associated with stroke also demonstrate an increased risk of bleeding, but the HAS-BLED score outperforms stroke risk scores such as $CHADS_2$ and CHA_2DS_2-VASc in predicting bleeding outcomes.[53]

Assessing a patient's bleeding risk is especially relevant to patients with HF because many patients will have renal disease, anemia, liver disease, and a history of bleeding. The decision to anticoagulate patients with HF should be done on a case-by-case basis, examining the patients' individual bleeding risk factor profile.

SUBTYPES OF ATRIAL FIBRILLATION AND HEART FAILURE

As previously mentioned, the ESC divides HF into 3 subtypes: HFpEF, HFmrEF, and HFrEF.[19] The HFmrEF group was created to further research the gray area of patients with EFs of 40% to 49%.

Although all types of HF have an increased risk of AF, HFpEF is associated with the greatest risk.[54–57] This is thought to be due to increased left atrial stiffness seen in HFpEF, whereas HFrEF is associated with eccentric left atrial remodeling.[54–56] Moreover, a prospective multinational cohort study of 6170 patients comparing patients with AF and HF showed that the HFpEF group on average have a higher CHA_2DS_2-VASc score compared with HFrEF and HFmrEF (4.7 vs 4.1 and 4.4, respectively.)[58] Despite the higher CHA_2DS_2-VASc score in the HFpEF group, there was a lower incidence in stroke in that group compared with the other 2

Table 2
Morbidity and mortality of atrial fibrillation and heart failure

Authors,[Ref.] Year	Study Type	N	Population	Findings
Wang et al,[24] 2003	Retrospective observational	1470	Patients with HF and AF	In AF patients who developed HF, mortality was increased: (men: hazard ratio [HR] 2.7; 95% confidence interval [CI] 1.9–3.7; women: HR 3.1; 95% CI 2.2–4.2) In HF patients who developed AF, mortality was also increased (men: HR 1.6; 95% CI 1.2–2.1; women: HR 2.7, 95% CI 2.0–3.6)
Miyasaka et al,[26] 2006	Prospective observational	3288	Patients with AF but without HF	Incidence of CHF was 44 per 1000 person-years (95% CI 41–47) Post-AF CHF was associated with increased mortality risk (HR 3.4, 95% CI 3.1–3.8, $P<.0001$)
Mamas et al,[47] 2009	Meta-analysis	53,969	HF patients with AF	AF is associated with an adverse prognosis in HF irrespective of left ventricular systolic function OR of 1.40 (95% CI 1.32–1.48, $P<.0001$) in randomized trials and an odds ratio (OR) of 1.14 (95% CI 1.03–1.26, $P<.05$) in observational studies
Wasywich et al,[48] 2010	Meta-analysis	32,946	HF patients	AF is associated with worse outcomes for patients with HF compared with those with sinus rhythm OR for mortality 1.33 (95% CI 1.12–1.59) for AF compared with sinus rhythm
Mountantonakis et al,[46] 2012	Prospective observational	31,555	HF patients with AF	In patients hospitalized with HF, AF patients were more likely to be hospitalized >4 d (48.8% vs 41.5%, $P<.001$), and had higher hospital mortality rate (4.0% vs 2.6%, $P<.001$)

(*continued on next page*)

Table 2
(continued)

Authors,[Ref.] Year	Study Type	N	Population	Findings
Zakeri et al,[56] 2013	Prospective observational	939	Patients with HFpEF with AF	Of HFpEF patients in sinus rhythm at diagnosis, 32% developed AF. AF in these patients had HR 2.1 (95% CI 1.4–3.0, $P<.001$) of mortality
Zafrir et al,[60] 2018	Prospective observational	14,964	HF patients with or without AF	HR of AF for HF hospitalizations was 1.036 (95% CI 0.888–1.208, $P = .652$) in HFrEF, 1.430 (95% CI 1.087–1.882, $P = .011$) in HFmrEF, and 1.487 (95% CI 1.195–1.851, $P < .001$) in HFpEF; and for combined all-cause death or HF hospitalizations: 0.957 (95% CI 0.843–1.087, $P = .502$), 1.302 (95% CI 1.055–1.608, $P = .014$), and 1.365 (95% CI 1.152–1.619, $P<.001$), respectively

groups (0.65% vs 1.71% in HFmrEF; 1.75% in HFrEF; $P = .014$.)[58] The investigators were also able to demonstrate that stroke risk increased on average by 0.054% per 1% decrease in EF (95% CI 0.013%–0.096%; $P = .031$), and in anticoagulated patients (90% of the cohort) it still showed an increased risk of 0.030% per 1% decrease in EF (95% CI 0.011%–0.048%; $P = .003$).[58] This is interesting because, despite a lower CHA_2DS_2-VASc score in these groups, they were associated with a higher risk of stroke.

In a previous meta-analysis from 2016, there was no difference in stroke risk between the 2 groups in the presence of AF.[59] Nevertheless, the definition of HFpEF does differ between experts, and there is, therefore, heterogeneity among HFpEF patients, which may explain the different results of these trials.[54–59] The predictors of thromboembolic risk in AF-HF patients were HF subgroup (explained earlier), NYHA class, and age. NYHA class showed an odds ratio (OR) of 2.92 (95% CI 1.60–5.30) for every increasing NYHA point. Age also showed an OR of 1.04 (95% CI 1.00–1.08) per 1 year of age.[58] A clear relationship is also demonstrated between HF subtype and all-cause mortality. A significantly higher all-cause mortality is seen in patients with HfrEF.[54–60]

Hypertrophic cardiomyopathy (HCM) constitutes a subset of patients who routinely fall into the HFpEF category. AF is the most common arrhythmia in these patients.[61] The guidance on HCM and AF is limited, owing to HCM patients being excluded from many randomized controlled trials (RCTs) in stroke prevention.[61] A recent study examined the Korean National Health Insurance Service database from January 1, 2005 to December 31, 2016, with a total of 979,784 patients, which demonstrated that 1.1% of AF patients had HCM. Importantly, there was a significant stroke risk in this patient group with a hazard ratio of 1.55 (95% CI 1.48–1.63; $P<.001$) compared with AF patients without HCM.[62] The investigators also reported that a patient with HCM and AF without any other risk factors for stroke were at a similar risk of stroke as an AF patient (without HCM) with a CHA_2DS_2-VASc score of 3.[62] Conversely, the prevalence of AF in HCM has not been fully determined.[63] Considering the significant stroke risk, the current guidance is to consider anticoagulation for all patients with HCM and AF.[18,63]

Table 3
Thromboembolism in heart failure (and its subtypes) and atrial fibrillation

Authors,[Ref.] Year	Study Type	N	Population	Findings
Melgaard et al,[50] 2015	Prospective observational	42,987	HF patients with or without AF	In HF patients with CHA2DS2-VASc SCORES 1–6 the risk of ischemic stroke with concomitant AF: 4.5%, 3.7%, 3.2%, 4.3%, 5.6%, and 8.4%; without concomitant AF: 1.5%, 1.5%, 2.0%, 3.0%, 3.7%, and 7% respectively. All-cause death with concomitant AF: 19.8%, 19.5%, 26.1%, 35.1%, 37.7%, and 45.5%; without concomitant AF: 7.6%, 8.3%, 17.8%, 25.6%, 27.9%, and 35.0%
Kotecha et al,[59] 2016	Meta-analysis	54,578	AF patients with HFpEF and HFrEF	There were no significant differences in incident stroke between groups (relative risk [RR] 0.85, 95% CI 0.70–1.03, $P = .094$; n = 33,773). Mortality was higher in HFrEF
Sartipy et al,[57] 2017	Prospective observational	41,446	HF patients with HFpEF, HFmrEF and HFrEF	Prevalence of AF was 65%, 60%, and 53% in HFpEF, HFmrEF, and HFrEF, respectively HR for AF vs sinus rhythm in HFpEF, HFmrEF, and HFrEF were the following: for death, 1.11 (95% CI 1.02–1.21), 1.22 (95% CI 1.12–1.33), and 1.17 (95% CI 1.11–1.23); for HF and stroke or TIA or death, 1.15 (95% CI 1.07–1.25), 1.23 (95% CI 1.13–1.34), and 1.19 (95% CI 1.14–1.26).
Sobue et al,[54] 2018	Prospective observational	301	AF patients with HFpEF or HFrEF	Crude annual rates of thromboembolism in HFrEF and HFpEF were 3.9% and 2.7% ($P = .47$), respectively

(continued on next page)

Table 3
(continued)

Authors,[Ref.] Year	Study Type	N	Population	Findings
Siller-Matula et al,[58] 2018	Retrospective observational	6170	AF patients with HFpEF, HFmrEF, and HFrEF	HFpEF had the highest CHA_2DS_2-VASc score lower stroke incidence than other HF groups (0.65%, compared with HFmrEF 1.71%; HFrEF 1.75%; trend $P = .014$). The incidence of major adverse cardiac and cerebrovascular events was also lower in HFpEF (2.0%) compared with other HF groups (range 3.8%–4.4%; $P = .001$)
Balsam et al,[49] 2018	Retrospective observational	3506	AF patients with or without HF	Patients with HF had a higher CHA_2DS_2-VASc score (3.8 ± 1.7 vs 2.6 ± 1.8, $P <.001$), and higher composite of stroke, TIA or systemic embolization (16.2% vs 10.7%, $P <.001$)
Jung et al,[62] 2019	Retrospective observational	979,784	AF patients	1.1% of AF patients had HCM. Increased stroke risk in AF and HCM (compared with AF no HCM) with HR of 1.55 (95% CI 1.48–1.63; $P < .001$) HCM and AF without any other risk factors for stroke were at a similar risk of stroke as an AF patient (without HCM) with a CHA_2DS_2-VASc score of 3

ANTITHROMBOTIC MANAGEMENT

All patients with AF and HF should be strongly considered for anticoagulation. Until recently, warfarin and vitamin K antagonists were the mainstay of antithrombotic management in AF.[64] Warfarin has been shown to reduce ischemic stroke by 65% and all-cause mortality by 26% compared with placebo or control, with absolute risk reductions by 2.7% in primary stroke and 8.4% in secondary stroke.[64]

In the older adult population, comorbidities and polypharmacy are common and, thus, the potential for drug interactions with warfarin increases, as well as the inconvenience of regular blood tests. This led to the development of other non–vitamin K antagonist oral anticoagulants (NOACs) (**Table 4**).

The NOACs are approved as antithrombotic management for nonvalvular AF.[18] The most commonly used NOACs are apixaban, edoxaban, rivaroxaban (factor Xa inhibitors), and dabigatran (direct thrombin antagonist).[65–68] All of the NOACs were shown to have noninferiority or superiority in stroke prevention, and noninferiority in bleeding profile compared with warfarin.[65–68] Therefore,

Table 4
Anticoagulation in atrial fibrillation and heart failure

Authors,[Ref.] Year	Study Type	N	Population	Findings
Lip et al,[13] 2012	Meta-analysis	2 RCTs	HF in sinus rhythm	Oral anticoagulant therapy does not modify mortality or vascular events in patients with HF and sinus rhythm
Ahmad et al,[73] 2012	Meta-analysis	3 RCTs	AF	Patients with HF and AF NOACs are noninferior to warfarin. With OR 0.91 (0.78, 1.06)
McMurray et al,[70] 2013	Prospective RCT	14,671	AF	HF had an increased risk of stroke, bleeding, and death, but this was all less so in the apixaban group vs warfarin (apixaban/warfarin HR for stroke or death was 0.89 [95% CI 0.81–0.98; $P = .02$]; for stroke, major bleed, or death it was 0.85 [95% CI 0.78–0.92; $P<.001$])
Xiong et al,[69] 2015	Meta-analysis	32,512	AF with HF	Single-/high-dose NOAC use had a significantly improved efficacy compared with warfarin, with an OR of 0.86 (95% CI 0.76–0.98) of thromboembolism NOACs shown to have an improved safety profile when compared with warfarin and with OR of 0.7 (95% CI 0.57–0.86) and 0.43 (95% CI 0.30–0.61) of major bleeding and intracranial hemorrhage, respectively
Magnani et al,[72] 2016	Prospective RCT	14,701	AF with or without HF	The efficacy of edoxaban compared with warfarin in preventing stroke was similar in patients without and with HF regardless of the severity of HF

(*continued on next page*)

Table 4
(continued)

Authors,[Ref.] Year	Study Type	N	Population	Findings
Savarese et al,[71] 2016	Meta-analysis	55,011	AF with or without HF	HF patients showed a thromboembolism RR of 0.98 (95% CI 0.90–1.07; $P = .68$) compared with non-HF. HF patients with major bleeding RR 0.95 (95% CI 0.88–1.03; $P = .21$) were comparable in patients with and without HF. HF patients had reduced rates of any bleeding (RR 0.86; 95% CI 0.81–0.91; $P<.01$) and intracranial bleeding (RR 0.74; 95% CI 0.63–0.88; $P<.01$) but increased rates of all-cause and CV death RR of 1.70 (95% CI 1.31–2.19; $P<.01$) and 2.05 (95% CI 1.66–2.55; $P<.01$), respectively
Jung et al,[75] 2019	Retrospective cohort	955	HCM and AF	NOACs were associated with significantly lower risk of all-cause mortality (HR 0.43%; 95% CI 0.32–0.57) and composite fatal cardiovascular events (HR 0.39%; 95% CI 0.18–0.82) compared with warfarin Both warfarin and NOACs had similar stroke risks of 8.33 vs 7.96 events per 100 person-years, respectively ($P = .725$)

NOACs are increasingly being used as first-line therapy for stroke prevention in AF unless contraindicated.[18]

A meta-analysis of 32,512 patients from 4 RCT studies compared the use of all 4 NOACs versus warfarin in AF-HF patients.[69] The results showed that single-dose/high-dose NOAC use had a significantly improved efficacy compared with warfarin, with an OR of 0.86 (95% CI 0.76–0.98) for thromboembolism.[69] Moreover, NOACs were shown to have an improved safety profile when compared with warfarin, with an OR of 0.7 (95% CI 0.57–0.86) and 0.43 (95% CI 0.30–0.61) for major bleeding and intracranial hemorrhage, respectively.[69]

Previous studies have demonstrated that HF is a risk factor for bleeding in patients anticoagulated with warfarin, and these results further affirm that

Table 5
Comparison of NOAC RCTs

	RE-LY (2009)[68]	ROCKET-AF (2011)[67]	ARISTOTLE (2011)[68]	ENGAGE-AF (2013)[65]
Trial design	Randomized open-label Dabigatran 110 mg/150 mg twice daily vs warfarin (INR 2.0–3.0)	Randomized double-blind Rivaroxaban (20 or 15 mg daily) vs warfarin	Randomized double-blind Apixaban 5 mg twice daily vs warfarin	Randomized double-blind Edoxaban 30 mg/60 mg vs warfarin
Primary study outcome	Stroke and systemic embolic events	Stroke and systemic embolic events	Stroke and systemic embolic events	Stroke and systemic embolic events
Primary safety outcome	Major hemorrhage	Major hemorrhage	Major hemorrhage	Major hemorrhage
No. of HF Patients	4904 (27.1%)	9033 (63.7%)	6451 (35.4%)	8145 (57.9%)
Definition of HF	LVEF <40%, NYHA class II or higher, or HF symptoms within 6 mo before screening	Clinical HF and/or LVEF ≤35%	Symptomatic HF within the previous 3 mo or left ventricular dysfunction with LVEF ≤40% by echocardiography, radionuclide study, or contrast angiography	Presence or previous history of HF at stage C or D according to the ACC/AHA definition

Abbreviations: ACC, American College of Cardiology; AHA, American Heart Association; INR, international normalized ratio; LVEF, left ventricular ejection fraction; NYHA, New York Heart Association.

perhaps NOACs should be the anticoagulants of choice in patients with AF and HF.[69–73] A further meta-analysis examined 55,011 patients in the aforementioned trials, and demonstrated that although patients with HF and AF had increased mortality, when anticoagulated there was no difference in thromboembolism or major bleeding between HF and non-HF patients.[74]

It is important that in the RE-LY, ROCKET-AF, ARISTOTLE, and the ENGAGE-AF trials, the definitions of HF did differ (**Table 5**). There is no clear evidence that one NOAC is better than others in the context of AF-HF. The choice of NOAC depends on multiple factors, and it is difficult to make direct comparisons because of the lack of head-to-head data and differences in trial designs of each NOAC. Indeed, current evidence would suggest that in nonvalvular AF and HF patients, all 4 NOACs are comparable.[69–73] However, when prescribing NOACs in clinical practice, the prescriber should consider the dose and renal function.[74] Given that chronic kidney disease frequently coexists with AF and HF, the use of NOACs should be carefully considered in the context of coexisting

renal disease. Thus, more evidence is needed in this context.[74]

When comparing the subtypes of HF and AF, there is also limited evidence in comparing NOACs. This is an area that could be further researched, especially with the relatively new category of HFmrEF. Current evidence would suggest that clinical practice should not differ between the subtypes. When considering HCM and AF, evidence is also limited in the use of NOACs and requires further assessment. A retrospective cohort study of 955 patients with AF and HCM demonstrated similar stroke rates in patients on warfarin and NOACs.[75]

SUMMARY

HF and AF commonly exist together, leading to an increased risk of thromboembolic disease. The evidence so far would suggest that regardless of HF subtype, there is a favorable outcome in anticoagulating these patients. In most cases, NOACs are optimal over warfarin; however, NOACs have not been evaluated in a dedicated RCT assessing patients with AF and HF (and its subtypes).

REFERENCES

1. Savarese G, Lund LH. Global public health burden of heart failure. Card Fail Rev 2017;3(1):7.
2. Anter E, Jessup M, Callans DJ. Atrial fibrillation and heart failure: treatment considerations for a dual epidemic. Circulation 2009;119(18):2516–25.
3. Lloyd-Jones DM, Wang TJ, Leip EP, et al. Lifetime risk for development of atrial fibrillation: the Framingham Heart Study. Circulation 2004;110(9):1042–6.
4. Chao T, Liu C, Tuan T, et al. Lifetime risks, projected numbers, and adverse outcomes in asian patients with atrial fibrillation: a report from the Taiwan Nationwide AF cohort study. Chest 2018;153(2): 453–66.
5. Lip G, Freedman B, De Caterina R, et al. Stroke prevention in atrial fibrillation: past, present and future. Comparing the guidelines and practical decision-making. Thromb Haemost 2017;117(7):1230–9.
6. Lamassa M, Di Carlo A, Pracucci G, et al. Characteristics, outcome, and care of stroke associated with atrial fibrillation in Europe: data from a multicenter multinational hospital-based registry (The European Community Stroke Project). Stroke 2001;32(2): 392–8.
7. Thygesen SK, Frost L, Eagle KA, et al. Atrial fibrillation in patients with ischemic stroke: A population-based study. Clin Epidemiol 2009;1:55–65.
8. Mackenzie J. Disease of the heart. 3rd edition. London: Oxford Medical Publications; 1914.
9. Ferreira JP, Santos M. Heart failure and atrial fibrillation: from basic science to clinical practice. Int J Mol Sci 2015;16(2):3133–47.
10. Santhanakrishnan R, Wang N, Larson MG, et al. Atrial fibrillation begets heart failure and vice versa: temporal associations and differences in preserved versus reduced ejection fraction. Circulation 2016; 133(5):484–92.
11. Ling L, Kistler PM, Kalman JM, et al. Comorbidity of atrial fibrillation and heart failure. Nat Rev Cardiol 2016;13(3):131–47.
12. Borre ED, Goode A, Raitz G, et al. Predicting thromboembolic and bleeding event risk in patients with non-valvular atrial fibrillation: a systematic review. Thromb Haemost 2018;118(12):2171–87.
13. Lip GY, Wrigley BJ, Pisters R. Anticoagulation versus placebo for heart failure in sinus rhythm. Cochrane Database Syst Rev 2012;(6):CD003336. https://doi.org/10.1002/14651858.CD003336.pub2.
14. Lip GYH, Nieuwlaat R, Pisters R, et al. Refining clinical risk stratification for predicting stroke and thromboembolism in atrial fibrillation using a novel risk factor-based approach: the euro heart survey on atrial fibrillation. Chest 2010;137(2):263–72.
15. Overview | Atrial fibrillation: management | Guidance | NICE. Available at: https://www.nice.org.uk/guidance/cg180. Accessed February 28, 2019.
16. Lip GYH, Banerjee A, Boriani G, et al. Antithrombotic therapy for atrial fibrillation: CHEST guideline and expert panel report. Chest 2018;154(5):1121–201.
17. Proietti M, Mujovic N, Potpara TS. Optimizing stroke and bleeding risk assessment in patients with atrial fibrillation: a balance of evidence, practicality and precision. Thromb Haemost 2018;118(12):2014–7.
18. Kirchhof P, Benussi S, Kotecha D, et al. 2016 ESC Guidelines for the management of atrial fibrillation developed in collaboration with EACTS. Eur Heart J 2016;37(38):2893–962.
19. Ponikowski P, Voors AA, Anker SD, et al. 2016 ESC Guidelines for the diagnosis and treatment of acute and chronic heart failure: the task force for the diagnosis and treatment of acute and chronic heart failure of the European Society of Cardiology (ESC) developed with the special contribution of the Heart Failure Association (HFA) of the ESC. Eur Heart J 2016;37(27):2129–200.
20. Balasubramaniam R, Kistler PM. Atrial fibrillation in heart failure: the chicken or the egg? Heart 2009; 95(7):535–9.
21. Clark DM, Plumb VJ, Epstein AE, et al. Hemodynamic effects of an irregular sequence of ventricular cycle lengths during atrial fibrillation. J Am Coll Cardiol 1997;30(4):1039–45.
22. Lee Park K, Anter E. Atrial fibrillation and heart failure: a review of the intersection of two cardiac epidemics. J Atrial Fibrillation 2013;6(1):751.
23. Shinbane JS, Wood MA, Jensen DN, et al. Tachycardia-induced cardiomyopathy: a review of animal models and clinical studies. J Am Coll Cardiol 1997;29(4):709–15.
24. Wang TJ, Larson MG, Levy D, et al. Temporal relations of atrial fibrillation and congestive heart failure and their joint influence on mortality: the Framingham Heart Study. Circulation 2003;107(23):2920–5.
25. Gronefeld GC, Hohnloser SH. Heart failure complicated by atrial fibrillation: mechanistic, prognostic, and therapeutic implications. J Cardiovasc Pharmacol Ther 2003;8(2):107–13.
26. Miyasaka Y, Barnes ME, Gersh BJ, et al. Incidence and mortality risk of congestive heart failure in atrial fibrillation patients: a community-based study over two decades. Eur Heart J 2006;27(8):936–41.
27. Melenovsky V, Hwang S, Redfield MM, et al. Left atrial remodeling and function in advanced heart failure with preserved or reduced ejection fraction. Circ Heart Fail 2015;8(2):295–303.
28. Zile MR, Gottdiener JS, Hetzel SJ, et al. Prevalence and significance of alterations in cardiac structure and function in patients with heart failure and a preserved ejection fraction. Circulation 2011;124(23): 2491–501.
29. Shah AM, Shah SJ, Anand IS, et al. Cardiac structure and function in heart failure with preserved ejection fraction: baseline findings from the

echocardiographic study of the Treatment of Preserved Cardiac Function Heart Failure with an Aldosterone Antagonist trial. Circ Heart Fail 2014;7(1): 104–15.

30. Cioffi G, Gerdts E, Cramariuc D, et al. Left atrial size and force in patients with systolic chronic heart failure: Comparison with healthy controls and different cardiac diseases. Exp Clin Cardiol 2010;15(3):e45.

31. Hartupee J, Mann DL. Neurohormonal activation in heart failure with reduced ejection fraction. Nat Rev Cardiol 2017;14(1):30–8.

32. Masuda M, Yamada T, Mizuno H, et al. Impact of atrial fibrillation ablation on cardiac sympathetic nervous system in patients with and without heart failure. Int J Cardiol 2015;199:65–70.

33. Florea VG, Cohn JN. The autonomic nervous system and heart failure. Circ Res 2014;114(11):1815–26.

34. Floras JS, Ponikowski P. The sympathetic/parasympathetic imbalance in heart failure with reduced ejection fraction. Eur Heart J 2015;36(30):1982b.

35. Ng J, Villuendas R, Cokic I, et al. Autonomic remodeling in the left atrium and pulmonary veins in heart failure: creation of a dynamic substrate for atrial fibrillation. Circ Arrhythm Electrophysiol 2011;4(3): 388–96.

36. Antoine S, Vaidya G, Imam H, et al. Pathophysiologic mechanisms in heart failure: role of the sympathetic nervous system. Am J Med Sci 2017;353(1): 27–30.

37. Perera RK, Sprenger JU, Steinbrecher JH, et al. Microdomain switch of cGMP-regulated phosphodiesterases leads to ANP-induced augmentation of β-adrenoceptor-stimulated contractility in early cardiac hypertrophy. Circ Res 2015;116(8): 1304–11.

38. Khan AA, Lip GYH. The prothrombotic state in atrial fibrillation: pathophysiological and management implications. Cardiovasc Res 2019;115(1):31–45.

39. Watson T, Shantsila E, Lip GYH. Mechanisms of thrombogenesis in atrial fibrillation: Virchow's triad revisited. Lancet 2009;373(9658):155–66.

40. Jafri SM, Ozawa T, Mammen E, et al. Platelet function, thrombin and fibrinolytic activity in patients with heart failure. Eur Heart J 1993;14(2):205–12.

41. Abe Y, Asakura T, Gotou J, et al. Prediction of embolism in atrial fibrillation: classification of left atrial thrombi by transesophageal echocardiography. Jpn Circ J 2000;64(6):411–5.

42. Lip GY. Does atrial fibrillation confer a hypercoagulable state? Lancet 1995;346(8986):1313–4.

43. Lip GY, Lowe GD, Rumley A, et al. Increased markers of thrombogenesis in chronic atrial fibrillation: effects of warfarin treatment. Br Heart J 1995; 73(6):527–33.

44. Mazurek M, Huisman M, Rothman K, et al. Regional differences in antithrombotic treatment for atrial

fibrillation: insights from the GLORIA-AF phase II registry. Thromb Haemost 2017;117(12):2376–88.

45. Triposkiadis F, Pieske B, Butler J, et al. Global left atrial failure in heart failure. Eur J Heart Fail 2016; 18(11):1307–20.

46. Mountantonakis SE, Grau-Sepulveda MV, Bhatt DL, et al. Presence of atrial fibrillation is independently associated with adverse outcomes in patients hospitalized with heart failure: an analysis of get with the guidelines-heart failure. Circ Heart Fail 2012;5(2): 191–201.

47. Mamas MA, Caldwell JC, Chacko S, et al. A meta-analysis of the prognostic significance of atrial fibrillation in chronic heart failure. Eur J Heart Fail 2009; 11(7):676–83.

48. Wasywich CA, Pope AJ, Somaratne J, et al. Atrial fibrillation and the risk of death in patients with heart failure: a literature-based meta-analysis. Intern Med J 2010;40(5):347–56.

49. Balsam P, Gawałko M, Peller M, et al. Clinical characteristics and thromboembolic risk of atrial fibrillation patients with and without congestive heart failure. Results from the CRATF study. Medicine (Baltimore) 2018;97(45):e13074.

50. Melgaard L, Gorst-Rasmussen A, Lane DA, et al. Assessment of the CHA2DS2-VASc score in predicting ischemic stroke, thromboembolism, and death in patients with heart failure with and without atrial fibrillation. JAMA 2015;314(10):1030–8.

51. Pisters R, Lane DA, Nieuwlaat R, et al. A novel user-friendly score (HAS-BLED) to assess 1-year risk of major bleeding in patients with atrial fibrillation: the Euro Heart Survey. Chest 2010;138(5):1093–100.

52. Lip GYH, Lane DA. Bleeding risk assessment in atrial fibrillation: observations on the use and misuse of bleeding risk scores. J Thromb Haemost 2016; 14(9):1711–4.

53. Apostolakis S, Lane DA, Buller H, et al. Comparison of the CHADS2, CHA2DS2-VASc and HAS-BLED scores for the prediction of clinically relevant bleeding in anticoagulated patients with atrial fibrillation: the AMADEUS trial. Thromb Haemost 2013; 110(5):1074–9.

54. Sobue Y, Watanabe E, Lip GYH, et al. Thromboembolisms in atrial fibrillation and heart failure patients with a preserved ejection fraction (HFpEF) compared to those with a reduced ejection fraction (HFrEF). Heart Vessels 2018;33(4):403–12.

55. Brouwers FP, de Boer RA, van der Harst P, et al. Incidence and epidemiology of new onset heart failure with preserved vs. reduced ejection fraction in a community-based cohort: 11-year follow-up of PREVEND. Eur Heart J 2013;34(19):1424–31.

56. Zakeri R, Chamberlain AM, Roger VL, et al. Temporal relationship and prognostic significance of atrial fibrillation in heart failure patients with preserved

ejection fraction: a community-based study. Circulation 2013;128(10):1085–93.

57. Sartipy U, Dahlström U, Fu M, et al. Atrial fibrillation in heart failure with preserved, mid-range, and reduced ejection fraction. JACC Heart Fail 2017; 5(8):565–74.

58. Siller-Matula JM, Pecen L, Patti G, et al. Heart failure subtypes and thromboembolic risk in patients with atrial fibrillation: The PREFER in AF-HF substudy. Int J Cardiol 2018;265:141–7.

59. Kotecha D, Chudasama R, Lane DA, et al. Atrial fibrillation and heart failure due to reduced versus preserved ejection fraction: a systematic review and meta-analysis of death and adverse outcomes. Int J Cardiol 2016;203:660–6.

60. Zafrir B, Lund LH, Laroche C, et al. Prognostic implications of atrial fibrillation in heart failure with reduced, mid-range, and preserved ejection fraction: a report from 14 964 patients in the European Society of Cardiology Heart Failure Long-Term Registry. Eur Heart J 2018;39(48):4277–84.

61. Guttmann OP, Rahman S, O'Mahony C, et al. Systematic review of atrial fibrillation and stroke in patients with hypertrophic cardiomyopathy. Eur Heart J 2013;34(suppl_1). https://doi.org/10.1093/eurheartj/eht309.P2965.

62. Jung H, Yang P, Sung J, et al. Hypertrophic cardiomyopathy in patients with atrial fibrillation: prevalence and associated stroke risks in a nationwide cohort study. Thromb Haemost 2019;119(2): 285–93.

63. Borer JS, Atar D, Marciniak T, et al. Atrial fibrillation and stroke in patients with hypertrophic cardiomyopathy: important new insights. Thromb Haemost 2019;119(3):355–7.

64. Hart RG, Pearce LA, Aguilar MI. Meta-analysis: antithrombotic therapy to prevent stroke in patients who have nonvalvular atrial fibrillation. Ann Intern Med 2007;146(12):857–67. Available at: https://www.ncbi.nlm.nih.gov/pubmed/?term=Meta-analysis%3A+antithrombotic+therapy+to+prevent+stroke+in+patients+who+have+nonvalvular+atrial+fibrillation. Accessed February 28, 2019.

65. Giugliano RP, Ruff CT, Braunwald E, et al. Edoxaban versus warfarin in patients with atrial fibrillation. N Engl J Med 2013;369(22):2093–104.

66. Granger CB, Alexander JH, McMurray JJV, et al. Apixaban versus warfarin in patients with atrial fibrillation. N Engl J Med 2011;365(11):981–92.

67. Patel MR, Mahaffey KW, Garg J, et al. Rivaroxaban versus warfarin in nonvalvular atrial fibrillation. N Engl J Med 2011;365(10):883–91.

68. Connolly S, Ezekowitz M, Yusuf S, et al. Dabigatran versus warfarin in patients with atrial fibrillation. N Engl J Med 2009;361(12):1139.

69. Xiong Q, Lau YC, Senoo K, et al. Non-vitamin K antagonist oral anticoagulants (NOACs) in patients with concomitant atrial fibrillation and heart failure: a systemic review and meta-analysis of randomized trials. Eur J Heart Fail 2015;17(11):1192–200.

70. McMurray JJV, Ezekowitz JA, Lewis BS, et al. Left ventricular systolic dysfunction, heart failure, and the risk of stroke and systemic embolism in patients with atrial fibrillation: insights from the ARISTOTLE trial. Circ Heart Fail 2013;6(3):451–60.

71. Savarese G, Giugliano RP, Rosano GMC, et al. Efficacy and safety of novel oral anticoagulants in patients with atrial fibrillation and heart failure: a meta-analysis. JACC Heart Fail 2016;4(11):870–80.

72. Magnani G, Giugliano RP, Ruff CT, et al. Efficacy and safety of edoxaban compared with warfarin in patients with atrial fibrillation and heart failure: insights from ENGAGE AF-TIMI 48. Eur J Heart Fail 2016; 18(9):1153–61.

73. Ahmad Y, Lip GYH, Apostolakis S. New oral anticoagulants for stroke prevention in atrial fibrillation: impact of gender, heart failure, diabetes mellitus and paroxysmal atrial fibrillation. Expert Rev Cardiovasc Ther 2012;10(12):1471–80.

74. Nielsen PB, Lane DA, Rasmussen LH, et al. Renal function and non-vitamin K oral anticoagulants in comparison with warfarin on safety and efficacy outcomes in atrial fibrillation patients: a systemic review and meta-regression analysis. Clin Res Cardiol 2015;104(5):418–29.

75. Jung H, Yang P, Jang E, et al. Effectiveness and safety of non-vitamin K antagonist oral anticoagulants in patients with atrial fibrillation with hypertrophic cardiomyopathy: a nationwide cohort study. Chest 2019;155(2):354–63.

Sex and Gender-Related Issues in Heart Failure

Giulio Francesco Romiti, MD[a], Fabrizio Recchia, MD[a], Andrea Zito, MS[a],
Giacomo Visioli, MD[b], Stefania Basili, MD[a], Valeria Raparelli, MD, PhD[c,d],*

KEYWORDS

• Sex • Gender • Pharmacology • Clinical outcomes • Sex-stratified analysis • Clinical trials

KEY POINTS

• Sex-based differences between clinical characteristics, comorbidities, and clinical outcomes in heart failure.
• A low participation of women in clinical trial testing the efficacy and safety of drugs and medical device among adults with heart failure limits the opportunity to manage differentially, if needed, men and women with heart failure.
• Beyond sex, gender (ie, psychosocial cultural factors) is a neglected yet relevant determinant of heart failure prognosis that should be considering in the management of men and women with heart failure.

INTRODUCTION

Heart failure (HF) is a major health care issue, given its high prevalence and incidence, the rate of comorbidities, the related high health care costs, and its poor outcomes. In the last decades, the integration of sex and gender perspectives in clinical research on adults with HF has improved our understanding of the disease and provided compelling findings on a more individualized approach to HF based on sex. Therefore, the present review aims to provide overview of the available evidence on sex- and gender-related differences in HF.

EPIDEMIOLOGY OF HEART FAILURE: A GLOBAL AND SEX-RELATED BURDEN

HF affects about 25 million people worldwide,[1] representing a major public health problem. The estimated prevalence varies between 1% and 3%, but a 46% increase is projected by 2030.[2] However, thanks to the improvements in primary prevention of HF, incidence is expected to decrease, so that the changing prevalence is probably related to the enhanced survival of patients.[3] More than 50% of patients with HF are women[4,5]; despite this, HF incidence remains lower in females compared with men,[6,7] except for people aged 80 years or more.[8]

Overall, women tend to be older than men at diagnosis.[9,10] One-half of patients with HF have a preserved ejection fraction (HFpEF); among these, female sex is over-reppresented.[11] This sex-related difference, given the more advanced age of patients with HFpEF, seems to be consistent with the specific age distribution of this phenotype; therefore, women are not at higher risk for HFpEF

This article originally appeared in *Heart Failure Clinics*, Volume 16, Issue 1, January 2020.
Disclosure Statement: Dr. Raparelli was supported by the Scientific Independence of Young Researchers Program (RBSI14HNVT), Italian Ministry of Education, University and Research (MIUR), Rome, Italy.
[a] Department of Translational and Precision Medicine, Sapienza University of Rome, Policlinico Umberto I, Viale Regina Elena 324, Rome 00161, Italy; [b] Department of Sense Organs, Sapienza University of Rome, Policlinico Umberto I, Viale Regina Elena 324, Rome 00161, Italy; [c] Department of Experimental Medicine, Sapienza University of Rome, Policlinico Umberto I, Viale Regina Elena 324, Rome 00161, Italy; [d] McGill University Health Centre Research Institute, Centre for Outcomes Research and Evaluation, Montreal, Quebec, Canada
* Corresponding author. Department of Experimental Medicine, Sapienza University of Rome, Viale Regina Elena 324, Rome 00161, Italy.
E-mail addresses: valeria.raparelli@uniroma1.it; valeria.raparelli@mcgill.ca

cardiology.theclinics.com

than men.[12] Moreover, Ho and colleagues[13] demonstrated that, in a multivariable analysis (including sex, age, obesity, blood pressure, current treatment for hypertension [HTN], and previous myocardial infarction) women did not have a significantly increased risk of HFpEF compared with men. Conversely, adjusting for the same risk factors plus left ventricular hypertrophy, left bundle branch block, and diabetes mellitus (DM), men were at much higher risk of HF with reduced ejection fraction (HFrEF).

COMORBIDITIES AND HEART FAILURE SEX-RELATED DIFFERENCES

Several risk factors, as shown by the Framingham Heart Study (FHS), are highly associated with an increased risk of developing HF such as HTN, DM, and coronary heart disease (CHD).[14,15] A sex-specific relation between risk factors and HF development has been observed. In women, HF is primarily associated with HTN and DM; in contrast, HF in men seems to have a strong association with CHD.[16]

- *HTN*: HTN is highly prevalent among the general population, but tends to be more common in women with HF compared with men.[17,18] Even though it is commonly associated with HF in both sexes, having the greatest population attributable risk among all risk factors,[14] the FHS demonstrated a stronger association in women compared with men, with a 3.4-fold and 2.0-fold increased risk of HF, respectively.[14] This evidence could be partly attributable to the higher prevalence of HTN in women and to their suboptimal blood pressure control, despite receiving adequate treatment.[19] In contrast, data from large European community based-studies[5] found a higher HF risk in men with elevated blood pressure when adjusting for antihypertensive medication. This observation may be related to an higher incidence of hypertensive-related cardiac diseases in men,[20] which could influence HF development in males.
- *DM*: DM also emerged as another important precursor of HF. Data about DM prevalence by sex in HF patients show conflicting results. In the Olmsted County Study, diabetic women were fewer than men, whereas other studies show a similar or even higher prevalence of DM in women with HF.[6,21,22] Overall, considering the risk for HF related to DM, significant differences exist. In the FHS, the population attributable risk leading to HF was 12% in women and 6% in men.[16] In an 18-year

follow-up study of patients with DM, women with DM were found to have a 5-fold increase in the risk of HF compared with women without DM, whereas DM is related to a 2-fold increase in the risk of HF in men.[15] Similar results are mirrored by a recent large cohort study[23] with a stronger risk of HF associated to DM in women of all ages. Notably, diabetic women are more likely than men to present with HFpEF.[1]

- *CHD*: CHD is a stronger predictor of HF in men than in women, who more commonly develop HF with no evidence of ischemic heart disease.[24] However, myocardial ischemia with no obstructive CHD, which is highly prevalent among women,[25] could be an underdiagnosed cause of cardiac damage that may affect the real incidence of ischemic heart disease in females with HF. Data from the FHS reveal a population attributable risk related to CHD for HF of 34% in men versus 13% in women.[14] However, the National Health and Nutrition Examination Survey study, which included more than 8000 women, points out that CHD still has a great impact on the risk of HF in females, showing a relative risk of 8.16 ($P<.001$), even higher than that for HTN (relative risk, 1.51; $P<.001$).[26] In addition to this, when considering HFrEF, CHD represents the most relevant risk factor for HF in women, with a prevalence of nearly 63%, although this remains smaller compared with that of men.[9]
- *Obesity:* Obesity is a common risk factor for HF in both men and women. Females with HF tend to have a higher body mass index (BMI) compared with men.[9,10] However, in the FHS, the prevalence of obesity emerged to be nearly identical between the 2 sexes (about 16%). After adjusting for common risk factors, women had a 7% additional HF risk for each increase of 1 kg/m^2 of BMI, whereas men had only a 5% increased risk. Compared with subjects of the same sex with normal BMI, overweight women (BMI of $\geq$25 kg/m^2) had a 50% greater risk of developing HF, whereas overweight men had no significantly increased risk. Obese women (BMI of $\geq$30 kg/m^2) had a doubled risk of HF compared with those with normal BMI, whereas the risk was 90% higher for men.[27]
- *Atrial fibrillation:* Atrial fibrillation (AF) represents both a consequence of HF and a risk factor for HF decompensation. Data from large population-based studies show that women with AF are more likely to have HF compared with men.[18,28] In particular, women

with AF have a greater risk of HFpEF compared with men[29]; moreover, a higher risk of developing AF has been observed in women with HF.[30]

Finally, it has been generally observed that women with HF tend to have a higher incidence of other comorbidities compared with men, such as chronic kidney disease, anemia, iron deficiency, depression, and thyroid dysfunction.[31] However, no significant difference was found between men and women with HF concerning the number of comorbidities simultaneously present.[32]

SEX DIFFERENCES IN CLINICAL PRESENTATION, DIAGNOSIS, AND OUTCOMES

On average, women present with higher left ventricular ejection fraction than men, and they tend to show a more severe clinical picture. This has been reported using both clinical scores (New York Heart Association functional class) and patient-reported scores (Kansas City Cardiomyopathy Questionnaire clinical summary score); in particular, the large difference (10 points) in the Kansas City Cardiomyopathy Questionnaire average score reported in women and men with HF is mainly owing to the "physical limitations" (frailty), which have a greater impact on women.[33,34]

Women report more symptoms than men, with a higher prevalence of dyspnea on effort, paroxysmal nocturnal dyspnea, and other signs of congestion (peripheral edema, jugular venous congestion, and rales). In addition, women develop anxiety or depression more often than men; this finding is supported by the state of health score (from the EQ-5D-3L) and might suggest that HF has a greater psychological impact on female patients.[34]

To diagnose HF, suspicion can arise with clinical features, which then leads the clinician to run other diagnostic tests, such as electrocardiogram, brain natriuretic peptide (BNP) or pro-BNP, echocardiography, and coronary angiography (when ischemic etiology is suspected). Moreover, these tests can be useful to stratify patients.[33] Currently, there is only limited evidence on sex differences in the diagnostic tests. However, an echocardiographic study compared cardiac structural adaptation in HTN between patients of both sexes and showed that premenopausal women had smaller left ventricle size and better systolic function than men of the same age; however, this difference was less pronounced in postmenopausal women.[35] These findings could suggest that the EF cut-off to define HFrEF may not be appropriate in women.

Sex-driven differences in both reference and cut-off values have already been described for several biomarkers, especially in cardiovascular diseases.[36–38] Likewise, BNP is a biomarker whose average reference values are normally higher in women.[33] This finding shows that, even in the diagnostic field, it may be important to keep the patient's sex under consideration.

Although women with HF have worse symptoms and worse quality of life than their male counterparts, they have a better prognosis and survival with lower rate of hospitalization, cardiovascular death and noncardiovascular death.[33] The reasons why such differences exist remain unclear, but they may be attributable to the sex differences in etiology (eg, women have a lower prevalence of myocardial ischemia, which is associated with a pattern of volume overload, eccentric hypertrophy of the heart, and cardiac dilation, all of which are associated with a worse prognosis) and in systolic function (eg, women are more likely to have HFpEF, which has a better prognosis and low mortality than HFrEF, as reported by the FHS).[33,34] However, regardless of etiology and left ventricular ejection fraction, female sex is intrinsically associated with a better prognosis.[1]

SEX DIFFERENCES IN MANAGEMENT: CLINICAL TRIALS AND PHARMACOLOGIC THERAPY

Even though women with HF present several differences in etiology, clinical condition, and prognosis compared with men, they are still underrepresented in most of the clinical trials studying the HF population and, generally, less than 20% to 30% are enrolled[39,40] (**Table 1**). Consequentially, medical and device therapies are mainly studied in men, resulting not only in a lack of information about pharmacologic safety and tolerance in women, but also about drug dosing, interaction with sexual hormones,[74,75] potential sex-related dissimilarities in pharmacokinetics, pharmacodynamics, and treatment response[76,77] and different gender behaviors (such as a poorer therapy adherence in women[78]).

In many trials, some sex-related differences in pharmacologic therapy have been found by conducting subgroup and post hoc analysis restricted to women, sometimes lacking in significance or potentially flawed by bias.[79,80]

Among the several drugs studied in HF, selective β-blockers and angiotensin-converting enzyme inhibitors have shown their efficacy in

Table 1
Participation of women in HF randomized controlled trials

Trial Name	Year	Treatment	Comparison	No. of Adults with HF	% Women	HFrEF vs HFpEF
A-HeFT[41]	2004	Isosorbide dinitrate/ hydralazine	Placebo	1050	40	HFrEF
ATMOSPHERE[42]	2016	Aliskiren	Enalapril	7016	22	HFrEF
BEAUTIFUL[43]	2008	Ivabradine	Placebo	10,917	17	HFrEF
BEST[44]	2001	Bucindolol	Placebo	2708	22	HFrEF
CARE-HF[45]	2005	CRT	No CRT	813	26	HFrEF
CHARM[46]	2003	Candesartan	Placebo	7601	32	HFrEF HFpEF
CIBIS-II[47]	1999	Bisoprolol	Placebo	2647	19	HFrEF
COMPANION[48]	2004	CRT ± ICD	No CRT ± ICD	1520	32	HFrEF
COMET[49]	2003	Carvedilol	Metoprolol	3029	20	HFrEF
CONSENSUS[50]	1987	Enalapril	Placebo	253	29	HFrEF
COPERNICUS[51]	2001	Bisoprolol	Placebo	2289	20	HFrEF
CORONA[52]	2007	Rosuvastatin	Placebo	5011	41	HFrEF
DIG[53]	1997	Digoxin	Placebo	6800	22	HFrEF
ELITE-II[54]	1997	Losartan	Captopril	722	31	HFrEF
EMPHASIS-HF[55]	2011	Eplerenone	Placebo	2737	22	HFrEF
EPHESUS[56]	2003	Eplerenone	Placebo	6642	29	HFrEF
I-PRESERVE[57]	2008	Irbesartan	Placebo	4128	60	HFpEF
MADIT-CRT[58]	2009	CRT + ICD	ICD	1820	25	HFrEF
MADIT-II[59]	2002	ICD	No ICD	1232	16	HFrEF
MERIT-HF[60]	1999	Metoprolol	Placebo	3991	23	HFrEF
PARADIGM-HF[61]	2014	Sacubitril/ valsartan	Enalapril	8442	21	HFrEF
PARAMOUNT[62]	2012	Sacubitril/ valsartan	Valsartan	301	57	HFpEF
PIOONER-HF[63]	2019	Sacubitril/ valsartan	Enalapril	881	26	HFrEF
RALES[64]	1999	Spironolactone	Placebo	1663	27	HFrEF
SENIORS[65]	2005	Nebivolol	Placebo	2128	37	HFrEF
SHIFT[66]	2010	Ivabradine	Placebo	6505	24	HFrEF
SOLVD-P[67]	1992	Enalapril	Placebo	4228	13	HFrEF
SOLVD-T[68]	1991	Enalapril	Placebo	2569	20	HFrEF
TOPCAT[69]	2014	Spironolactone	Placebo	3445	51	HFpEF
U.S. CARVEDILOL[70]	1996	Carvedilol	Placebo	1094	23	HFrEF
Val-HeFT[71]	2001	Valsartan	Placebo	5010	20	HFrEF
V-HeFT I[72]	1986	Isosorbide dinitrate/ hydralazine or prazosin	Placebo	642	0	HFrEF
V-HeFT II[73]	1991	Isosorbide dinitrate/ hydralazine	Enalapril	804	0	HFrEF

Abbreviations: CRT, cardiac resynchronization therapy; ICD, implantable cardioverter defibrillator.

both sexes.[51,70] Furthermore, some trials like Metoprolol CR/XL Randomized Intervention Trial-HF (MERIT-HF)[60] or Cardiac Insufficiency Bisoprolol Study II (CIBIS-II),[47] registered a lower mortality and hospitalization in women compared with men when selective β-blockers were used in HF. When patients are intolerant to angiotensin-converting enzyme inhibitors, the risk of angioedema and cough is greater in women than in men,[76,81] and angiotensin receptor blockers are prescribed instead. Angiotensin receptor blockers showed clear beneficial effects in men like in Valsartan Heart Failure Trial (Val-HeFT),[71] but there is not the same evidence in women yet.[46,82] Regarding the new combination sacubitril/valsartan, its efficacy has been highlighted in both sexes, but the sex-related adverse events have not been analyzed yet.[1] Digoxin, sometimes used to decrease the risk of hospitalization, showed a higher death rate in women, probably linked to a different tolerance of its serum concentration than man.[83,84] Finally, spironolactone in HFpEF has recently shown a decrease in all-cause mortality in women.[85]

Some sex-related differences have also been found in devices therapies like the implantable cardioverter-defibrillator,[86] where men are associated with higher survival benefit, or like cardiac resynchronization therapy, where women register less all-cause mortality and HF events than men.[45,48,87]

Overall, as shown in a recent systematic review that included 81 trials with subgroup analyses, no significant differences between men and women regarding treatment efficacy have been observed in most studies. However, when differences were detected, they usually tended to benefit women. Presumably, more studies specifically designed to assess sex-based disparities are required to obtain individually tailored indications for HF therapy.[88]

Table 2 summarizes the main sex differences actually highlighted in HF.[8]

GENDER-RELATED FACTORS AND IMPACT ON HEART FAILURE

Beyond sex, gender is an important frequently neglected determinant of human health. Clinical outcomes as well as the efficacy and the safety of common used drugs may be tremendously influenced not only by sex, but also by gender-related factors.[89,90] Gender is a complex construct that captures the socially constructed roles, behaviors, expressions and identities of girls, women, boys, men, and gender-diverse people. According to the Women Health Research Network of the Canadian Institutes of Health Research,[91,92] the concept of gender includes 4 interrelated aspects that encompass the gender construct: gender roles (eg, child care), gender identity (eg, personality traits), gender relationships (eg, social support), and what is termed "institutionalized gender" (eg, education level, personal income) (**Fig. 1**).

So far, the assessment of impact of gender domains in the clinical outcomes of adults with HF has been only partially explored. Some gender-related factors seem to have an association with HF outcomes even though data are conflicting. The marital status, and particularly living without a spouse, have been reported to be associated with a major risk of rehospitalization for HF, and that it could account for around one-third of the total risk.[93,94] However, other studies have not found a significant connection between the marital status

---

Table 2
Main sex differences in HF

	Women	Men
Age at diagnosis	Commonly in elderly patients	Younger than women
Phenotype	Mostly HFpEF	Mostly HFrEF
Comorbidities	HTN, DM, obesity, AF	CHD
Symptoms	More signs of congestion and depression/anxiety	Milder symptoms than women
Prognosis	Good	Poor
Management	β-Blockers: lower risk of mortality and hospitalization Digoxin is associated with higher death rate CRT contributes to lower all-cause mortality	ACE inhibitors are associated with lower incidence of cough and angioedema ICD confers better survival benefit

Abbreviations: ACE, angiotensin-converting enzyme; CRT, cardiac resynchronization therapy; ICD, implantable cardioverter defibrillator.

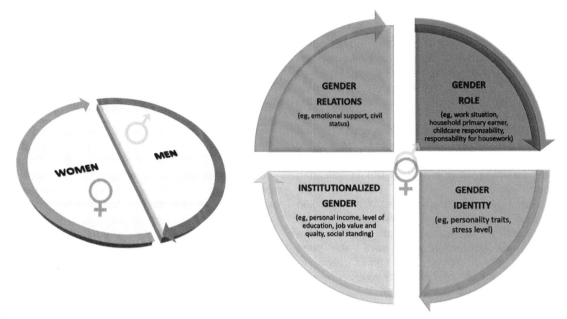

Fig. 1. Sex and gender domains in health. Sex and gender are not interchangeable terms; sex is used as biological variable whereas gender is a complex construct that includes different domains: gender identity, gender role, gender relations, and institutionalized gender.

and HF clinical outcomes. Of note, Watkins and colleagues[95] reported significantly lower levels of the BNP in married patients, which has been associated with a better prognosis.[96,97]

An association between gender role or institutionalized gender and survival in adults with HF has been investigated: unemployment,[98] no activity, and low educational level seem to be correlated to a worse prognosis.[94,99] Conversely, larger observational studies, even noting slight differences in treatment depending on socioeconomic status, have not highlighted significant differences in clinical outcomes.[100] Despite that, when social support is considered in combination with physical frailty, it could predict 30-day outcome after a hospital admission for HF.[101]

Finally, some studies have explored the gender identity domain, in particular Makowska and colleagues[102] observed that men with HF tend to have lack of masculine tracts, suggesting a psychological adaptation to carry the burden of the disease.

SUMMARY

Health care providers and scientists should define their clinical and research questions starting from the already available evidence on sex differences in clinical, comorbidities, response to treatment, and outcomes in adults with HF. An increased awareness of such differences can favor a more

personalized approach to the management of women and men with HF. Beyond sex, gender-related factors should also be investigated because they might play an important role along the lifespan of HF and to avoid missing opportunities for improving the outcomes women and men with HF.

REFERENCES

1. Levinsson A, Dubé MP, Tardif JC, et al. Sex, drugs, and heart failure: a sex-sensitive review of the evidence base behind current heart failure clinical guidelines. ESC Heart Fail 2018. https://doi.org/10.1002/ehf2.12307.

2. Benjamin EJ, Muntner P, Alonso A, et al. Heart disease and stroke statistics-2019 update: a report from the American Heart Association. Circulation 2019;139(10):e56–66. https://doi.org/10.1161/CIR.0000000000000659.

3. Roger VL. Epidemiology of heart failure. Circ Res 2013;113(6):646–59.

4. Levy D, Kenchaiah S, Larson MG, et al. Long-term trends in the incidence of and survival with heart failure. N Engl J Med 2002;347(18):1397–402.

5. Magnussen C, Niiranen TJ, Ojeda FM, et al. Sex-specific epidemiology of heart failure risk and mortality in Europe. JACC Hear Fail 2019;7(3):204–13.

6. Roger VL, Weston SA, Redfield MM, et al. Trends in heart failure incidence and survival in a community-based population. JAMA 2004;292(3):344.

7. Barker WH, Mullooly JP, Getchell W. Changing incidence and survival for heart failure in a well-defined older population, 1970–1974 and 1990–1994. Circulation 2006;113(6):799–805.

8. Marra AM, Salzano A, Arcopinto M, et al. The impact of gender in cardiovascular medicine: lessons from the gender/sex-issue in heart failure. Monaldi Arch Chest Dis 2018;88(3):988.

9. Daubert MA, Douglas PS. Primary prevention of heart failure in women. JACC Hear Fail 2019;7(3): 181–91.

10. Meyer S, Van Der Meer P, Van Deursen VM, et al. Neurohormonal and clinical sex differences in heart failure. Eur Heart J 2013;34(32):2538–47.

11. Dunlay SM, Roger VL, Redfield MM. Epidemiology of heart failure with preserved ejection fraction. Nat Rev Cardiol 2017;14(10):591–602.

12. Pandey A, Omar W, Ayers C, et al. Sex and race differences in lifetime risk of heart failure with preserved ejection fraction and heart failure with reduced ejection fraction. Circulation 2018; 137(17):1814–23.

13. Ho JE, Enserro D, Brouwers FP, et al. Predicting heart failure with preserved and reduced ejection fraction. Circ Heart Fail 2016;9(6).

14. Levy D, Larson MG, Vasan RS, et al. The progression from hypertension to congestive heart failure. JAMA 1996;275(20):1557–62.

15. Kannel WB, Hjortland M, Castelli WP. Role of diabetes in congestive heart failure: the Framingham study. Am J Cardiol 1974;34(1):29–34.

16. Lundberg G, Walsh MN, Mehta LS. Sex-specific differences in risk factors for development of heart failure in women. Heart Fail Clin 2019;15(1):1–8.

17. Lenzen MJ, Rosengren A, op Reimer WJMS, et al. Management of patients with heart failure in clinical practice: differences between men and women. Heart 2008;94(3):e10.

18. Shafazand M, Schaufelberger M, Lappas G, et al. Survival trends in men and women with heart failure of ischaemic and non-ischaemic origin: data for the period 1987-2003 from the Swedish Hospital Discharge Registry. Eur Heart J 2008;30(6): 671–8.

19. Wenger NK, Arnold A, Bairey Merz CN, et al. Hypertension across a woman's life cycle. J Am Coll Cardiol 2018;71(16):1797–813.

20. Albrektsen G, Heuch I, Løchen M-L, et al. Lifelong gender gap in risk of incident myocardial infarction. JAMA Intern Med 2016;176(11):1673.

21. Frazier CG, Alexander KP, Newby LK, et al. Associations of gender and etiology with outcomes in heart failure with systolic dysfunction. J Am Coll Cardiol 2007;49(13):1450–8.

22. Simon T, Mary-Krause M, Funck-Brentano C, et al. Sex differences in the prognosis of congestive heart failure: results from the Cardiac Insufficiency Bisoprolol Study (CIBIS II). Circulation 2001;103(3): 375–80.

23. Uijl A, Koudstaal S, Direk K, et al. Risk factors for incident heart failure in age- and sex-specific strata: a population-based cohort using linked electronic health records. Eur J Heart Fail 2019. https://doi.org/10.1002/ejhf.1350.

24. Franke J, Lindmark A, Hochadel M, et al. Gender aspects in clinical presentation and prognostication of chronic heart failure according to NT-proBNP and the Heart Failure Survival Score. Clin Res Cardiol 2015;104(4):334–41.

25. Raparelli V, Proietti M, Lenzi A, et al. Sex and gender differences in ischemic heart disease: endocrine vascular disease approach (EVA) study design. J Cardiovasc Transl Res 2018. https://doi.org/10.1007/s12265-018-9846-5.

26. He J, Ogden LG, Bazzano LA, et al. Risk factors for congestive heart failure in US men and women: NHANES I epidemiologic follow-up study. Arch Intern Med 2001;161(7):996–1002.

27. Kenchaiah S, Evans JC, Levy D, et al. Obesity and the risk of heart failure. N Engl J Med 2002;347(5): 305–13.

28. Marzona I, Proietti M, Farcomeni A, et al. Sex differences in stroke and major adverse clinical events in patients with atrial fibrillation: a systematic review and meta-analysis of 993,600 patients. Int J Cardiol 2018;269:182–91.

29. Santhanakrishnan R, Wang N, Larson MG, et al. Atrial fibrillation begets heart failure and vice versa. Circulation 2016;133(5):484–92.

30. Benjamin EJ, Levy D, Vaziri SM, et al. Independent risk factors for atrial fibrillation in a population-based cohort. The Framingham Heart Study. JAMA 1994;271(11):840–4.

31. Hopper I, Kotecha D, Chin KL, et al. Comorbidities in heart failure: are there gender differences? Curr Heart Fail Rep 2016;13(1):1–12.

32. Chamberlain AM, St. Sauver JL, Gerber Y, et al. Multimorbidity in heart failure: a community perspective. Am J Med 2015;128(1):38–45.

33. Hsich EM, Piña IL. Heart failure in women. A need for prospective data. J Am Coll Cardiol 2009. https://doi.org/10.1016/j.jacc.2009.02.066.

34. Dickstein K, Solomon SD, Dewan P, et al. Differential impact of heart failure with reduced ejection fraction on men and women. J Am Coll Cardiol 2019. https://doi.org/10.1016/j.jacc.2018.09.081.

35. Garavaglia GE, Messerli FH, Schmieder RE, et al. Sex differences in cardiac adaptation to essential hypertension. Eur Heart J 1989. https://doi.org/10.1093/oxfordjournals.eurheartj.a059434.

36. Romiti GF, Cangemi R, Toriello F, et al. Sex-specific cut-offs for high-sensitivity cardiac troponin: is less more? Cardiovasc Ther 2019;2019:1–12.

37. Hamada M, Shigematsu Y, Takezaki M, et al. Plasma levels of atrial and brain natriuretic peptides in apparently healthy subjects: effects of sex, age, and hemoglobin concentration. Int J Cardiol 2017;228:599–604.

38. Slagman A, Searle J, Vollert JO, et al. Sex differences of troponin test performance in chest pain patients. Int J Cardiol 2015;187:246–51.

39. Heiat A, Gross CP, Krumholz HM. Representation of the elderly, women, and minorities in heart failure clinical trials. Arch Intern Med 2002;162(15):1682–8.

40. Tahhan AS, Vaduganathan M, Greene SJ, et al. Enrollment of older patients, women, and racial and ethnic minorities in contemporary heart failure clinical trials: a systematic review. JAMA Cardiol 2018;3(10):1011–9.

41. Taylor AL, Ziesche S, Yancy C, et al. Combination of isosorbide dinitrate and hydralazine in blacks with heart failure. N Engl J Med 2004;351(20):2049–57.

42. McMurray JJV, Krum H, Abraham WT, et al. Aliskiren, enalapril, or aliskiren and enalapril in heart failure. N Engl J Med 2016;374(16):1521–32.

43. Fox K, Ford I, Steg PG, et al. Ivabradine for patients with stable coronary artery disease and left-ventricular systolic dysfunction (BEAUTIFUL): a randomised, double-blind, placebo-controlled trial. Lancet 2008;372(9641):807–16.

44. Beta-Blocker Evaluation of Survival Trial Investigators, Eichhorn EJ, Domanski MJ, Krause-Steinrauf H, et al. A trial of the beta-blocker bucindolol in patients with advanced chronic heart failure. N Engl J Med 2001;344(22):1659–67.

45. Cleland JGF, Daubert J-C, Erdmann E, et al. The effect of cardiac resynchronization on morbidity and mortality in heart failure. N Engl J Med 2005;352(15):1539–49.

46. Pfeffer MA, Swedberg K, Granger CB, et al. Effects of candesartan on mortality and morbidity in patients with chronic heart failure: the CHARM-Overall programme. Lancet 2003;362(9386):759–66.

47. CIBIS-II Investigators and Committees. The Cardiac Insufficiency Bisoprolol Study II (CIBIS-II): a randomised trial. Lancet 1999;353(9146):9–13.

48. Bristow MR, Saxon LA, Boehmer J, et al. Cardiac-resynchronization therapy with or without an implantable defibrillator in advanced chronic heart failure. N Engl J Med 2004;350(21):2140–50.

49. Poole-Wilson PA, Swedberg K, Cleland JG, et al. Comparison of carvedilol and metoprolol on clinical outcomes in patients with chronic heart failure in the Carvedilol Or Metoprolol European Trial (COMET): randomised controlled trial. Lancet 2003;362(9377):7–13.

50. CONSENSUS Trial Study Group. Effects of enalapril on mortality in severe congestive heart failure. N Engl J Med 1987;316(23):1429–35.

51. Packer M, Coats AJ, Fowler MB, et al. Effect of carvedilol on survival in severe chronic heart failure. N Engl J Med 2001;344(22):1651–8.

52. Kjekshus J, Apetrei E, Barrios V, et al. Rosuvastatin in older patients with systolic heart failure. N Engl J Med 2007;357(22):2248–61.

53. Digitalis Investigation Group. The effect of digoxin on mortality and morbidity in patients with heart failure. N Engl J Med 1997;336(8):525–33.

54. Pitt B, Segal R, Martinez FA, et al. Randomised trial of losartan versus captopril in patients over 65 with heart failure (Evaluation of Losartan in the Elderly Study, ELITE). Lancet 1997;349(9054):747–52.

55. Zannad F, McMurray JJV, Krum H, et al. Eplerenone in patients with systolic heart failure and mild symptoms. N Engl J Med 2011;364(1):11–21.

56. Pitt B, Remme W, Zannad F, et al. Eplerenone, a selective aldosterone blocker, in patients with left ventricular dysfunction after myocardial infarction. N Engl J Med 2003;348(14):1309–21.

57. Massie BM, Carson PE, McMurray JJ, et al. Irbesartan in patients with heart failure and preserved ejection fraction. N Engl J Med 2008;359(23):2456–67.

58. Moss AJ, Hall WJ, Cannom DS, et al. Cardiac-resynchronization therapy for the prevention of heart-failure events. N Engl J Med 2009;361(14):1329–38.

59. Moss AJ, Zareba W, Hall WJ, et al. Prophylactic implantation of a defibrillator in patients with myocardial infarction and reduced ejection fraction. N Engl J Med 2002;346(12):877–83.

60. MERIT-HF Study Group. Effect of metoprolol CR/XL in chronic heart failure: metoprolol CR/XL Randomised Intervention Trial in Congestive Heart Failure (MERIT-HF). Lancet 1999;353(9169):2001–7.

61. McMurray JJV, Packer M, Desai AS, et al. Angiotensin–neprilysin inhibition versus enalapril in heart failure. N Engl J Med 2014;371(11):993–1004.

62. Solomon SD, Zile M, Pieske B, et al. The angiotensin receptor neprilysin inhibitor LCZ696 in heart failure with preserved ejection fraction: a phase 2 double-blind randomised controlled trial. Lancet 2012;380(9851):1387–95.

63. Velazquez EJ, Morrow DA, DeVore AD, et al. Angiotensin–neprilysin inhibition in acute decompensated heart failure. N Engl J Med 2019;380(6):539–48.

64. Pitt B, Zannad F, Remme WJ, et al. The effect of spironolactone on morbidity and mortality in patients with severe heart failure. N Engl J Med 1999;341(10):709–17.

65. Flather MD, Shibata MC, Coats AJS, et al. Randomized trial to determine the effect of nebivolol on

mortality and cardiovascular hospital admission in elderly patients with heart failure (SENIORS). Eur Heart J 2005;26(3):215–25.

66. Swedberg K, Komajda M, Böhm M, et al. Ivabradine and outcomes in chronic heart failure (SHIFT): a randomised placebo-controlled study. Lancet 2010;376(9744):875–85.

67. Investigators TS. Effect of enalapril on mortality and the development of heart failure in asymptomatic patients with reduced left ventricular ejection fractions. N Engl J Med 1992;327(10):685–91.

68. Investigators TS. Effect of enalapril on survival in patients with reduced left ventricular ejection fractions and congestive heart failure. N Engl J Med 1991;325(5):293–302.

69. Pitt B, Pfeffer MA, Assmann SF, et al. Spironolactone for heart failure with preserved ejection fraction. N Engl J Med 2014;370(15):1383–92.

70. Packer M, Bristow MR, Cohn JN, et al. The effect of carvedilol on morbidity and mortality in patients with chronic heart failure. U.S. Carvedilol Heart Failure Study Group. N Engl J Med 1996;334(21):1349–55.

71. Cohn JN, Tognoni G. A randomized trial of the angiotensin-receptor blocker valsartan in chronic heart failure. N Engl J Med 2001;345(23):1667–75.

72. Cohn JN, Archibald DG, Ziesche S, et al. Effect of vasodilator therapy on mortality in chronic congestive heart failure. N Engl J Med 1986;314(24):1547–52.

73. Cohn JN, Johnson G, Ziesche S, et al. A comparison of enalapril with hydralazine–isosorbide dinitrate in the treatment of chronic congestive heart failure. N Engl J Med 1991;325(5):303–10.

74. Shin JJ, Hamad E, Murthy S, et al. Heart failure in women. Clin Cardiol 2012;35(3):172–7.

75. Saitta A, Altavilla D, Cucinotta D, et al. Randomized, double-blind, placebo-controlled study on effects of raloxifene and hormone replacement therapy on plasma no concentrations, endothelin-1 levels, and endothelium-dependent vasodilation in postmenopausal women. Arterioscler Thromb Vasc Biol 2001;21(9):1512–9.

76. Tamargo J, Rosano G, Walther T, et al. Gender differences in the effects of cardiovascular drugs. Eur Heart J Cardiovasc Pharmacother 2017;3(3):163–82.

77. Cangemi R, Romiti GF, Campolongo G, et al. Gender related differences in treatment and response to statins in primary and secondary cardiovascular prevention: the never-ending debate. Pharmacol Res 2017;117:148–55.

78. Raparelli V, Proietti M, Romiti GF, et al. The sex-specific detrimental effect of diabetes and gender-related factors on pre-admission medication adherence among patients hospitalized for

ischemic heart disease: insights from EVA study. Front Endocrinol (Lausanne) 2019;10. https://doi.org/10.3389/fendo.2019.00107.

79. D'Agostino RBS, Grundy S, Sullivan LM, et al. Validation of the Framingham coronary heart disease prediction scores: results of a multiple ethnic groups investigation. JAMA 2001;286(2):180–7.

80. Rathore SS, Wang Y, Krumholz HM. Sex-based differences in the effect of digoxin for the treatment of heart failure. N Engl J Med 2002;347(18):1403–11.

81. Yancy CW, Jessup M, Bozkurt B, et al. 2016 ACC/AHA/HFSA focused update on new pharmacological therapy for heart failure: an update of the 2013 ACCF/AHA Guideline for the Management of Heart Failure: A report of the American College of Cardiology/American Heart Association Task Force on Clinic. Circulation 2016;134(13):e282–93.

82. Konstam MA, Neaton JD, Dickstein K, et al. Effects of high-dose versus low-dose losartan on clinical outcomes in patients with heart failure (HEAAL study): a randomised, double-blind trial. Lancet 2009;374(9704):1840–8.

83. Adams KFJ, Patterson JH, Gattis WA, et al. Relationship of serum digoxin concentration to mortality and morbidity in women in the digitalis investigation group trial: a retrospective analysis. J Am Coll Cardiol 2005;46(3):497–504.

84. Rathore SS, Curtis JP, Wang Y, et al. Association of serum digoxin concentration and outcomes in patients with heart failure. JAMA 2003;289(7):871–8.

85. Merrill M, Sweitzer NK, Lindenfeld JA, et al. Sex differences in outcomes and responses to spironolactone in heart failure with preserved ejection fraction: a secondary analysis of TOPCAT trial. JACC Hear Fail 2019. https://doi.org/10.1016/j.jchf.2019.01.003.

86. Santangeli P, Pelargonio G, Dello Russo A, et al. Gender differences in clinical outcome and primary prevention defibrillator benefit in patients with severe left ventricular dysfunction: a systematic review and meta-analysis. Hear Rhythm 2010;7(7):876–82.

87. Barsheshet A, Brenyo A, Goldenberg I, et al. Sex-related differences in patients' responses to heart failure therapy. Nat Rev Cardiol 2012. https://doi.org/10.1038/nrcardio.2012.10.

88. Vaduganathan M, Tahhan AS, Alrohaibani A, et al. Do women and men respond similarly to therapies in contemporary heart failure clinical trials? JACC Hear Fail 2019. https://doi.org/10.1016/j.jchf.2018.12.016.

89. Clayton JA, Tannenbaum C. Reporting sex, gender, or both in clinical research? JAMA 2016;316(18):1863–4.

90. Legato MJ, Johnson PA, Manson JE. Consideration of sex differences in medicine to improve health

care and patient outcomes. JAMA 2016;316(18): 1865–6.

91. Canadian Institutes of Health Research. What is gender? What is sex?. Available at: http://www.cihr-irsc.gc.ca/e/48642.html. Accessed September 26, 2018.

92. Johnson JL, Greaves L, Repta R. Better science with sex and gender: a primer for health research. Vancouver (Canada): Women's Health Research Network; 2007.

93. Georgiopoulou VV, Velayati A, Burkman G, et al. Comorbidities, sociodemographic factors, and hospitalizations in outpatients with heart failure and preserved ejection fraction. Am J Cardiol 2018. https://doi.org/10.1016/j.amjcard.2018.01. 040.

94. Schockmel M, Agrinier N, Jourdain P, et al. Socioeconomic factors and mortality in diastolic heart failure. Eur J Clin Invest 2014;44(4):372–83.

95. Watkins T, Mansi M, Thompson J, et al. Effect of marital status on clinical outcome of heart failure. J Investig Med 2013;61(5):835–41. https://doi.org/10.2310/JIM.0b013e31828c823e.

96. Braunwald E. Biomarkers in heart failure. N Engl J Med 2008;358(20):2148–59.

97. Neuhold S, Huelsmann M, Strunk G, et al. Prognostic value of emerging neurohormones in chronic heart failure during optimization of heart failure-specific therapy. Clin Chem 2010;56(1):121–6.

98. Rørth R, Fosbøl EL, Mogensen UM, et al. Employment status at time of first hospitalization for heart failure is associated with a higher risk of death and rehospitalization for heart failure. Eur J Heart Fail 2018. https://doi.org/10.1002/ejhf.1046.

99. Capdevila C, Bilal U, Farre N, et al. Individual income, mortality and healthcare resource use in patients with chronic heart failure living in a universal healthcare system: a population-based study in Catalonia, Spain. Int J Cardiol 2018. https://doi. org/10.1016/j.ijcard.2018.10.099.

100. Hawkins NM, Scholes S, Bajekal M, et al. Community care in England. Circulation 2012;126(9): 1050–7.

101. Pauws SC, Sokoreli I, Clark AL, et al. Added value of frailty and social support in predicting risk of 30-day unplanned re-admission or death for patients with heart failure: an analysis from OPERA-HF. Int J Cardiol 2018. https://doi.org/10.1016/j.ijcard. 2018.12.030.

102. Makowska A, Rydlewska A, Krakowiak B, et al. Psychological gender of men with systolic heart failure: a neglected strategy to cope with the disease? Am J Mens Health 2014;8(3):249–57. https://doi.org/10.1177/1557988313508429.

Psychological Disorders in Heart Failure

Katherine E. Di Palo, PharmD

KEYWORDS

- Heart failure • Depression • Anxiety • Insomnia • Screening • Prognosis • Outcomes

KEY POINTS

- Depression, anxiety, and insomnia are common psychological comorbidities in patients with heart failure and are associated with poor clinical outcomes.
- Routine recognition, possibly owing to overlapping symptomatology, is suboptimal despite screening tools that can facilitate early detection.
- Treatment modalities such as exercise training and psychotherapy have demonstrated positive findings; data to support psychopharmacologic interventions are lacking.

INTRODUCTION

Heart failure (HF) is a chronic, progressive cardiovascular disease punctuated by hospitalizations and associated with high morbidity, mortality, and economic costs. In US adults, the prevalence of HF is greater than 6 million and up to one-third of the population carries a risk factor.[1] As the population ages, the impact of HF is expected to increase substantially; however, despite advances in management 5-year mortality remains high and rivals that of many cancers.[2] From a patient perspective, quality of life dramatically decreases as disease worsens and health burden is significantly greater than other chronic diseases.[3]

Depression, anxiety, and insomnia are common comorbid psychological disorders that influence care in patients with HF. Although the bidirectional link between mental illness and cardiovascular disease is well-established,[4–6] pathophysiologic pathways are complex[7,8] and not completely understood. Furthermore, clinical trial data supporting antidepressant pharmacotherapy to improve symptoms and hard clinical end points in patients with HF is absent.[8] Therefore, little progress has been made to shift prognosis and outcomes. The purpose of this review is to describe relevant mood disorders, with an emphasis on presentation and identification, and to examine current information on treatment.

PREVALENCE AND RECOGNITION

Depression

Clinical depression is a mood disorder consisting of a combination of elements that interfere with a person's ability to perform day-to-day functioning.[9] Depressive symptoms correlate to health status and predict poor clinical outcomes in patients with HF.[10] Although the rate of depression in the general US population is 8.1%,[11] the prevalence among patients with HF is alarmingly high at an estimated rate of 21.6% and varies by setting and functional class.[12] A pivotal meta-analysis by Rutledge and colleagues[12] reported a range of 11% to 35% among outpatients and 35% to 70% among inpatients depending on how depression is defined and assessed. Not surprisingly, depression rates increase drastically as symptoms progress and range from 11% in patients with New York Heart Association functional class I symptoms to 42% in patients with New York Heart Association functional class IV

This article originally appeared in *Heart Failure Clinics*, Volume 16, Issue 1, January 2020.
Disclosure Statement: The author has nothing to disclose.
Office of the Medical Director, Montefiore Medical Center, 111 East 210th Street, Bronx, NY 10467, USA
E-mail address: kdipalo@montefiore.org

Cardiol Clin 40 (2022) 269–276
https://doi.org/10.1016/j.ccl.2021.12.014

symptoms.[12] Findings from an analysis of the Rehabilitation Therapy in Older Acute Heart Failure Patients (REHAB-HF) noted differences by ejection fraction (EF) subtype with depression observed as more common and severe in patients with preserved EF.[13]

Despite high occurrence, depression can easily go undiagnosed given the overlap of symptoms, such as a loss of energy, increased fatigability, weight loss or gain, and sleep disturbances. Clinicians should also pay attention to risk factors, which include female gender, lack of social support, a previous history of depression, family history of depression, and loss of function or major life role.[14] The 9-item Patient Health Questionnaire (PHQ-9) can be used to both diagnose depression and grade severity (**Table 1**).

Depression in patients with HF is significantly related to reduced functional status,[10,15] greater symptom severity,[16] and poorer health-related quality of life[17–19] and contributes to nonadherence[9,16] and participation in high-risk behaviors such as smoking and alcohol use.[20,21] Additionally, it drives higher use across the care continuum, including emergency department visits, hospitalizations, readmissions, and outpatient office visits.[22–24] The relationship to cardiovascular mortality and all-cause mortality is well-documented with depression linked to poor survival in both men and women.[24,25] Depression should be considered a cardiac risk factor, similar to diabetes and smoking, because it is an independent predictor of future cardiac events in patients with HF.[7,24]

Anxiety

Anxiety is a future-oriented mood state resulting from an individual's perception and preparation for possible, upcoming negative events.[26] Frequently comorbid with depression, anxiety prevalence ranges from 18.4%[27] to 36.7%,[28] although when compared with healthy elders levels of anxiety may be up to 60% higher.[9] Anxiety may be more common in outpatients with HF than inpatients.[29] There are numerous sources of anxiety for patients with HF including symptom progression, social isolation, health care system navigation, financial burden, and complicated treatment regimens. Similar to the PHQ-9, the Generalized Anxiety Disorder 7-item Questionnaire can be used as a screener to support the diagnosis of anxiety (**Table 2**).

Although depression is acknowledged as an important and independent predictor of mortality in patients with HF, a systematic review and meta-analysis of 17,214 patients with anxiety was inconclusive of any link.[30] However, other HF outcomes such as repeated hospitalizations,[31] quality of life,[32] and functional status[33] are adversely impacted by anxiety.

Insomnia

The most commonly encountered sleep disorder is insomnia. As many as 73% of patients with HF report sleep disturbance symptoms,[34] which may be related to Cheyne-Stokes respiration, adverse drug effects, or other mood disorders.[35] A large community study found that HF was associated with more than a 2-fold increased risk of self-reported insomnia.[36] Drugs used to treat HF symptoms, particularly diuretics, can contribute by causing nocturia. Illustrated in **Box 1**, diagnosis requires associated daytime dysfunction in addition to appropriate symptomatology and is considered chronic when lasting at least 3 months.

Insomnia symptoms correlate with impaired functional performance, including decreased exercise capacity[39] and 6-minute walk test distance,[40] increased daytime fatigue, and excessive daytime sleepiness.[41] In a large, prospective, population-based cohort study of patients free from HF at baseline, insomnia was associated with an increased risk of incident HF.[42] Evidence connecting the prognostic significance of insomnia to HF outcomes is emerging. Kanno and colleagues[43] compared cardiac event rates, including death and worsening HF, in 1011 patients with and without insomnia. In the insomnia group, patients with HF had more cardiac events, which was contributed to impaired exercise capacity and renin–angiotensin–aldosterone system activation.

TREATMENT
Exercise

Exercise training (ET) is frequently related to improvements in depression and is an appealing treatment modality in complex patients with HF with multiple comorbidities and complicated drug regimens. In the Heart Failure: A Controlled Trial Investigating Outcomes of Exercise Training (HF-ACTION) trial, patients with HF with reduced EF randomized to aerobic exercise 3 times per week had a modest but statistically significant decline in depressive symptoms at 3 months.[44] A meta-analysis and systematic review of 19 randomized controlled trials in 3447 patients showed that ET was associated with a significant decrease in depressive symptoms irrespective of age, duration of exercise intervention, or exercise setting.[45] Survival benefits have also been observed in depressed patients with HF with coronary heart disease that completed ET.[46]

Table 1
Assessment of depression

Diagnostic Symptoms	Criteria	PHQ-9 Questionnaire
Depressed mood most of the day, nearly every day, as indicated by either subjective report (eg, feels sad, empty, hopeless) or observation made by others (eg, appears tearful)	5 or more symptoms Must be present nearly every day for a 2-week period At least one of the symptoms must be either depressed mood or loss of interest or pleasure	1. Little interest or pleasure doing things
		2. Feeling down, depressed, or hopeless
		3. Trouble falling asleep, staying asleep or sleeping too much
Markedly diminished interest or pleasure in all, or almost all, activities most of the day, nearly every day (as indicated by either subjective account or observation)	Must represent a change from previous functioning resulting in social occupational or other life impairment	4. Feeling tired or having too little energy
		5. Poor appetite or overeating
		6. Feeling bad about yourself – or that you are a failure or have let yourself or your family down
Significant weight loss when not dieting or weight gain (eg, a change of >5% of body weight in a month), or decrease or increase in appetite nearly every day	Cannot be the direct result of a substance, medical condition or bereavement There has never been a manic or hypomanic episode	7. Trouble concentrating on things, such as reading the newspaper or watching television
Insomnia or hypersomnia nearly every day	Occurrence of major depressive episode is not better explained by another psychiatric or psychotic disorder	8. Feeling bad about yourself— or that you are a failure or have let yourself or your family down
Psychomotor agitation or retardation nearly every day (observable by others, not merely subjective feelings of restlessness or being slowed down)		9. Thoughts that you would be better off dead or of hurting yourself in some way
Fatigue or loss of energy nearly every day		
Feelings of worthlessness or excessive or inappropriate guilt (which may be delusional) nearly every day (not merely self-reproach or guilt about being sick)		
Diminished ability to think or concentrate, or indecisiveness, nearly every day (either by subjective account or as observed by others)		
Recurrent thoughts of death (not just fear of dying), recurrent suicidal ideation without a specific plan, or a suicide attempt or a specific plan for committing suicide		

Data from American Psychiatric Association. Diagnostic and statistical manual of mental disorders (DSM-5®). American Psychiatric Pub; 2013; and Löwe B, Gräfe K, Zipfel S, et al. Diagnosing ICD-10 depressive episodes: superior criterion validity of the Patient Health Questionnaire. Psychother Psychosom. 2004;73(6):386–90.

Small studies have also noted decreased anxiety levels after cardiac rehabilitation[47] and improved sleep quality after a 12-week ET program in patients recently hospitalized with HF.[48]

Cognitive–Behavioral Therapy

Cognitive–behavioral therapy (CBT) refers to a class of therapeutic strategies that share the

Table 2
Assessment of anxiety

Diagnostic Symptoms	Criteria	Generalized Anxiety Disorder 7-item Questionnaire
Being easily fatigued Difficulty concentrating or mind going blank Irritability Muscle tension Sleep disturbance (difficulty falling or staying asleep, or restless, unsatisfying sleep)	Three or more symptoms (with at least some symptoms having been present for more days than not for the past 6 mo) Difficult to control the worry Excessive anxiety and worry (apprehensive expectation), occurring more days than not for $\geq$6 mo, about a number of events or activities (such as work or school performance) Anxiety, worry, or physical symptoms cause clinically significant distress or impairment in social, occupational, or other important areas of functioning. Disturbance is not attributable to the physiologic effects of a substance or another medical condition Disturbance is not better explained by another mental disorder	1. Feeling nervous, anxious, or on edge 2. Not being able to stop or control worrying 3. Worrying too much about different things 4. Trouble relaxing 5. Being so restless that it is hard to sit still 6. Becoming easily annoyed or irritable 7. Feeling afraid as if something awful might happen

Data from American Psychiatric Association. Diagnostic and statistical manual of mental disorders (DSM-5®). American Psychiatric Pub; 2013; and Spitzer RL, Kroenke K, Williams JB, Löwe B. A brief measure for assessing generalized anxiety disorder: the GAD-7. Arch Intern Med. 2006;166(10):1092–7.

essential principle that maladaptive cognitions contribute to the maintenance of emotional distress and behavioral problems. With emphasis on short-term, problem-focused skill development, patients actively participate and collaborate to test, challenge, and modify dysfunctional patterns. CBT protocols are effective in symptom reduction, functional improvement, and remission for a variety of psychological disorders.[49] A randomized clinical trial conducted by Freedland and colleagues[50] noted lower 6-month depression scores, decreased anxiety and fatigue, improved social functioning, and fewer hospitalizations in depressed patients with HF receiving CBT compared with usual care. However, there was no difference in HF self-care or physical functioning between groups. CBT intervention also demonstrated positive effects on insomnia and

Box 1
Assessment of insomnia

Insomnia symptomatology	Perceived difficulty with sleep initiation, consolidation, duration or quality
Daytime dysfunction	Problems with attention, concentration or memory Fatigue, malaise, energy reduction or daytime sleepiness Error or accidents at work, while driving Headaches or gastrointestinal symptoms owing to sleep loss Mood disturbances, irritability, or specific worrying about sleep

Data from Refs.[34,37,38]

fatigue in a small, pilot randomized controlled trial of patients with HF.[51] Results from a larger clinical trial are forthcoming.[52]

Psychoeducation

Another evidence-based therapeutic intervention for depression and anxiety is psychoeducation, which partners providers with patients and caregivers in treatment and uses techniques to remove comprehension barriers thus allowing for the development proactive strategies based on enhanced knowledge.[53,54] The Support, Education, and Research in Chronic Heart Failure (SEARCH) study found that after an 8-week psychoeducational intervention that included mindfulness meditation, coping skills, and support group discussion, anxiety and depression were decreased in patients with HF with reduced EF compared with the control group.[55] Although there were no treatment effects on death or rehospitalization, the intervention led to symptomatic HF improvement at 1 year. Psychoeducational interventions have also demonstrated positive results in decreasing anxiety and depression in patients with implantable cardioverter defibrillators.[56]

Psychopharmacology

Evidence-based antidepressant and antianxiety drug classes include selective serotonin reuptake inhibitors (SSRIs) and serotonin and norepinephrine reuptake inhibitors. Drugs within these classes have nuisances in regard to metabolism, drug–drug interactions, and cardiovascular side effects and are described in depth in a contemporary state-of-the art review by Piña and colleagues.[57] Older agents such as tricyclic antidepressants should not be used because their proarrhythmic and hypotensive risks outweigh potential benefits. Atypical agents, such as buspirone, mirtazapine, and bupropion, have not been studied formally.

Although the results from Sertraline Against Depression and Heart Disease in Chronic Heart Failure (SADHART-CHF) demonstrated SSRI safety, there was no greater decrease in depression or improved cardiovascular status compared with placebo.[58] Similar findings were observed in Morbidity, Mortality and Mood in Depressed Heart Failure Patients (MOOD-HF), which evaluated escitalopram, a SSRI considered superior to sertraline in the treatment of primary depression.[59] Compared with placebo, there was no significant improvement in depression or decrease in all-cause mortality or hospitalization.[60] Recent findings from a meta-analysis of 21 randomized controlled trials comparing treatment options for depression in HF confirmed that antidepressant therapy did not provide significant therapeutic benefit in the reduction of depressive symptoms compared with placebo or usual care.[61] Conversely, ET and CBT demonstrated a superior effect.

A different pathophysiologic target is omega-3 fatty acids. Low concentrations have been observed in both depression and cardiovascular disease[62,63] and are associated with worse outcomes as evidenced in SADHART-CHF.[64] Recently, the Omega-3 Supplementation for Co-Morbid Depression and Heart Failure Treatment (OCEAN) trial observed positive changes in cognitive depressive symptoms and social function in a small sample of patients randomized to 400/200 EPA/DHA fish oil.[65]

The use of sedative hypnotics, such as zolpidem, may provide short-term insomnia respite; however, they should be prescribed with caution. In a qualitative study evaluating the perceptions of patients with HF of insomnia, the use of hypnotics or anxiolytics were viewed as necessary but not without consequence such as dependency, daytime drowsiness, and acute cognitive effects.[66] Benzodiazepines, such as alprazolam and clonazepam, are highly habit forming and several major organizations, including the American Geriatrics Society, advise against their use in older adults.[67]

Cardiovascular and health status outcomes may improve in patients who do respond to pharmacotherapy and achieve remission. In an analysis of SADHART-CHF, patients whose depression remitted had significantly fewer fatal and nonfatal cardiovascular events compared with those who depression remained,[68] whereas a separate analysis found greater improvement in physical function, social function, and quality of life.[69]

PRACTICE CONSIDERATIONS

Given the frequency of comorbid psychological disorders in patients with HF, coupled with the strong implication on outcomes, screening should be routinely integrated into clinical practice. The American Heart Association recommends routine screening for depression among cardiac patients using the PHQ-2, an abbreviated version of the PHQ-9, which asks patients if they had (1) little interest or pleasure in doing things and (2) feeling down, depressed, or hopeless over the past 2 weeks.[70,71] However, HF guidelines provide no further recommendations for treatment. In a review by Newhouse and Jiang,[7] a care algorithm for depression is offered that incorporates psychoeducation, ET, omega-3 supplementation, and considerations for choosing an antidepressant agent as well as criteria for psychiatry referral.

As with most aspects of HF patient care, an interdisciplinary team, with shared decision making between cardiology, primary care, and psychiatry, should be used. Patients and caregivers should also be included in the discussion. Although CBT and psychoeducation are efficacious, there is a time commitment that may not be feasible for patients with busy work schedules. Adding omega-3 or psychotropic agents may not be desirable for patients with high pill burdens at risk for nonadherence. ET and cardiac rehabilitation are currently not reimbursable for patients with HF with preserved EF and require transportation, which may be difficult for older patients who rely on caregivers. Despite these barriers, the treatment of comorbid psychological disorders is imperative and care plans that are patient tailored are more likely to achieve success.

SUMMARY

Though the impact of comorbid psychological disorders on HF morbidity and mortality is well-recognized, diagnostic gaps remain. While data to support psychopharmacologic interventions are lacking, treatment modalities such as CBT, psychoeducation and ET can be safely and effectively implemented. Future clinical trials examining atypical antidepressants, which can be used for depression, anxiety, and insomnia, are warranted. If habitually addressed in clinical practice, there is potential to improve quality of life, the cost effectiveness of care, and cardiovascular outcomes in patients with HF.

REFERENCES

1. Benjamin Emelia J, Muntner P, Alonso A, et al. Heart disease and stroke statistics—2019 update: a report from the American Heart Association. Circulation 2019;139(10):e56–528.
2. Bui AL, Horwich TB, Fonarow GC. Epidemiology and risk profile of heart failure. Nat Rev Cardiol 2010;8: 30.
3. Hobbs FD, Kenkre JE, Roalfe AK, et al. Impact of heart failure and left ventricular systolic dysfunction on quality of life: a cross-sectional study comparing common chronic cardiac and medical disorders and a representative adult population. Eur Heart J 2002; 23(23):1867–76.
4. Cohen S, Janicki-Deverts D, Miller GE. Psychological stress and disease. JAMA 2007;298(14):1685–7.
5. Hare DL, Toukhsati SR, Johansson P, et al. Depression and cardiovascular disease: a clinical review. Eur Heart J 2013;35(21):1365–72.
6. Van der Kooy K, Van Hout H, Marwijk H, et al. Depression and the risk for cardiovascular diseases: systematic review and meta analysis. Int J Geriatr Psychiatry 2007;22(7):613–26.
7. Newhouse A, Jiang W. Heart failure and depression. Heart Fail Clin 2014;10(2):295–304.
8. Angermann CE, Ertl G. Depression, anxiety, and cognitive impairment: comorbid mental health disorders in heart failure. Curr Heart Fail Rep 2018;15(6): 398–410.
9. Konstam V, Moser DK, De Jong MJ. Depression and anxiety in heart failure. J Card Fail 2005;11(6): 455–63.
10. Rumsfeld JS, Havranek E, Masoudi FA, et al. Depressive symptoms are the strongest predictors of short-term declines in health status in patients with heart failure. J Am Coll Cardiol 2003;42(10): 1811–7.
11. Brody DJ, Pratt LA, Hughes JP. Prevalence of depression among adults aged 20 and over: United States, 2013-2016. NCHS Data brief 2018;(303): 1–8.
12. Rutledge T, Reis VA, Linke SE, et al. Depression in heart failure a meta-analytic review of prevalence, intervention effects, and associations with clinical outcomes. J Am Coll Cardiol 2006;48(8):1527–37.
13. Warraich Haider J, Kitzman Dalane W, Whellan David J, et al. Physical function, frailty, cognition, depression, and quality of life in hospitalized adults ≥60 years with acute decompensated heart failure with preserved versus reduced ejection fraction. Circ Heart Fail 2018;11(11):e005254.
14. Guck TP, Elsasser GN, Kavan MG, et al. Depression and congestive heart failure. Congest Heart Fail 2003;9(3):163–9.
15. Vaccarino V, Kasl SV, Abramson J, et al. Depressive symptoms and risk of functional decline and death in patients with heart failure. J Am Coll Cardiol 2001;38(1):199–205.
16. Morgan AL, Masoudi FA, Havranek EP, et al. Difficulty taking medications, depression, and health status in heart failure patients. J Card Fail 2006; 12(1):54–60.
17. Bekelman DB, Havranek EP, Becker DM, et al. Symptoms, depression, and quality of life in patients with heart failure. J Card Fail 2007;13(8):643–8.
18. Mårtensson J, Dracup K, Canary C, et al. Living with heart failure: depression and quality of life in patients and spouses. J Heart Lung Transplant 2003; 22(4):460–7.
19. Carels RA. The association between disease severity, functional status, depression and daily quality of life in congestive heart failure patients. Qual Life Res 2004;13(1):63–72.

20. Havranek EP, Spertus JA, Masoudi FA, et al. Predictors of the onset of depressive symptoms in patients with heart failure. J Am Coll Cardiol 2004;44(12):2333–8.

21. Rumsfeld JS, Jones PG, Whooley MA, et al. Depression predicts mortality and hospitalization in patients with myocardial infarction complicated by heart failure. Am Heart J 2005;150(5):961–7.

22. Freedland KE, Carney RM, Rich MW, et al. Depression and multiple rehospitalizations in patients with heart failure. Clin Cardiol 2016;39(5):257–62.

23. Moraska Amanda R, Chamberlain Alanna M, Shah Nilay D, et al. Depression, healthcare utilization, and death in heart failure. Circ Heart Fail 2013;6(3):387–94.

24. Jiang W, Alexander J, Christopher E, et al. Relationship of depression to increased risk of mortality and rehospitalization in patients with congestive heart failure. Arch Intern Med 2001;161(15):1849–56.

25. Sherwood A, Blumenthal JA, Hinderliter AL, et al. Worsening depressive symptoms are associated with adverse clinical outcomes in patients with heart failure. J Am Coll Cardiol 2011;57(4):418–23.

26. Craske MG, Rauch SL, Ursano R, et al. What is an anxiety disorder? Focus 2011;9(3):369–88.

27. Haworth JE, Moniz-Cook E, Clark AL, et al. Prevalence and predictors of anxiety and depression in a sample of chronic heart failure patients with left ventricular systolic dysfunction. Eur J Heart Fail 2005;7(5):803–8.

28. Friedmann E, Thomas SA, Liu F, et al. Relationship of depression, anxiety, and social isolation to chronic heart failure outpatient mortality. Am Heart J 2006;152(5):940.e1-8.

29. Jiang W, Kuchibhatla M, Cuffe MS, et al. Prognostic value of anxiety and depression in patients with chronic heart failure. Circulation 2004;110(22):3452–6.

30. Sokoreli I, De Vries J, Pauws S, et al. Depression and anxiety as predictors of mortality among heart failure patients: systematic review and meta-analysis. Heart Fail Rev 2016;21(1):49–63.

31. Volz A, Schmid JP, Zwahlen M, et al. Predictors of readmission and health related quality of life in patients with chronic heart failure: a comparison of different psychosocial aspects. J Behav Med 2011;34(1):13–22.

32. Uchmanowicz I, Gobbens RJ. The relationship between frailty, anxiety and depression, and health-related quality of life in elderly patients with heart failure. Clin Interv Aging 2015;10:1595.

33. Shen B-J, Eisenberg SA, Maeda U, et al. Depression and anxiety predict decline in physical health functioning in patients with heart failure. Ann Behav Med 2010;41(3):373–82.

34. Javaheri S, Redline S. Insomnia and risk of cardiovascular disease. Chest 2017;152(2):435–44.

35. Parati G, Lombardi C, Castagna F, et al. Heart failure and sleep disorders. Nat Rev Cardiol 2016;13:389.

36. Katz DA, McHorney CA. Clinical correlates of insomnia in patients with chronic illness. Arch Intern Med 1998;158(10):1099–107.

37. Edinger JD, Bonnet MH, Bootzin RR, et al. Derivation of research diagnostic criteria for insomnia: report of an American Academy of Sleep Medicine Work Group. Sleep 2004;27(8):1567–96.

38. Schutte-Rodin S, Broch L, Buysse D, et al. Clinical guideline for the evaluation and management of chronic insomnia in adults. J Clin Sleep Med 2008;4(05):487–504.

39. Mayou R, Blackwood R, Bryant B, et al. Cardiac failure: symptoms and functional status. J Psychosom Res 1991;35(4–5):399–407.

40. Redeker NS, Hilkert R. Sleep and quality of life in stable heart failure. J Card Fail 2005;11(9):700–4.

41. Redeker NS, Jeon S, Muench U, et al. Insomnia symptoms and daytime function in stable heart failure. Sleep 2010;33(9):1210–6.

42. Vatten LJ, Strand LB, Laugsand LE, et al. Insomnia and the risk of incident heart failure: a population study. Eur Heart J 2013;35(21):1382–93.

43. Kanno Y, Yoshihisa A, Watanabe S, et al. Prognostic significance of insomnia in heart failure. Circ J 2016;80(7):1571–7.

44. Blumenthal JA, Babyak MA, O'connor C, et al. Effects of exercise training on depressive symptoms in patients with chronic heart failure: the HF-ACTION randomized trial. JAMA 2012;308(5):465–74.

45. Tu R-H, Zeng Z-Y, Zhong G-Q, et al. Effects of exercise training on depression in patients with heart failure: a systematic review and meta-analysis of randomized controlled trials. Eur J Heart Fail 2014;16(7):749–57.

46. Milani RV, Lavie CJ, Mehra MR, et al. Impact of exercise training and depression on survival in heart failure due to coronary heart disease. Am J Cardiol 2011;107(1):64–8.

47. Kulcu D, Kurtais Y, Tur B, et al. The effect of cardiac rehabilitation on quality of life, anxiety and depression in patients with congestive heart failure. A randomized controlled trial, short-term results. Eura Medicophys 2007;43(4):489–97.

48. Suna JM, Mudge A, Stewart I, et al. The effect of a supervised exercise training programme on sleep quality in recently discharged heart failure patients. Eur J Cardiovasc Nurs 2014;14(3):198–205.

49. Hofmann SG, Asnaani A, Vonk IJ, et al. The efficacy of cognitive behavioral therapy: a review of meta-analyses. Cognit Ther Res 2012;36(5):427–40.

50. Freedland KE, Carney RM, Rich MW, et al. Cognitive behavior therapy for depression and self-care in heart failure patients: a randomized clinical trial. JAMA Intern Med 2015;175(11):1773–82.

51. Redeker NS, Jeon S, Andrews L, et al. Feasibility and efficacy of a self-management intervention for insomnia in stable heart failure. J Clin Sleep Med 2015;11(10):1109–19.

52. Redeker NS, Knies AK, Hollenbeak C, et al. Cognitive behavioral therapy for insomnia in stable heart failure: protocol for a randomized controlled trial. Contemp Clin trials 2017;55:16–23.

53. Donker T, Griffiths KM, Cuijpers P, et al. Psychoeducation for depression, anxiety and psychological distress: a meta-analysis. BMC Med 2009;7(1):79.

54. Lukens EP, McFarlane WR. Psychoeducation as evidence-based practice: considerations for practice, research, and policy. Brief Treat Crisis Interv 2004;4(3):205.

55. Sullivan MJ, Wood L, Terry J, et al. The Support, Education, and Research in Chronic Heart Failure Study (SEARCH): a mindfulness-based psychoeducational intervention improves depression and clinical symptoms in patients with chronic heart failure. Am Heart J 2009;157(1):84–90.

56. Dunbar SB, Langberg JJ, Reilly CM, et al. Effect of a psychoeducational intervention on depression, anxiety, and health resource use in implantable cardioverter defibrillator patients. Pacing Clin Electrophysiol 2009;32(10):1259–71.

57. Piña IL, Di Palo KE, Ventura HO. Psychopharmacology and cardiovascular disease. J Am Coll Cardiol 2018;71(20):2346–59.

58. O'Connor CM, Jiang W, Kuchibhatla M, et al. Safety and efficacy of sertraline for depression in patients with heart failure: results of the SADHART-CHF (Sertraline Against Depression and Heart Disease in Chronic Heart Failure) trial. J Am Coll Cardiol 2010;56(9):692–9.

59. Cipriani A, Furukawa TA, Salanti G, et al. Comparative efficacy and acceptability of 12 new-generation antidepressants: a multiple-treatments meta-analysis. Lancet 2009;373(9665):746–58.

60. Angermann CE, Gelbrich G, Störk S, et al. Effect of escitalopram on all-cause mortality and hospitalization in patients with heart failure and depression: the MOOD-HF randomized clinical trial. JAMA 2016;315(24):2683–93.

61. Das A, Roy B, Schwarzer G, et al. Comparison of treatment options for depression in heart failure: a network meta-analysis. J Psychiatr Res 2019;108:7–23.

62. Frasure-Smith N, Lespérance F, Julien P. Major depression is associated with lower omega-3 fatty acid levels in patients with recent acute coronary syndromes. Biol Psychiatry 2004;55(9):891–6.

63. Kromhout D, Bosschieter EB, Coulander CDL. The inverse relation between fish consumption and 20-year mortality from coronary heart disease. N Engl J Med 1985;312(19):1205–9.

64. Jiang W, Oken H, Fiuzat M, et al. Plasma omega-3 polyunsaturated fatty acids and survival in patients with chronic heart failure and major depressive disorder. J Cardiovasc Transl Res 2012;5(1):92–9.

65. Jiang W, Whellan DJ, Adams KF, et al. Long-chain omega-3 fatty acid supplements in depressed heart failure patients: results of the OCEAN trial. JACC Heart Fail 2018;6(10):833–43.

66. Andrews LK, Coviello J, Hurley E, et al. "I'd eat a bucket of nails if you told me it would help me sleep:" perceptions of insomnia and its treatment in patients with stable heart failure. Heart Lung 2013;42(5):339–45.

67. By the American Geriatrics Society 2015 Beers Criteria Update Expert Panel. American Geriatrics Society 2015 updated beers criteria for potentially inappropriate medication use in older adults. J Am Geriatr Soc 2015;63(11):2227–46.

68. Jiang W, Krishnan R, Kuchibhatla M, et al. Characteristics of depression remission and its relation with cardiovascular outcome among patients with chronic heart failure (from the SADHART-CHF Study). Am J Cardiol 2011;107(4):545–51.

69. Xiong GL, Fiuzat M, Kuchibhatla M, et al. Health status and depression remission in patients with chronic heart failure: patient-reported outcomes from the SADHART-CHF trial. Circ Heart Fail 2012;5(6):688–92.

70. Lichtman JH, Bigger JT Jr, Blumenthal JA, et al. Depression and coronary heart disease: recommendations for screening, referral, and treatment: a science advisory from the American Heart Association Prevention Committee of the Council on Cardiovascular Nursing, Council on Clinical Cardiology, Council on Epidemiology and Prevention, and Interdisciplinary Council on Quality of Care and Outcomes Research: endorsed by the American Psychiatric Association. Circulation 2008;118(17):1768–75.

71. Kroenke K, Spitzer RL, Williams JB. The Patient Health Questionnaire-2: validity of a two-item depression screener. Med Care 2003;41(11):1284–92.

Printed and bound by CPI Group (UK) Ltd, Croydon, CR0 4YY

03/10/2024

01040367-0008